Foundations Of Nutritional Medicine

A SourceBook of Clinical Research

Also by Melvyn R. Werbach

SourceBooks of Clinical Research

Botanical Influences on Illness (Michael T. Murray, co-author)

Nutritional Influences on Illness

Nutritional Influences on Mental Illness

———————————————

Healing Through Nutrition:
A Natural Approach to Treating 50 Common Illnesses with Diet and Nutrients

Third Line Medicine:
Modern Treatment for Persistent Symptoms

Foundations of Nutritional Medicine

A sourcebook of clinical research

Melvyn R. Werbach, M.D.
Assistant Clinical Professor
School of Medicine, UCLA
Los Angeles, California

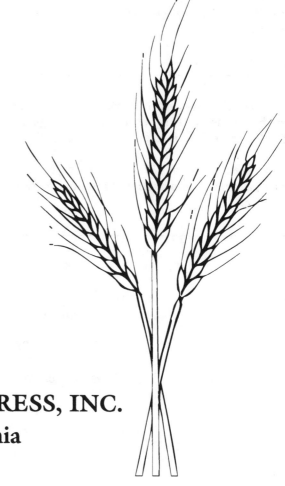

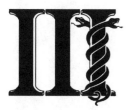 **THIRD LINE PRESS, INC.**
Tarzana, California

**To my wife, Gail,
and my sons, Kevin and Adam,
for their love and support
that made this book possible.**

Information presented in this book changes rapidly and is subject to differing interpretations. It is up to you to check it thoroughly before relying on it. Neither the author nor the publisher makes any guarantees regarding the outcome of the uses to which this book is put.

The treatment of illness should be supervised by a physician or other licensed health professional. Information presented herein does not contain treatment recommendations for the public.

Printed in the United States of America

ISBN 0-9618550-6-1

Library of Congress Catalog Card Number: 96-90623

FOUNDATIONS OF
NUTRITIONAL MEDICINE

TABLE OF CONTENTS

INTRODUCTION

Health practitioners familiar with the contributions that nutritional medicine can make to the prevention and treatment of illness have long had to content themselves with a paucity of reference books to assist them in applying the scientific literature concerning nutritional factors to their work with individual patients. This has been a serious limitation, since the large number of nutrients makes it nearly impossible for clinicians to memorize most of the voluminous data in order to recognize which may be relevant to a particular case.

Foundations of Nutritional Medicine attempts to reduce that problem by providing detailed information on dozens of nutrients in a format especially designed to make that information easily and quickly accessible. A desktop reference book designed to provide frequent guidance to the busy practitioner, it is designed to serve as a companion to Nutritional Influences on Illness and Nutritional Influences on Mental Illness, reference books by the same author that concern the influences of nutritional factors on specific disorders.

Like the other books in this series, Foundations of Nutritional Medicine is a sourcebook of clinical research; that is, it is neither a typical textbook nor a single author's pronouncements. Rather it is a compilation of current scientific knowledge curried from the work of thousands of research scientists from around the world.

The book is divided into nine chapters, each of which provides information on an aspect of nutritional medicine relevant to clinical practice. The contributions of the material in each chapter to clinical work are as follows:

EVALUATION

● History

Chapter One suggests whether the patient's symptoms could be related to specific nutritional abnormalities.

If the dietary history raises the suspicion that the diet may be nutritionally inadequate, Chapter Two suggests which nutrient deficiencies are most likely to be present.

Chapter Three suggests how bioavailable current nutritional supplements may be.

Chapter Four suggests whether adverse effects of these supplements could be contributing to the current illness.

Chapter Five suggests which other nutrients these supplements may be affecting.

Chapter Six suggests which nutrients prescribed medications may be affecting, and whether current nutritional supplements may be affecting drug bioavailability.

Chapter Seven suggests whether the patient's symptoms could be promoted by heavy metal toxicity.

If heavy metal toxicity appears to be relevant, <u>Chapter Eight</u> explores the relationship between the implicated metal and nutrients.

● Physical Examination

<u>Chapter One</u> suggests whether the physical findings could be related to specific nutrient abnormalities.

<u>Chapter Seven</u> suggests whether the physical findings could be promoted by heavy metal toxicity.

● Laboratory Testing

If, based on the history, physical examination and the information presented in chapters one to eight, the clinician concludes that the patient's nutriture should be directly evaluated by laboratory testing, <u>Chapter Nine</u> suggests the best method(s) of doing so.

TREATMENT

● Nutritional Supplements

If the clinician decides to prescribe specific nutritional supplements, <u>Chapter Three</u> suggests how to prescribe the supplements that will be most effective.

<u>Chapter Four</u> warns of potential adverse effects from the supplements being considered.

<u>Chapter Five</u> warns of potential interactions of the supplements being considered with other nutrients.

<u>Chapter Eight</u> summarizes relevant interactions between nutrients and toxic metals.

● Medications

If the clinician decides to prescribe medications, <u>Chapter Six</u> warns of known interactions of those medications that may affect the patient's nutritional status.

I compiled <u>Foundations of Nutritional Medicine</u> in order to assist health practitioners in integrating nutritional medicine into their practices. Nutrition is basic to life; thus, nutritional medicine should not be considered an 'alternative' or a 'complement' to conventional medicine, but an essential component of good medical practice. It is my hope that readers will benefit their patients by learning to refer to this book regularly.

Melvyn R. Werbach, M.D.
Tarzana, California

Chapter One

DISORDERS DUE TO ABNORMAL NUTRITURE

This chapter summarizes current knowledge concerning the possible contribution of nutrient deficiencies and excesses to various disorders. It is designed to suggest relevant abnormalities in nutriture that should be confirmed by history, physical examination and testing procedures.

```
KEY:   ↓ = possible effect of deficiency
       ↑ = possible effect of excess
```

ALLERGY

ANGIOEDEMA (hives)

↑ Iodine
        with laryngeal swelling
↑ Selenium

SERUM SICKNESS

↑ Iodine

AUTOIMMUNE DISORDERS

↓ Copper

BLOOD PRESSURE

HYPERTENSION

↓ Calcium
↓ Magnesium
↑ Manganese
↑ Phenylalanine
↑ Sodium
↑ Vitamin E (*exacerbates*)

HYPOTENSION

↑ <u>Magnesium</u>
↓ <u>Magnesium</u>
↑ <u>Niacin</u>
↓ <u>Pantothenic Acid</u>
↓ <u>Potassium</u>
↓ <u>Thiamine</u> (*beriberi*)

BONES and JOINTS

ARTHRITIS, GOUTY

↑ <u>Vitamin A</u> (*chronic*)

BONE ABNORMALITIES

↓ <u>Iron</u>
↑ <u>Vitamin A</u> (*chronic*)
↓ <u>Vitamin C</u> (*scurvy*)

BONE FRAGILITY

↓ <u>Manganese</u>

BONE PAIN

↓ <u>Calcium</u>
↓ <u>Phosphorus</u>
↑ <u>Vitamin A</u> (*chronic*)
↓ <u>Vitamin C</u> (*scurvy*)
↓ <u>Vitamin D</u>

BONE TENDERNESS

↑ <u>Vitamin A</u> (*chronic*)
      (long bones)

CHONDROCALCINOSIS (*calcification of cartilage*)

↑ <u>Iron</u>

GROWTH IMPAIRMENT

↓ <u>Zinc</u>

JOINT PAIN

↓ Copper
↑ Vitamin A (*chronic*)
↓ Vitamin C (*scurvy*)

JOINT SWELLING

↓ Vitamin C (*scurvy*)

OSTEOMALACIA (soft bones)

↓ Calcium
↓ Phosphorus
↓ Vitamin D
also painless epiphyseal enlargement, beading of ribs, bowed legs, skull bossing, thoracic deformaties

OSTEOPOROSIS

↓ Calcium
↓ Copper
↓ Vitamin D

RICKETS (softened, deformed bones)

↓ Calcium
↓ Vitamin D

EARS

NYSTAGMUS

↓ Magnesium

VERTIGO

↓ Magnesium

EYES

BITOT'S SPOTS (frothy white/yellow spots under bulbar conjunctivae)

↓ Vitamin A

BLURRED VISION

↑ <u>S-Adenosyl-methionine</u>
↑ <u>Vitamin A</u>

CATARACTS

↓ <u>Riboflavin</u>

CONJUNCTIVITIS

↓ <u>Iron</u> (pale)
↓ <u>Riboflavin</u>
↑ <u>Vitamin A</u>
↓ <u>Vitamin B$_6$</u>

CORNEAL ULCERATION

↓ <u>Riboflavin</u>
↓ <u>Vitamin A</u>

CORNEAL VASCULARIZATION

↓ <u>Riboflavin</u>

DIPLOPIA

↓ <u>Magnesium</u>
↑ <u>Vitamin A</u>

EXOPHTHALMOS

↑ <u>Vitamin A</u>

KERATOMALACIA *(corneal softening)*

↓ <u>Vitamin A</u>

decreased LACRIMATION

↓ <u>Vitamin A</u>

MYOPIA

↓ <u>Vitamin D</u>

NIGHT BLINDNESS

↓ Molybdenum
↓ Vitamin A
↓ Zinc

OCULAR PALSY

↓ Vitamin B$_{12}$

OPHTHALMOPLEGIA

↓ Thiamine
↓ Vitamin E

OPTIC NEURITIS

↓ Thiamine
↓ Vitamin B$_{12}$

PAPILLEDEMA

↑ Vitamin A

PHOTOPHOBIA

↓ Riboflavin
↓ Vitamin A
↓ Zinc

SCOTOMATAS

↓ Molybdenum

***poor* VISUAL ACUITY**

↓ Essential Fatty Acids
↓ Omega-3 Fatty Acids
↓ Riboflavin

XEROPHTHALMIA *(extreme conjunctival dryness)*

↓ Vitamin A

EYELIDS

BLEPHARITIS

↓ <u>Riboflavin</u> (*angular*)
↓ <u>Vitamin B$_6$</u>

PALLOR

↓ <u>Folic Acid</u>
↓ <u>Iron</u>

FACE

MOON FACIES

↓ <u>Protein-Calorie</u>

GALLBLADDER

GALLSTONES

↓ <u>Essential Fatty Acids</u>

GASTROINTESTINAL

GENERAL SYMPTOMS

↑ <u>L-Carnitine</u>
↑ <u>Choline</u>
↓ <u>Folic Acid</u>
↑ <u>Iron</u>
↓ <u>Iron</u>
↓ <u>Para-aminobenzoic Acid</u> (<u>PABA</u>)
↓ <u>Vitamin B$_{12}$</u>
↑ <u>Vitamin E</u>

ABDOMINAL PAIN

↓ <u>Pantothenic Acid</u>
↑ <u>Selenium</u>
↓ <u>Sodium</u>
↑ <u>Vitamin A</u>
↓ <u>Vitamin B$_6$</u>
↑ <u>Vitamin C</u>

↑ Vitamin D
↑ Vitamin E

ACHLORHYDRIA *(lack of stomach acid)*

↓ Vitamin B$_{12}$

ANOREXIA

↓ Biotin *(rare)*
↑ Calcium
↓ Chloride
↑ Folic Acid
↓ Folic Acid
↑ Iron
↓ Iron
↓ Magnesium
↓ Niacin
↓ Pantothenic Acid
↑ Para-aminobenzoic Acid (PABA)
↓ Phosphorus
↑ Sodium
↓ Sodium
↓ Thiamine *(mild)*
↑ Vitamin A
↓ Vitamin B$_6$
↓ Vitamin B$_{12}$
↓ Vitamin C
↑ Vitamin D
↓ Zinc *(moderate)*

CONSTIPATION

↓ Folic Acid
↓ Inositol
↓ Iron
↓ Para-aminobenzoic Acid (PABA)
↓ Potassium
↓ Thiamine *(atony)*
↑ Vitamin A
↓ Vitamin B$_{12}$
↑ Vitamin D

DIARRHEA

↑ Bismuth
↑ Choline
↓ Copper

↓ Essential Fatty Acids
↓ Folic Acid
↑ L-5-Hydroxytryptophan
↑ Iodine
↑ Lithium
↑ Niacin
↓ Niacin (*pellagra*)
      due to mucous membrane lesions in the colon
↓ Protein-Calorie
↑ Vitamin A
↓ Vitamin B$_{12}$
↑ Vitamin C
↓ Vitamin D
↑ Vitamin E
↓ Zinc (*severe*)

DYSPHAGIA

↓ Iron
↓ Magnesium
↑ Potassium

FLATULENCE

↑ Folic Acid
↑ S-Adenosyl-methionine
↓ Sodium
↓ Vitamin B$_{12}$
↑ Vitamin E

HYPOGEUSIA (*loss of taste*)

↓ Zinc (*moderate*)

INDIGESTION

↓ Niacin
↓ Thiamine

MELENA (*black stools due to blood loss*)

↓ Vitamin C (*scurvy*)

NAUSEA

↓ Biotin (*rare*)
↑ Folic Acid
↑ L-5-Hydroxytryptophan

↑ <u>Magnesium</u>
↓ <u>Magnesium</u>
↑ <u>Niacin</u> (*lactic acidosis*)
↓ <u>Niacin</u>
↓ <u>Pantothenic Acid</u>
↑ <u>Para-aminobenzoic Acid</u> (PABA)
↑ <u>S-Adenosyl-methionine</u>
↑ <u>Selenium</u>
↓ <u>Sodium</u>
↓ <u>Thiamine</u> (*mild*)
↑ <u>L-Tryptophan</u>
↑ <u>Vitamin A</u> (*acute*)
↓ <u>Vitamin B$_6$</u>
↑ <u>Vitamin D</u>
↑ <u>Vitamin E</u>
↑ <u>Zinc</u>

ULCERS

↑ <u>Chromium</u>

VOMITING

↑ <u>Choline</u>
↑ <u>L-5-Hydroxytryptophan</u>
↑ <u>Magnesium</u>
↓ <u>Magnesium</u>
↑ <u>Niacin</u> (*lactic acidosis*)
↓ <u>Pantothenic Acid</u>
↑ <u>Selenium</u>
↓ <u>Sodium</u>
↓ <u>Thiamine</u>
↑ <u>Vitamin A</u> (*acute*)
↓ <u>Vitamin B$_6$</u>
↑ <u>Vitamin D</u>

WEIGHT GAIN

↓ <u>Iodine</u>
↑ <u>Lithium</u>
↑ <u>Sodium</u>

GUMS

BLEEDING

↓ <u>Vitamin C</u>

BRIGHT RED
   (marginal)

   ↑ Vitamin A (*chronic*)

GINGIVAL HYPERTROPHY

   ↓ Vitamin C (*scurvy*)

GINGIVITIS

   ↓ Niacin
   ↓ Riboflavin
   ↓ Vitamin A
   ↓ Vitamin C (*scurvy*)
      Hemorrhages may precede a hyperplastic hemorrhagic gingivitis with reddish-blue edematous, friable gums and localized necrotic lesions.

HAIR

ALOPECIA (*hair loss*)

   ↓ Biotin (*rare*)
   ↓ Copper
   ↓ Essential Fatty Acids
   ↓ Inositol
   ↓ Pantothenic Acid
   ↓ Protein- Calorie
      also thin, coarse, dull, brittle, stiff, straight and easily pluckable.
         In blacks, hair becomes reddish; in whites, there is horizontal depigmentation ('flag sign').
   ↓ Riboflavin
   ↑ Selenium
   ↑ Vitamin A
   ↓ Vitamin B_6
   ↓ Zinc (*severe*)

COILED (*"corkscrew"*)

   ↓ Vitamin A
   ↓ Vitamin C (*scurvy*)

DRY & STIFF

   ↓ Essential Fatty Acids
   ↑ Selenium

GREYING (premature)

↓ Para-aminobenzoic Acid (PABA)

PAINFUL WHEN PULLED

↓ Vitamin D

HEART

ARRHYTHMIAS (general)

↓ Copper
↑ Magnesium
↓ Magnesium
↓ Potassium

ATRIAL FIBRILLATION

↑ Niacin

BRADYCARDIA (at rest)

↓ Potassium
↓ Protein-Calorie
↓ Thiamine (*beriberi*)

CARDIOMYOPATHY

↓ Selenium

CONGESTIVE HEART FAILURE

↑ Sodium
↓ Thiamine (*beriberi*) (*high-output*)

DYSPNEA (shortness of breath)

↑ Thiamine
↓ Thiamine (*beriberi*) (*on exertion*)

MYOCARDIAL INFARCTION

↓ Copper

MYOCARDITIS

↓ Thiamine (*beriberi*)

PALPITATIONS

↓ Calcium
↓ Iron (*exertional*)
↓ Thiamine
↓ Vitamin B$_{12}$

PERICARDIAL PAIN (*pseudoangina*)

↓ Thiamine (*beriberi*) (*on exertion*)

TACHYCARDIA

↓ Magnesium
↓ Molybdenum
↓ Pantothenic Acid
↑ Thiamine
↓ Thiamine (*beriberi*) (*on exertion*)

HEMATOLOGY

ANEMIA

↓ Biotin (*rare*)
↓ Copper (*early*)
  (hypochromic, microcytic)
↓ Essential Fatty Acids (*general*)
↓ Folic Acid
  (megaloblastic)
↓ Iron
  (hypochromic, microcytic)
↓ Magnesium
  (hemolytic)
↓ Phosphorus
  (hemolytic)
↓ Riboflavin
  (normochromic, normocytic)
↓ Selenium (hemolytic)
↑ Vitamin A
↓ Vitamin B$_6$
  (microcytic)
↓ Vitamin B$_{12}$
  (megaloblastic)

↓ Vitamin C (*scurvy*)
↓ Vitamin E
      (hemolytic)
↓ Vitamin K
      (hypoprothrombinemia)

LEUKOPENIA

↓ Copper

LYMPHOPENIA

↓ Folic Acid
↓ Vitamin B_6

NEUTROPENIA

↓ Copper (*early*)

THROMBOCYTOPENIA

↑ Omega-3 Fatty Acids
↓ Phosphorus

KIDNEY

DYSFUNCTION

↑ Chromium
↓ Essential Fatty Acids
↓ Potassium (*proteinuria; salt retention*)
↑ Selenium
↑ Sodium
↑ Vitamin D

DYSURIA (*painful urination*)

↑ Vitamin A

POLYURIA (*frequent urination*)

↑ Lithium
↑ Vitamin A
↑ Vitamin D

STONES

↑ L-Cystine
↓ Magnesium

URINARY DELAY

↑ S-Adenosyl-methionine

LIPS

CHEILITIS (angular stomatitis; inflammation, with fissures radiating from the corners of the mouth)

↓ Folic Acid
↓ Iron
↓ Niacin
↓ Pantothenic Acid
↓ Protein
↓ Riboflavin
↑ Vitamin A
↓ Vitamin B$_6$

DRY & FISSURED

↓ Niacin (*pellagra*)
↓ Riboflavin
        also smooth
↑ Vitamin A

LIVER

DYSFUNCTION

↓ Choline
↑ Chromium
↑ Niacin *or* Niacinamide
↑ Para-aminobenzoic Acid (PABA)
↑ Selenium
↓ Selenium
↑ Vitamin A

FATTY

↓ Choline
↓ Essential Fatty Acids

↓ Protein

HEMOCHROMATOSIS (iron accumulation with tissue damage)

↑ Iron

HEMOSIDEROSIS (iron accumulation)

↑ Iron

HEPATOMEGALY

↑ Vitamin A

MUCUS MEMBRANES

GENERAL

DRYNESS

↑ Vitamin A

ORAL MUCOSA

APHTHOUS STOMATITIS (canker sores; ulcerative inflammation of the mucous membranes)

↓ Folic Acid
↓ Niacin
↓ Vitamin B$_{12}$ *(early)*

BURNING & SORENESS

↑ Iodine
↓ Riboflavin
    with hyperemia and edema of the pharyngeal mucous membranes
↓ Vitamin B$_{12}$ *(early)*
↓ Vitamin D

DRYNESS

↑ Magnesium
↑ S-Adenosyl-methionine

DRYNESS & REDNESS

↓ <u>Biotin</u> (*rare*)
↓ <u>Niacin</u> (*pellagra*)
    also smooth
    with numerous, sometimes large, aphthous lesions

STOMATITIS

↓ <u>Folic Acid</u>
↓ <u>Vitamin B$_6$</u>
↓ <u>Vitamin B$_{12}$</u> (*early*)

MUSCLES *(see also NEUROPSYCHIATRY)*

ATROPHY

↓ <u>Thiamine</u>

FASCICULATIONS

↓ <u>Magnesium</u>

HYPOTONIA

↓ <u>Copper</u>
↓ <u>Vitamin D</u>

MYALGIA *(muscle pain)*
see also PERIPHERAL NEUROPATHY under NEUROPSYCHIATRY

↓ <u>Biotin</u> (*rare*)
↓ <u>Copper</u>
↓ <u>Magnesium</u>
↓ <u>Selenium</u>
↑ <u>Vitamin A</u>

MYOPATHY

↓ <u>Magnesium</u>
↓ <u>Phosphate</u>
↓ <u>Vitamin E</u>

MYOSITIS

↓ <u>Selenium</u>

SPASMS

↓ Calcium
↓ Chloride
↓ Magnesium
↓ Pantothenic Acid
↓ Sodium

STIFFNESS

↑ Vitamin A

TENDERNESS
see also *PERIPHERAL NEUROPATHY*

↓ Thiamine (*beriberi*)
     (calf muscles)
↓ Vitamin D
     (calf muscles)

TREMORS

↓ Magnesium (coarse)
↑ Thiamine

TWITCHES

↓ Magnesium

WASTING
see also *PERIPHERAL NEUROPATHY*

↓ Magnesium
↓ Protein-Calorie

WEAKNESS
see *PERIPHERAL NEUROPATHY and WEAKNESS under*
NEUROPSYCHIATRY

NAILS

BRITTLE

↓ Calcium
↓ Essential Fatty Acids
↓ Iron
↑ Selenium
     also thickened

↑ <u>Vitamin A</u>
↓ <u>Zinc</u>

HYPERPIGMENTATION (sub-ungual)

↓ <u>Vitamin B$_{12}$</u> (brown, reticular)

KOILONYCHIA (spooning)

↓ <u>Chromium</u>
↓ <u>Iron</u>
      with ridging, brittleness, thinness and lack of luster
↓ <u>Vitamin C</u> (*scurvy*)
      with other ungual alterations

LEUKONYCHIA (white spots on nails)

↓ <u>Zinc</u>

SPLINTER HEMORRHAGES

↓ <u>Vitamin C</u> (*scurvy*) (*rare*)
      Extensive hemorrhages in a semicircular lattice

NEUROPSYCHIATRY (see also MUSCLES)

AGITATION

↓ <u>Calcium</u>
↓ <u>Magnesium</u>
↓ <u>Thiamine</u>

AMNESIA

↓ <u>Zinc</u>

ANXIETY

↓ <u>Chromium</u>
↓ <u>Magnesium</u>
↓ <u>Niacin</u> (*pellagra*) (*mild*)
↑ <u>Phenylalanine</u>
↓ <u>Phosphorus</u>
↑ <u>S-Adenosyl-methionine</u>
↑ <u>L-Tyrosine</u>

APATHY

↓ Folic Acid
↓ Magnesium
↓ Niacin (*pellagra*)
↓ Protein (*kwashiorkor*)
↓ Zinc

APHASIA

↑ Calcium (*transient*)

APHONIA

↓ Thiamine

AREFLEXIA

↓ Vitamin E

ASTHENIA

↑ Vitamin A

ATAXIA
        see also PERIPHERAL NEUROPATHY

↑ Calcium
↓ Copper
↓ Magnesium
↓ Sodium
↓ Thiamine
↑ Vitamin A
↓ Vitamin B$_{12}$

AUTONOMIC DYSFUNCTION

↓ Thiamine

BEHAVIORAL DISTURBANCES

↓ Magnesium

BURNING FEET

↓ Pantothenic acid
↓ Thiamine
↓ Vitamin B$_{12}$

COGNITIVE IMPAIRMENT (confusion, disorientation, memory loss)

↑ Calcium
↓ Calcium
↑ Copper
↓ Folic Acid
↓ Iron
↑ Magnesium
↓ Magnesium
↓ Niacin (*pellagra*)
↓ Phosphorus
↑ Potassium
↓ Potassium
↑ Sodium
↓ Sodium
↓ Thiamine
↑ L-Tyrosine
↑ Vitamin B_6
↓ Vitamin B_6
↓ Vitamin B_{12}
↓ Zinc

COMA

↓ Magnesium
↓ Thiamine
   WARNING: Give thiamine hydrochloride IV before administering glucose. (*Since thiamine is a cofactor in glucose metabolism, remaining thiamine stores will be utilized.*)

depressed DEEP TENDON REFLEXES

↑ Calcium
↓ Folic Acid
↑ Sodium

DELIRIUM

↓ Magnesium

DEMENTIA

↓ Niacin (*pellagra*) (*late*)
↓ Thiamine
↓ Vitamin B_6
↓ Vitamin B_{12}

DEPRESSION

↓ Biotin (*rare*)
↑ Calcium
↓ Calcium
↑ Copper
↓ Copper
↓ Folic acid
↓ Iron
↑ Magnesium
↓ Magnesium
↓ Niacin (*pellagra*) (*mild*)
↓ Pantothenic Acid
↓ Para-aminobenzoic Acid (PABA)
↓ Potassium
↓ Riboflavin
↑ Selenium
↓ Sodium
↓ Thiamine
↓ Vitamin B_6
↓ Vitamin B_{12}
↓ Vitamin C (*mild*)
↑ Zinc
↓ Zinc

DIZZINESS

↑ Bismuth
↑ Iron
↓ Iron
↑ Magnesium (hypotension)
↓ Niacin (*pellagra*) (*mild*)
↓ Phosphorus
↓ Riboflavin
↓ Sodium
↓ Vitamin B_6
↓ Vitamin B_{12}

DYSARTHRIA

↑ Potassium

EMOTIONAL LABILITY (*moodiness*)

↓ Niacin
↓ Sodium
↓ Vitamin B_{12}

EPILEPSY (seizures)

↑ Folic Acid (*exacerbation*)
↑ Gamma-Linolenic Acid (*exacerbation*)
↓ Magnesium
↑ Sodium
↓ Sodium
↓ Vitamin B$_6$
     (infantile, drug-resistant)
↑ Zinc (*exacerbation of grand mal*)

EXCITABILITY

↑ Folic Acid

EXTENSOR PLANTAR RESPONSES ('Babinski's sign')

↓ Vitamin B$_{12}$

FAINTNESS

↑ Magnesium (*hypotension*)
↓ Pantothenic Acid

FATIGUE

↓ Biotin (*rare*)
↓ Calories
↓ Chromium
↑ Copper
↓ Copper
↓ Folic Acid
↓ Iodine
↑ Iron
↓ Iron
↑ Magnesium
↓ Magnesium
↓ Niacin (*mild*)
↓ Pantothenic Acid
↓ Para-aminobenzoic Acid (PABA)
↓ Phosphorus
↓ Potassium
↑ Selenium
↓ Sodium
↓ Thiamine
↑ Vitamin A
↓ Vitamin A
↓ Vitamin B$_6$

↓ Vitamin B$_{12}$
↓ Vitamin C *(mild)*
↑ Vitamin E
↓ Zinc

GAIL DISTURBANCE

↓ Vitamin E

GAIT, HIGH STEPPING

↓ Riboflavin
↓ Vitamin B$_6$
↓ Vitamin B$_{12}$

HEADACHE

↑ Bismuth
↓ Folic Acid
↑ Iron
↓ Iron
↓ Niacin *(pellagra)* *(mild)*
↓ Pantothenic Acid
↓ Para-aminobenzoic Acid (PABA)
↑ Phenylalanine
↑ S-Adenosyl-methionine
↓ Sodium
↑ Thiamine
↑ Vitamin A *(acute)*
↓ Vitamin B$_{12}$

HYDROCELPHALUS

↑ Vitamin A

HYPERACTIVITY

↓ Calcium
↑ Folic Acid
↓ Magnesium
↑ Sodium

HYPERESTHESIA *(increased sensitivity to touch)*

↓ Biotin *(rare)*

HYPERTONIA

↑ <u>Sodium</u>

HYPOESTHESIA (*decreased sensitivitty to touch*)

↓ <u>Folic Acid</u> (*"stocking" distribution*)

HYPOREFLEXIA

↓ <u>Potassium</u>

INCOORDINATION

↓ <u>Pantothenic acid</u>
↓ <u>Thiamine</u>

INSOMNIA

↓ <u>Biotin</u> (*rare*)
↓ <u>Calcium</u>
↑ <u>Chromium</u>
↑ <u>Copper</u>
↑ <u>Folic Acid</u>
↓ <u>Folic Acid</u>
↓ <u>Magnesium</u>
↓ <u>Niacin</u> (*pellagra*) (*mild*)
↓ <u>Pantothenic acid</u>
↓ <u>Potassium</u>
↑ <u>Thiamine</u>
↑ <u>L-Tyrosine</u>
↑ <u>Vitamin A</u>
↓ <u>Vitamin A</u>
↓ <u>Vitamin D</u>

IRRITABILITY

↑ <u>Calcium</u>
↓ <u>Calcium</u>
↑ <u>Chromium</u>
↓ <u>Copper</u>
↑ <u>Folic Acid</u>
↓ <u>Iron</u>
↓ <u>Magnesium</u>
↓ <u>Molybdenum</u>
↓ <u>Niacin</u> (*early*)
↓ <u>Pantothenic Acid</u>
↓ <u>Para-aminobenzoic Acid (PABA)</u>

↓ Phosphorus
↓ Protein-Calorie (*marasmus*)
↑ Selenium
↑ Sodium
↑ Thiamine
↓ Thiamine
↑ L-Tyrosine
↑ Vitamin A
↓ Vitamin B_6
↓ Vitamin B_{12}
↓ Vitamin C
↓ Zinc

KORSAKOFF'S PSYCHOSIS (confabulation & amnesia)

↓ Thiamine

LETHARGY

↓ Folic acid
↓ Magnesium
↑ Selenium
↓ Sodium
↑ Vitamin A
↓ Zinc (*moderate*)

LHERMITTE'S SIGN   (an 'electric shock' sensation upon bending the neck)

↓ Vitamin B_{12}

MALAISE

↑ Folic Acid
↑ Vitamin A
↓ Vitamin C

MANIA

↑ Folic Acid
↑ Gamma-Linolenic Acid (*exacerbation*)
↑ L-Glutamine
↑ L-5-Hydroxytryptophan
↑ S-Adenosyl-methionine

MOVEMENT DISORDERS

↑ Manganese

NERVOUSNESS

    ↓ Calcium
    ↓ Copper
    ↓ Magnesium
    ↓ Niacin *(mild)*
    ↓ Pantothenic Acid
    ↓ Potassium
    ↑ Thiamine
    ↓ Thiamine
    ↑ L-Tyrosine
    ↓ Vitamin B_6
    ↓ Vitamin D

NEUROMUSCULAR EXCITABILITY

    ↓ Calcium
    ↓ Magnesium

NUMBNESS OF LIMBS

    ↓ Thiamine

PAIN SENSITIVITY

    ↓ Thiamine

PARALYSIS

    ↑ Selenium

PERIPHERAL NEUROPATHY
    with *PARESTHESIAS (abnormal sensations such as burning, tingling or aching);*
        later with SENSORY and MOTOR DEFICITS, including MUSCLE WEAKNESS and
        REDUCED TENDON REFLEXES

    ↓ Calcium
    ↓ Folic Acid
    ↓ Magnesium
    ↓ Niacin *(pellagra)*
    ↓ Pantothenic Acid
    ↓ Phosphorus
    ↑ Selenium
    ↓ Thiamine *(beriberi) (late)*
    ↑ Vitamin B_6
    ↓ Vitamin B_6 *(sensory)*
    ↓ Vitamin B_{12}
    ↓ Vitamin C *(scurvy)*

↓ Vitamin E

PSEUDOTUMOR CEREBRI *(increased intracranial pressure)*

↑ Vitamin A (*acute*)

PSYCHOSIS

↑ Calcium
↓ Calcium
↑ Folic Acid (*exacerbation*)
↓ Folic Acid
↓ Magnesium
↓ Niacin (*pellagra*)
↓ Sodium
↓ Vitamin B$_{12}$
↑ Zinc (hallucinations)
↓ Zinc

RESTLESS LEGS

↓ Folic Acid

RESTLESSNESS

↑ S-Adenosyl-methionine
↑ L-Tyrosine
↑ Vitamin A

RETROBULBAR NEUROPATHY *(increased pallor of the temporal aspect of the optic disc accompanied by pain behind the eyeball, photophobia and visual field defects)*

↓ Thiamine
↓ Vitamin B$_{12}$

RIGIDITY

↓ Niacin (*pellagra*) (*late*)

SEDATION

↑ Niacinamide

SOMNOLENCE *(sleepiness)*

↑ Vitamin A
↓ Vitamin B$_6$

SONOPHOBIA

    ↓ Magnesium
    ↓ Thiamine

SUBACUTE COMBINED SPINAL CORD DEGENERATION

    ↓ Folic Acid
    ↓ Vitamin B_{12}

TETANY

    ↓ Calcium
    ↓ Magnesium
        causing hypocalcemia
    ↓ Vitamin D

TREMOR

    ↑ Lithium
    ↓ Magnesium
    ↓ Niacin (*pellagra*) (*late*)
    ↑ Sodium

TREMULOUSNESS

    ↓ Phosphorus

WEAKNESS

    ↓ Biotin (*rare*)
    ↑ Calcium
    ↑ Copper
    ↓ Copper
    ↓ Folic Acid
    ↑ Magnesium
    ↓ Magnesium
    ↓ Niacin
    ↓ Pantothenic Acid
    ↓ Phosphorus
    ↓ Potassium
    ↓ Protein
    ↑ Selenium
    ↓ Sodium
    ↑ Thiamine
    ↓ Thiamine
    ↑ Vitamin A

↓ Vitamin B$_6$
↓ Vitamin D
↑ Vitamin E

WERNICKE'S ENCEPHALOPATHY
(initially disorientation, drowsiness, inattentiveness; later oculomotor disturbances, cerebellar ataxia and confusion)

↓ Thiamine

NOSE

EPISTAXIS *(nosebleeds)*

↑ Vitamin A
↓ Vitamin C (*scurvy*)

PANCREAS

INSUFFICIENCY

↓ Selenium

PARATHYROIDS

HYPERPARATHYROIDISM

↑ Calcium
↓ Phosphorus

HYPOPARATHYROIDISM

↓ Calcium
↑ Phosphorus

PAROTID GLANDS

ENLARGEMENT

↓ Protein-Calorie

REPRODUCTIVE SYSTEM

AMENORRHEA

↑ <u>Vitamin A</u>

BREAST SORENESS

↑ <u>Vitamin E</u>

GYNECOMASTIA

↑ <u>Iodine</u>

HYPOGONADISM

↓ <u>Zinc</u> *(severe)*

HYPOSPERMIA

↓ <u>Zinc</u>

IMPOTENCE

↓ <u>Zinc</u>

INFERTILITY

↓ <u>Essential Fatty Acids</u>
↓ <u>Selenium</u> *(males)*
↓ <u>Zinc</u> *(males)*

MENSTRUAL ABNORMALITIES

↑ <u>Vitamin A</u>

OLIGOSPERMIA

↓ <u>Zinc</u> *(mild)*

delayed SEXUAL MATURATION

↓ <u>Zinc</u>

decreased TESTOSTERONE

↓ <u>Zinc</u> *(mild)*

RESPIRATORY SYSTEM

BRONCHIAL ASTHMA

↑ L-Tryptophan (*aggravation*)

COUGH, PRODUCTIVE

↑ Iodine

EMPHYSEMA

↓ Copper

IRREGULAR BREATHING

↓ Phosphorus

RESPIRATORY DISTRESS (*shortness of breath*)

↓ Potassium
↓ Thiamine

RESPIRATORY INSUFFICIENCY

↑ Magnesium

TACHYPNEA (*rapid breathing*)

↓ Molybdenum

SALIVARY GLANDS

EXCESSIVE SALIVATION

↑ Iodine

SIALADENITIS (*inflammation*)

↑ Iodine

SKIN

ACNE

↓ Essential Fatty Acids
↑ Iodine
↓ Potassium
↓ Vitamin A
↑ Vitamin B$_6$
↓ Vitamin B$_6$
↑ Vitamin B$_{12}$
↑ Vitamin E
↓ Zinc

ATROPHY

↓ Riboflavin *(localized)*

BROWN MOTTLING

↓ Folic acid
    (nape extending to the neck, axillae and lateral abdominal areas)
↓ Protein-Calorie
    (cheeks)
↓ Vitamin B$_{12}$
    (nape and extending to the neck, axillae and lateral abdominal areas)

BULLAE *(large vesicles)*
↓ Niacin *(pellagra)*

CASAL'S NECKLACE *(a reddish-purple, scaly band or collar of dermatosis running around the neck and down the sternum)*
↓ Niacin *(pellagra)*

DERMATOSIS

↑ Chromium
↓ Copper
↓ Essential Fatty Acids
    with scaling
↓ Niacin *(pellagra)*
    vesicles, blisters, fissures and scales (primarily seen in areas exposed to light
    or chronically irritated)
↓ Protein (*"flaky-paint"*)
↓ Riboflavin *(scrotal)*
↑ Selenium
↓ Sodium
↑ Vitamin A *(facial)*

↓ Zinc (*severe*)
      bullous and pustular

ECZEMATOID LESIONS

↓ Calcium
↓ Essential Fatty Acids
↓ Inositol
↓ Pantothenic Acid
↓ Zinc (*severe*)
      distal distribution (face, hands, feet, anogenital region)

EDEMA (*smoothness due to fluid retention*)

↓ Magnesium
↓ Niacin (*pellagra*)
      with scaly desquamation followed by a wizened, glazed skin
↓ Potassium
↓ Protein
      Pitting edema
↑ Sodium
↓ Thiamine (*beriberi*)
      Pitting edema
↑ Vitamin A
↓ Vitamin B_6
↓ Vitamin C (*scurvy*)
      Firm, painful edema
      sometimes with pigmentary alterations that resemble scleroderma

ERYTHEMA (*redness*)

↓ Essential Fatty Acids
      Glazed erythema around the nose, eyes and ears
↓ Niacin (*pellagra*) (*early*)
      with burning and pruritis (especially nose and cheekbones)
      Ears are silvery.
      Often better in the winter.
↓ Thiamine (*beriberi*) (*mild*)
↑ Vitamin A

EXANTHEMA (*eruptions*)

↑ Iodine
↑ Niacin
↑ Para-aminobenzoic Acid (PABA)
↑ Vitamin A

FLUSHING

↑ Magnesium
↑ Niacin
↑ Thiamine

HYPERHYDROSIS (excess sweatiness)

↑ S-Adenosyl-methionine
↑ Choline
↑ Thiamine
↓ Vitamin D
      (scalp only)
↑ Zinc

HYPERKERATOSIS (skin thickened, dry and wrinkled)

↓ Protein-Calorie
↓ Vitamin A

HYPERKERATOSIS, PERIFOLLICULAR ('gooseflesh'; 'sharkskin')

↓ Essential Fatty Acids
↓ Protein-Calorie
↓ Riboflavin
↓ Vitamin A
↓ Vitamin C (*scurvy*)
      with fragmented corkscrew-like hairs buried in a hyperkeratotic follicle
           with perifollicular hemorrhages within the hyperkeratotic areas on the
           posterior side of the thighs, on the anterior side of the forearms, and on the
           abdomen

HYPERPIGMENTATION

↓ Folic Acid
      especially palms and soles
↑ Niacin
↓ Niacin (*pellagra*) (late)
      also hard, rough and cracked with a marginated darker edge
      (due to fibrous deposition)
↓ Protein-Calorie
↓ Riboflavin
      (scrotal or vulvar area)
↓ Vitamin B$_{12}$
      especially palms and soles

ICTERUS (jaundice)

> ↑ <u>Vitamin A</u>
> ↓ <u>Vitamin B$_{12}$</u>

NIGHT SWEATS

> ↑ <u>Vitamin A</u>

PALLOR

> ↓ <u>Biotin</u> (rare)
> ↓ <u>Copper</u>
> ↓ <u>Folic Acid</u> (*lemon-yellow*)
> ↓ <u>Iron</u>
> ↓ <u>Vitamin B$_{12}$</u> (*lemon-yellow*)
> ↑ <u>Vitamin D</u>

PRESSURE SORES

> ↓ <u>Protein-Calorie</u>

PRURITIS

> ↑ <u>Niacin</u>
> ↑ <u>Selenium</u>
> ↑ <u>Thiamine</u>
> ↑ <u>Vitamin A</u>

PURPURA (bleeding into the skin)

> ↑ <u>Vitamin A</u>
> ↓ <u>Vitamin C</u> (*scurvy*)
>> *especially* at a site of trauma, pressure, or irritation, such as on the buttock or the posterior side of the thighs
> ↓ <u>Vitamin K</u>

RASH, BROWNISH-RED

> ↓ <u>Niacin</u> (*pellagra*)
>> Papules on the dorsum of the hands which may be pruriginous (itchy)

SEBORRHEIC DERMATOSIS (eczema; a scaly eruption covered with a slightly adherent oily scale)

> ↓ <u>Biotin</u> (*rare*)
> ↓ <u>Essential Fatty Acids</u>
> ↓ <u>Riboflavin</u>

(around the nose, eyes and ears)
↓ Thiamine
↓ Vitamin B$_6$ (rare)
    (around the nose, eyes and ears)
↓ Zinc
    (around the nose, eyes and ears)

SLATE GREY

↑ Iron

THICKENING

↓ Essential Fatty Acids

ULCERATIONS

↓ Vitamin C (*scurvy*) (*late*)

VITILIGO *(patchy depigmentation)*

↓ Copper
↑ Para-aminobenzoic Acid (PABA)

XEROSIS *(dryness)*

↓ Biotin (*rare*) (*greyish*)
    with scaly desquamation
↓ Essential Fatty Acids
↓ Iron
    with scales around the mouth and lips
↓ Potassium
↓ Protein-Calorie
↓ Riboflavin
↑ Vitamin A (*acute*)
    with scaly desquamation
↓ Vitamin A
    with roughness.
        Changes are prominent on the extensor surface of the limbs, the back, the posterior neck, and the shoulders.
↓ Zinc (*moderate*)
    with glazed erythema around the nose, eyes and ears

YELLOW-ORANGE COLOR
especially in palms, soles and nasolabial folds (sclerae remain clear, in contrast to jaundice)

↑ Beta-Carotene

SPLEEN

SPLENOMEGALY

↓ Iron (*common in iron-deficiency anemia*)
↑ Vitamin A

TEETH

CARIES

↓ Calcium
↓ Fluorine
↓ Phosphorus
↓ Protein-Calorie

LOOSE

↓ Vitamin C (*scurvy*)

MOTTLING OF ENAMEL

↑ Fluorine

PERIODONTAL DISEASE

↓ Calcium

TEMPERATURE

FEVER

↑ Para-aminobenzoic Acid (PABA)
↑ Vitamin A (*chronic*)
↑ Vitamin D

THYROID

GOITER

↓ <u>Iodine</u>

HYPOTHYROIDISM

↑ <u>Lithium</u>

TONGUE

Ignore tongue color in evaluating patients whose hemoglobins are below 8 g/dl because severe anemia will make tongue color normal *(Friedman PJ, Hodges RE. Tongue colour and B-vitamin deficiencies. Letter. <u>Lancet</u> i:1159-60, 1977)*.

ACUTE GLOSSITIS (bright scarlet red, painful, inflammed tongue with prominent papillae)

↓ <u>Folic Acid</u> *(mild)*
↓ <u>Iron</u> *(mild)*
↓ <u>Niacin</u> *(pellagra) (mild)*
↓ <u>Riboflavin</u> *(mild)*
↓ <u>Vitamin B$_6$</u> *(mild)*
↓ <u>Vitamin B$_{12}$</u> *(mild)*

ATROPHIC GLOSSITIS (smooth, small, glistening, non-painful tongue with atrophy of the filiform papillae)

Patients tend to have multiple nutritional deficiencies *(Drinka PJ, Langer EH, Voeks SK, et al. Nutritional correlates of atrophic glossitis: possible role of vitamin E in papillary atrophy. <u>J Am Coll Nutr</u> 12(1):14-20, 1993)*.

"The thin epithelium of the 'bald' tongue seems to be a poor veil over the capillary bed, thereby yielding an abnormally blue or cyanotic tongue. Patients with severe anaemia and papillary atrophy may retain a normal tongue colour because the capillary bed is pale rather than cyanotic" *(Friedman PJ, Hodges RE. Tongue colour and B-vitamin deficiencies. Letter. <u>Lancet</u> i:1159-60, 1977)*.

There is an 80% chance of a <u>niacin</u> or <u>riboflavin</u> deficiency in a patient without hypoxemia or severe anemia whose tongue shows papillary atrophy along with an abnormal color *(Leevy CM, Baker H, TenHove W, et al. <u>Am J Clin Nutr</u> 16:339, 1964)*.

↓ <u>Biotin</u> *(rare)*
↓ <u>Folic Acid</u> *(chronic or in remission)*
↓ <u>Iron</u> *(chronic)*
↓ <u>Niacin</u> *(chronic)*

↓ Protein
↓ Riboflavin
↓ Vitamin B$_6$
↓ Vitamin B$_{12}$ (*chronic or in remission*)
↓ Vitamin C
↓ Vitamin E

- with MAGENTA color (*deep, purplish-red tongue*)

"The cyanotic tongue colour in hypoxaemia cannot be distinguished clinically from that produced by nutritional deficiencies. Hypoxaemia, however, does not lead to papillary atrophy, so a bald tongue is a clue to underlying B-vitamin deficiencies" (*Friedman PJ, Hodges RE. Tongue colour and B-vitamin deficiencies. Letter. Lancet i:1159-60, 1977*).

↓ Biotin (*rare*)
    also swollen and painful
↓ Niacin (*pellagra*) (*more common*)
    also swollen, raw and fissured
↓ Pantothenic Acid
    usually painless
↓ Riboflavin (*more common*)
    also dry; painless or sore; may be swollen

- with BLACK color

↓ Niacin (*pellagra*) (*less common*)
↓ Riboflavin (*less common*)

VASCULAR

ANEURYSMS

↓ Copper

THROMBOPHLEBITIS

↑ Vitamin E

OTHER

BODY ODOR

↑ L-Carnitine

easy BRUISING

↓ Vitamin C

CACHEXIA

↓ Protein-Calorie

COLD SENSITIVITY

↓ Iron
↓ Magnesium

CRETINISM

↓ Iodine

DYSGEUSIA (taste impairment)

↓ Sodium
↓ Zinc (*mild*)

DYSOSMIA (smell impairment)

↓ Vitamin A
↓ Zinc (*mild*)

GLUCOSE INTOLERANCE

↓ Biotin (*rare*)
↓ Chromium
↓ Phosphorus
↓ Potassium
↓ Zinc

GROWTH IMPAIRMENT

↓ Calcium
↓ Chromium
↓ Essential Fatty Acids
↓ Folic Acid
↓ Iron
↓ Magnesium
↓ Potassium
↓ Protein-Calorie
↓ Riboflavin
↓ Selenium
↓ Vitamin A

↓ Vitamin B$_6$
↓ Vitamin D
↓ Zinc

HALITOSIS (breath odor)

↓ Niacin
↑ Selenium ("garlic" odor)

HEMORRHAGING

↓ Vitamin K

HYPERAMMONEMIA

↓ Zinc (mild)

HYPERCALCEMIA

↑ Vitamin D

HYPERCHOLESTEROLEMIA

↓ Biotin (rare)
↓ Chromium
↓ Copper
↓ Inositol
↓ Potassium
↓ Selenium
↓ Zinc

HYPOCHOLESTEROLEMIA

↓ Choline

reduced IMMUNE FUNCTION

↓ Essential Fatty Acids
↑ Omega-3 Fatty Acids (cell-mediated immunity)
↑ Selenium (phagocyte and natural killer cell activities)
↓ Selenium (leukocyte bactericidal activity and cell-mediated immunity)
↑ Zinc (phagocytic chemotaxis & T-cell function)

frequent INFECTIONS

↓ Copper
↓ Essential Fatty Acids
↓ Linoleic Acid

↓ Pantothenic Acid
↓ Selenium
↓ Vitamin A
↓ Zinc

KWASHIORKOR (edema, fatty liver, sparse & light hair, skin color changes, dermatosis)

↓ Protein

MARASMUS (wasting)

↓ Protein-Calorie

PAROTID SWELLING

↓ Protein-Calorie

POLYDIPSIA (excessive thirst)

↓ Essential Fatty Acids
↑ Lithium
↑ Magnesium
↓ Potassium
↑ S-Adenosyl-methionine
↑ Sodium
↑ Vitamin A
↑ Vitamin D

POLYURIA (frequent urination)

↓ Essential Fatty Acids

"SICCA" syndrome (lack of salivary and tear gland secretions)

↓ Vitamin C

bad TASTE

↑ Iodine ("brassy")
↑ Selenium ("metallic")

WEIGHT LOSS

↓ Sodium
↑ Vitamin A (chronic)
↓ Vitamin A
↓ Vitamin B$_6$

poor WOUND HEALING

↓ Essential Fatty Acids
↓ Protein-Calorie
↓ Vitamin B$_6$
↓ Vitamin C
↓ Zinc

SELECTED REFERENCES

Barthelemy H, Chouvet B, Cambazard F. Skin and mucosal manifestations in vitamin deficiency. J Am Acad Dermatol 15(4-6):1263-74, 1986

Buist RA. Editorial: Vitamin toxicities, side effects and contraindications. Int Clin Nutr Rev 4(4):159-71, 1984

Christakis G. How to make a nutritional diagnosis without really trying. A. Adult nutritional diagnosis. J Florida Med Assoc 66(4):34956, 1979

Hathcock JN, Hattan DG, Jenkins MY, et al. Evaluation of vitamin A toxicity. Am J Clin Nutr 52:183-202, 1990

McLaren DS. A Colour Atlas of Nutritional Disorders. London, Wolfe Medical Publications, Ltd., 1981

Prasad AS. Clinical, endocrinologic, and biochemical effects of zinc deficiency. Spec Top Endocrinol Metab 7:45-76, 1985

Prendiville JS, Manfredi LN. Skin signs of nutritional disorders. Semin Dermatol 11(1):88-97, 1992

Skelton WP III, Skelton NK. Deficiency of vitamins A, B, and C. Something to watch for. Postgrad Med 87(4):293-310, 1990

Skelton WP, Skelton NK. Thiamine deficiency neuropathy: it's still common today. Postgrad Med 85(8):301-6, 1989

Chapter Two

COMMON NUTRITIONAL DEFICIENCIES

Despite their adverse effects on health, nutritional deficiencies are frequently undiagnosed. This chapter reviews the deficiencies that are most frequently discovered when a proper nutritional work-up is performed and notes which population groups are most likely to develop them.

GENERAL

Hospitalized patients are frequently nutritionally deficient.

> *Note: Albumin and other negative acute-phase proteins fall after any episode resulting in a rise in release of cytokines; they may therefore be inappropriate as a measure of malnutrition for acutely ill patients (Fleck A, Smith G. Assessment of malnutrition in elderly patients. Letter. Lancet 337:793, 1991).*

Observational Study: 40% of 100 consecutive admissions from each of 5 departments (general surgery, medicine, respiratory medicine, orthopedic surgery, geriatric medicine) at a British hospital were undernourished (body mass index <20). Only 96 of the 200 undernourished pts. (48%) had any nutritional information documented in their charts by the time of discharge. At discharge, the 112 pts. who were reassessed had a mean wt. loss of 5.4%, with the greatest wt. loss occurring in those initially most undernourished. 10 pts. were referred for nutritional support, and these pts. had a mean wt. gain of 7.9% (*McWhirter JP, Pennington CR. Incidence and recognition of malnutrition in hospital. BMJ 308:945-8, 1994*).

Observational Study: 133 pts. were evaluated and stratified into 2 gps.: medical (n=64) or surgical (n=69). Age range was 16-97 yrs. (mean 48 ± 14). Nutritional assessment included serum albumin, total lymphocyte count, weight for height, triceps skinfold, and arm-muscle circumference. The overall prevalence of malnutrition as defined by at least one abnormal parameter was 72%. 29% of pts. had 2 or more abnormal nutritional parameters; 61% had recent weight loss, with an ave. loss of 12%. 81% of the medical pts. and 64% of the surgical pts. were malnourished based on the assessment. In the evaluable malnourished gp., 55/79 (70%) had no referral to a nutrition professional; 16% of that gp. was receiving a sub-optimal diet (*Vitello JM, Olree K. Prevalence of malnutrition in hospitalized patients remains high. Abstract. J Am Coll Nutr 12:599, 1993*).

Experimental Controlled Study: Elderly patients with fractured neck of the femur are frequently nutritionally deficient and, despite being offered adequate quantities of food to satisfy their nutritional needs, they are likely to fail to meet their nutritional requirements during their hospital stay. The use of an oral nutritional supplement (250 ml, 20 g protein, 30 g carbohydrate, 5.8 g lipid, 254 kcal, vitamins & minerals) may significantly improve the clinical outcome. In this study, following a mean of 32 days of supplementation, the clinical outcome was significantly better in the supplemented gp. of 27 elderly pts. vs. 32 controls (56% favorable course vs. 13%), the median duration of hospital stay was significantly shorter (24 vs. 40 days) and the rates of complications and death were significantly lower (44% vs. 87%). Moreover, 6 mo. after the fracture, the rates of complications and mortality were significantly lower (40% vs. 74%) *(Delmi M, Rapin CH, Bengoa JM, et al. Dietary supplementation in elderly patients with fractured neck of the femur. Lancet 335:1013-6, 1990).*

Observational Study: "Between 25 and 50% of patients admitted to an acute medical service are malnourished. Physicians are often unaware which patients are admitted at nutritional risk and make no attempt to arrest further nutritional decline until a dramatic deterioration has occurred. We studied all patients admitted to an acute medical ward before and after their physicians were taught to recognize nutritional deficiency early and to intervene appropriately. During the initial period, the house staff correctly identified two (12.5%) of 16 patients as being malnourished. During the posteducation period, physicians correctly identified all 14 patients admitted at nutritional risk (100%)" *(Roubenoff R, Roubenoff RA, Preto J, Balke CW. Malnutrition among hospitalized patients. A problem of physician awareness. Arch Intern Med 147(8):1462-5, 1987).*

Observational Study: In a 30 mo. study of records of 800 pts. admitted to two American hospitals with pneumonia, hip fracture, or inflammatory bowel disease, or in order to have hip, bowel or abdominal surgery, some degree of malnutrition was found in 55% of all pts. (based on: serum albumin below 3.4 g/dl; weight <90% of ideal body weight; total lymphocyte count <1400/mm^3; history of recent weight loss). Among the nonsurgical gps., malnourished pts. stayed in the hospital an ave. of 2 days longer than well-nourished pts. while, among the surgical gps., malnourished pts. stayed 5 days longer *(Nutritional therapy saves lives, costs. Med World News February 24, 1986, p. 99).*

Observational Study: 583/15,876 pts. (3.67%) were suffering from malnutrition or had nutritional risk factors (NRFs) (cancer, nothing by mouth for 3 or more days, loss of appetite, difficulty chewing or swallowing, persistent fever, cancer chemotherapy or radiation therapy) upon admission. 182/583 received nutritional support and were excluded from the study. After 3 wks., the remaining pts. were reassessed and had significant decreases in nutritional parameters: 622 pts. with deficits in one parameter on admission had a significant decrease in all parameters (p<0.001) and there was a deterioration in nutritional status in those pts. entering the hospital with NRFs only or with one low parameter *(Pinchcofsky GD, Kaminski MV Jr. Increasing malnutrition during hospitalization: Documentation by a nutritional screening program. J Am Coll Nutr 4(4):471-9, 1985).*

Observational Study: In a study of 3172 hospitalized American pts., 58% were malnourished according to at least one of the following indicators: serum albumin, total lymphocyte count, hemoglobin values, and weight-for-height measurement *(S Kamath - reported in Am Med News May 24/31, 1985).*

Observational Study: In a private American community hospital, 33% of pts. were found to be malnourished at a subclinical level, and clear clinical signs of malnutrition were prevalent in 17% of cases *(Willcutts - reported in Wright RA. Nutritional assessment. Commentary. JAMA 244(6):559-60, 1980).*

Observational Study: 3 single-day nutrition surveys were conducted on pts. in the general medical wards of the Boston City Hospital. By standard criteria, more than 44% of pts. were malnourished, and the majority had definite protein-calorie malnutrition (*Bistrian BR, Blackburn GL, Vitale J, et al. Prevalence of malnutrition in general medical patients. JAMA 235:1567-70, 1976*).

Review Article: More than 50% of pts. in the medical wards of private and public hospitals are at various states of starvation (*Butterworth CE. The skeleton in the hospital closet. Nutr Today 9:4-8, 1974*).

Consumption of foods from hospital diets may be nutritionally inadequate.

Observational Study: 28 hospitalized elderly French pts. were evaluated. Based on a 5-day duplicate-diet analysis, mean caloric intakes (1310 kcal/day) were insufficient. Mean vitamin C (25.3 mg) and tocopherol (3.9 mg TE/day) were also insufficient; 79% of pts. had vitamin C intakes <2/3 RDA, while 86% had tocopherol intakes <2/3 RDA. Concerning retinol, 71% had intakes >2/3 RDA. While 18% had low blood vitamin C levels, none exhibited biochemical evidence of retinol or tocopherol deficiency based on plasma levels and the ratio of α-tocopherol to cholesterol, suggesting that blood vitamin levels are poor indicators of insufficient dietary intakes (*Schmuck A, Ravel A, Franco A, et al. Antioxidant vitamin intake and status in hospitalized elderly subjects. Abstract. J Am Coll Nutr 1495):551, 1995*).

Observational Study: In a random sample of the diets of 93 adult hospitalized non-surgical pts. from 5 Beirut hospitals, the caloric and protein content was adequate; however they were low in fiber and high in cholesterol. Food consumed was low in folic acid, vitamin B_6, vitamin B_{12}, ascorbic acid, vitamin D, calcium, copper, iron and zinc (*Baba N, Shaar K, Jammal W. Nutritional assessment of patients and adequacy of diet in selected hospitals. J Nutr Med 4:297-310, 1994*).

Observational Study: Compared to a prospective evaluation of general medical pts. at the U. of Alabama at Birmingham performed in 1976, a similar evaluation performed in 1988 was performed on 228 consecutive pts. using plasma folate, plasma ascorbate, weight for height, triceps skinfold, arm muscle circumference, lymphocyte count, albumin, and hematocrit combined to form a likelihood of malnutrition (LOM) score. Both evaluations found that high LOM scores on admission predicted longer lengths of stay and increased mortality. LOM scores paired from admission to follow-up worsened with stay in 1976 but improved in 1988. The number of pts. with high LOM scores at follow-up at the 14th day of hospitalization was 62% in 1976 and declined to 46% in 1988. Findings indicate that identification of malnutrition indicators has improved; however, further improvement is desirable (*Coats KG, Morgan S, Bartolucci AA, et al. Hospital-associated malnutrition: a reevaluation 12 years later. J Am Diet Assoc 93:2-33, 1993*).

Observational Study: The ave. daily intake of energy, protein, iron and vitamins of pts. on a surgical, medical, accident and elective orthopedic ward of an English hospital was studied over 5 consecutive days. Daily energy intake was less than the predicted basal metabolic rate in 13/55 (24%) pts., and daily protein intake was < 0.8 g/kg body weight in 9/55 (16%). Many of the pts. had daily intakes of iron and of vitamins less than those recommended for healthy adults (*Todd EA, Hunt P, Crowe PJ, Royle GT. What do patients eat in hospital? Hum Nutr Appl Nutr 38(4):294-7, 1984*).

<u>Parenteral nutrition</u> (TPN) often causes nutritional deficiencies. Within the first week, there are severe deficiencies of phosphorus, potassium, sodium, magnesium and essential fatty acids, while long-term TPN often leads to depletion of vitamins A and E, folic acid, biotin and vitamin B_6 as well as zinc, copper, chromium and selenium *(Chipponi J. Total parenteral nutrition (TPN) often causes nutrient deficiencies. <u>Am J Clin Nutr</u> 35:1112-16, 1982).*

<u>Pregnant women</u> are frequently nutritionally deficient.

Observational Study: Of 76 healthy pregnant American women, 78% had one or more glaring vitamin deficiencies *(Dostalova L. Correlation of the vitamin status between mother and newborn during delivery. <u>Dev Pharmacol Ther</u> 4 (Suppl 1):45-57, 1982).*

Observational Study: In a gp. of 174 pregnant women evaluated at parturition, compared to norms developed by the authors, hypovitaminemia of folic acid, thiamine, vitamin A, vitamin C, vitamin B_{12}, vitamin B_6 and niacin, in descending order, was common, while vitamin supplementation reduced its incidence *(Baker H, Frank O, Thomson AD, et al. Vitamin profile of 174 mothers and newborns at parturition. <u>Am J Clin Nutr</u> 28(1):59-65, 1975).*

<u>The elderly</u> frequently fail to ingest adequate amounts of certain nutrients.

Observational Study: 474 people freeliving seniors aged 54-98 in 355 households were interviewed. More than 40% of the men consumed less than 2/3 of the RDAs for vitamin A, vitamin E, calcium, and zinc. More than 2/3 of the women consumed less than 2/3 of the RDAs for vitamin E, calcium, and zinc. More than 1/5 people skipped at least one meal, especially lunch *(Ryan A, Craig L, Finn S. Nutrient intakes and dietary patterns of older Americans: A national study. <u>J Gerontol</u> 47:M145-50, 1992).*

Observational Study: 403 elderly Europeans residing at home were interviewed in regard to their vitamin and mineral intake. Compared to the Recommended Dietary Allowances, the Joint Nordic Recommendations and the Absolute Minimal Necessary Amounts, folacin intake was low in 100%, cholecalciferol in 62%, pyridoxine in 83%, and zinc in 87% (although the risk of zinc deficiency was only present in 0.5%). Intakes of the other major vitamins and minerals were sufficient. In conclusion, the diet of the elderly, possibly with the exception of folacin, is well above their absolute minimal requirements, but the margin towards malnutrition is small *(Elsborg L et al. The intake of vitamins and minerals by the elderly at home. <u>Int J Vitam Nutr Res</u> 53(3):321-9, 1983).*

Observational Study: The nutrient content of meals planned for elderly Americans in 14 nursing homes were deficient in energy, niacin, magnesium, zinc, vitamin B_6, and total folate. Their actual intakes were low, not only for these nutrients, but also for 9 others. Approx. 30% consumed fewer than 1,200 Kcal *(Sempos CT et al. A dietary survey of 14 Wisconsin nursing homes. <u>J Am Diet Assoc</u> 81(1):35-40, 1982).*

<u>The elderly</u> are frequently nutritionally deficient.

Note: Nutritional deficiencies among the elderly are frequently due to physical disorders interfering with normal dietary intake (Stanton BR, Exton-Smith AN. A longitudinal study of the dietary of elderly women. London, King Edward's Hospital Fund, 1970) or to malabsorption

(Montgomery RD, Haeney MR, Ross IN, et al. The ageing gut: A study of intestinal absorption in relation to nutrition in the elderly. Quart J Med 47(186):197-211, 1978).

Experimental Double-blind Study: 175 elderly subjects living at home and 110 in hospital with normal serum vitamin concentrations received an IM vitamin supplement containing 1 mg vitamin B_{12}, 1.1 mg folate, and 5 mg vitamin B_6 or placebo administered 8 times over a 3-wk. period. Vitamin supplements but not placebo significantly reduced the concentrations of methylmalonic acid, homocysteine, 2-methylcitric acid, and cystathionine in both study gps., with the maximal effects usually occurring within 5-12 days. Initially elevated metabolite concentrations returned to normal in a higher proportion of the vitamin than of the placebo group. Results suggest that "metabolic evidence of vitamin deficiency is common in the elderly, even in the presence of normal serum vitamin levels" *(Naurath HJ, Joosten E, Riezler R, et al. Effects of vitamin B_{12}, folate, and vitamin B_6 supplements in elderly people with normal serum vitamin concentrations. Lancet 346:85-9, 1995).*

Observational Study: Despite eating supervision and assistance, the majority of eating-dependent nursing home residents have inadequate intakes of numerous macro- and micronutrients. While these intakes could be normalized by administration of a daily multivitamin/trace mineral supplement, only a minority of these residents in US Veterans Administration nursing homes receive such a supplement *(Rudman D, Abbasi AA, Issacson K, Karpiuk E. Observations on the nutrient intake of eating-dependent nursing home residents: underutilization of micronutrient supplements. J Am Coll Nutr 14(6):604-13, 1995).*

DIETARY FACTORS

Calories

Adolescent female gymnasts frequently consume inadequate calories.

Observational Study: 22 Swedish teenage girls involved in elite gymnastic training who showed signs of delayed pubertal development including growth rate were compared to 22 girls not participating in sport. There was no difference in food intake between the 2 groups. While the reference gp. fell within the limits of the Swedish Nutritional Recommendations, >50% of the gymnasts had energy intakes below the SNR due to their higher physical activity *(Lindholm C, Hagenfeldt K, Hagman U. A nutrition study in juvenile elite gymnasts. Acta Paediatr 84:273-7, 1995).*

Patient intakes from hospital diets are frequently inadequate.

Observational Study: Dietary registration was undertaken in 56 consecutive pts. admitted to a department of general medicine ward for an ave. of 10.2 days. In 40 pts. (71.4%) the energy intake was less than the corresponding energy requirement as assessed from the ave. requirement for sick adults *(Stellfeld M, Gyldendorf B. [Dietary investigation in a general medical ward: The energy, protein and zinc intakes of 56 patients during a period of hospitalization.] Ugeskr Laeg 150(25):1537-40, 1988).*

Observational Study: The ave. daily energy intake of pts. on a surgical, medical, accident and elective orthopedic ward of an English hospital studied over 5 consecutive days was less than the predicted basal metabolic rate in 13/55 (24%) pts. (*Todd EA, Hunt P, Crowe PJ, Royle GT. What do patients eat in hospital? Hum Nutr Appl Nutr 38(4):294-7, 1984*).

<u>Nursing home</u> diets are frequently inadequate.

Observational Study: The nutrient content of meals planned for elderly Americans in 14 nursing homes were deficient in energy. Approx. 30% of pts. consumed fewer than 1,200 Kcal (*Sempos CT et al. A dietary survey of 14 Wisconsin nursing homes. J Am Diet Assoc 81(1):35-40, 1982*).

> *Note: The RDA (1989) for this age group (> age 51) is 1,280 Kcal for women and 1,530 Kcal for men although, beyond age 75, it is noted that the requirements are "somewhat less" due to reduced body size, resting energy expenditure and activity* (*National Research Council. Recommended Dietary Allowances. 10th Edition. Washington, DC, National Academy Press, 1989:33*).

Protein

Intake by <u>the elderly</u> is often inadequate.

Observational Study: The ave. daily protein intake of pts. on a surgical, medical, accident and elective orthopedic ward of an English hospital studied over 5 consecutive days was < 0.8 g/kg body weight in 9/55 (16%) (*Todd EA, Hunt P, Crowe PJ, Royle GT. What do patients eat in hospital? Hum Nutr Appl Nutr 38(4):294-7, 1984*).

Observational Study: The second National Health and Nutrition Examination Survey (NHANES II) found that the diets of 10-25% of American women above age 55 contain less than 30 gm of protein daily (*National Center for Health Statistics. NCHS dietary intake source data: United States 1976-80. Washington, DC: US Department of Health, 1980; 231:149-51*).

> *Note: The RDA (1989) for this population group is 50 gm daily.*

<u>The elderly</u> accommodate to a low-protein diet with losses of body cell mass, muscle function, and immune response (*Castaneda C, Charnley JM, Evans WJ, Crim MC. Elderly women accommodate to a low-protein diet with losses of body cell mass, muscle function, and immune response. Am J Clin Nutr 62:30-9, 1995*).

Protein-Calorie

The <u>nursing-home elderly</u> are frequently deficient.

Review Article: Protein-calorie malnutrition of the nursing-home elderly is widespread, with substandard body weight, midarm muscle circumference, and serum albumin levels in 30-50% (*Arora VD, Rudman D. Protein-calorie undernutrition in the nursing home. Geriatr Med Today 7(7):66, 1988*).

Nursing home patients are frequently deficient.

Observational Study: In a study of male residents in a 400 bed VA nursing home, protein-calorie undernutrition was found in 30% of residents requiring partial or total assistance. Mortality rates rose from 10% to 60% per year with each decrement in body weight as % of ideal from 100% to 70%. The prevalence of protein-calorie undernutrition increased in direct proportion to degree of functional impairment, and to frequency of intercurrent infection. Serum cholesterol and hemoglobin were the most sensitive nutritional indicators (*Rudman D. Nutritional status of nursing home men. Abstract. J Am Coll Nutr 6(5):420, 1987*).

NUTRIENTS

Amino Acids

Plasma levels of essential amino acids may be suboptimal in the elderly.

Observational Study: The fasting plasma amino acid profile in 22 healthy young men aged 25-35 was compared to the profile in 21 healthy independent elderly men aged 65-85, in 23 orally-fed nursing home men with dementia aged 65-92, and in 17 tube-fed nursing home men with dementia aged 65-88. Compared to the young men, all 3 gps. of elderly men had significantly ($p<0.05$) lower levels of methionine and branched-chain amino acids than the healthy young men and the ratio of essential to nonessential amino acids was significantly lower. Methionine was significantly lower in the elderly men with dementia than in the elderly men without dementia (*Rudman D et al. Fasting plasma amino acids in elderly men. Am J Clin Nutr 49:559-66, 1989*).

Calcium   1.5 gm. daily for postmenopausal women (1 gm. daily for premenopausal women over 35)

Note: Based on long-term metabolic balance studies, the ideal ratio of calcium to magnesium intake appears to be 2- or 2.5-to-1 (*Mildred Seelig, M.D., Ph.D. - interviewed by Zucker M in Let's Live, April, 1996:36-8*).

Women who ingest less than the above amounts are in negative calcium balance (*Heaney RP et al. Menopausal changes in calcium balance performance. J Lab Clin Med 92(6):953-63, 1978*).

Observational Study: Based on data gathered from the NHANES II study, many children between the ages of 3 and 18 consume calcium-poor diets. Boys consumed more calcium than girls, and their calcium intakes approached or exceeded minimal RDA levels. Black youths, however, consumed calcium-poor diets as early as age 3. Calcium intake dropped during the adolescent age for both blacks and females of both races. Calcium intake tended to correlate with calorie intake; as girls and young children restricted calories, calcium intake also dropped below acceptable levels (*Eck L, Hackett-Renner C. Calcium intake in youth: sex, age, and racial differences in NHANES II. Prev Med 21:473-82, 1992*).

NIH Consensus Conference: Calcium intake is commonly insufficient and insufficient intake is associated with decreased bone mineral density. The typical American diet supplies about 450-550 mg daily, well below the RDA. "It seems likely that an increase in calcium intake to 1,000 to 1,500 mg/day beginning well before the menopause will reduce the incidence of osteoporosis in postmenopausal women. Increased calcium intake may prevent age-related bone loss in men as well" *(NIH Consensus Conference: Osteoporosis. JAMA 252(6):799-802, 1984).*

Observational Study: Daily calcium intakes based on 3-day dietary records from the USDA's 1977-8 Nationwide Food Consumption Survey were below the Recommended Dietary Allowance for the majority of the U.S. population, particularly for adult women *(Morgan KJ et al. Magnesium and calcium dietary intakes of the U.S. population. J Am Coll Nutr 4:195, 1985).*

Calcium is the only mineral whose requirement doubles during <u>pregnancy</u> *(Truswell AS. Nutrition for pregnancy. Br Med J [Clin Res] July, 1985).*

Intake by the general population is often inadequate.

Review Article: "Dietary calcium intake fails to meet recommended levels in virtually all categories of Americans. . . . In virtually all age, sex, and ethnic categories . . . , median calcium intake is equal to or less than the minimum recommendation, leaving more than 50% of individuals consuming inadequate amounts of calcium" *(McCarron DA, Hatton D. Dietary calcium and lower blood pressure. We can all benefit. Editorial. JAMA 275(14):1128-9, 1996).*

Observational Study: 22.5% of 1,450 French-Canadian adults had insufficient intakes of calcium relative to the Canadian Recommended Nutrient Intake. Of this sub-gp., 69.6% were females *(Shatenstein B, Ghadirian P. Nutrient patterns, nutritional adequacy, and comparisons with nutrition recommendations among French-Canadian adults in Montreal. J Am Coll Nutr 15(3):255-63, 1996).*

Observational Study: 28 American college females consumed slightly more than half of the RDA for calcium *(Meacham SL, Taper LK, Volpe SL. Effect of boron supplementation on blood and urinary calcium, magnesium, and phosphorus, and urinary boron in athletic and sedentary women. Am J Clin Nutr 61:341-5, 1995).*

Observational Study: 30% of 2151 Americans, whether or not they were taking nutritional supplements, were found to be consuming <67% of the RDA for calcium *(Bock MA et al. Contribution of diet versus supplements to selected nutrient intake in the Western region. Nutr Res 13:189-96, 1993).*

Intake by <u>children</u> is often inadequate.

Observational Study: An American study of >1,000 children found that their intakes at all ages were low in calcium *(Nicklas TA, Farris RP, Myers L, Gerenson GS. Dietary intakes of electrolytes, minerals and trace metals in children's' diets: The Bogalusa Heart Study. J Advancement Med 8(4):241-58, 1995).*

Observational Study: In an American study of children aged 2-10 in 4,000 households, calcium intake was below the RDA in over 50% of the population *(Albertson AM, Tobelmann RC, Engstom A, Asp EH. Nutrient intakes of 2- to 10-year-old American children: 10-year trends. J Am Diet Assoc 92(12):1492-6, 1992).*

Intake by <u>young women following surgical menopause</u> is often inadequate.

Observational Study: Following a surgically induced menopause, young Chinese women living in Hong Kong had a mean dietary calcium intake of 397.6 mg using the 24-hr. recall method or 390.9 mg using a food frequency questionnaire, a level that is inadequate for postmenopausal females *(Haines CJ, Chung TKH, Leung PC, et al. Dietary calcium intake in postmenopausal Chinese women. Eur J Clin Nutr 48:591-4, 1994).*

Intake by <u>the elderly</u> is often inadequate.

Observational Study: Only 43% of American women over 65 yrs. of age consume more than 70% of the RDA for calcium *(Wright ES, Guthrie HA, Wang MQ, Bernardo V. The 1987-88 Nationwide Food Consumption Survey: an uptake on the nutrient intake of respondents. Nutr Tod 26:21-7, 1991).*

Experimental and Observational Study: Almost 2/3 of older French adults studied consumed less than 500 mg calcium daily compared to the U.S. RDA of 800 mg daily as well as less than the RDA for vitamin D. Blood levels of calcium and vitamin D were low and blood indicators of tissue and bone loss were high. When their diets were supplemented with calcium and vitamin D, blood levels increased and bone loss was reversed *(Chapuy M et al. Calcium and vitamin D supplements: Effect on calcium metabolism in elderly people. Am J Clin Nutr 46:324-8, 1987).*

Chromium

Normal dietary chromium intake in the United States and other westernized countries is roughly 50-60% of the minimal Estimated Safe and Adequate Daily Dietary Intake of 50 µg established by the National Research Council (US) *(Anderson RA. Chromium and its role in lean body mass and weight reduction. Nutr Rep 11(6), 1993).*

Observational Study: 22 well-balanced daily diets prepared by nutritionists were found to contain only a fraction of the Estimated Safe and Adequate Dietary Intake of chromium (8.4-23.7 µg/1000 cal; mean 13.4 µg) *(Anderson RA, Bryden NA, Polansky MM. Dietary chromium intake. Freely chosen diets, institutional diet and individual foods. Biol Trace Elem Res 32:117-21, 1992).*

Observational Study: In a study of the self-selected diets of 10 males and 22 females (ages 25-65), chromium intake was only 33 µg/d for men and 25 µg/d for women; over 90% of the diets were below the US Recommended Dietary Allowance of 50-200 µg/d and 25% contained <20 µg/d *(Anderson RA, Kozlovsky AS. Chromium intake, absorption and excretion of subjects consuming self-selected diets. Am J Clin Nutr 41:1177-83, 1985).*

See Also:

Gibson R, Scythes C. Chromium, selenium and other trace element intakes of a selected sample of Canadian premenopausal women. Biol Trace Elem Res 6:105-16, 1984

Kumpulainen JT, Wolf WR, Veillon C, Mertz W. Determination of chromium in selected United States diets. J Agric Food Chem 27(3):490-4, 1979

Schroeder HA. The role of chromium in mammalian nutrition. Am J Clin Nutr 21(3):230-44, 1968

The elderly often ingest less than recommended levels. Moreover, urinary excretion increases with aging, suggesting that the body is less able to retain chromium (*Offenbacher E. Chromium and the elderly. Biol Trace Elem Res 32:123-31, 1992*).

See Also:

Bunker W et al. The uptake and excretion of chromium by the elderly. Am J Clin Nutr 39:799-802, 1984

Copper

The average daily intake by individuals consuming typical Western diets (1.0-1.5 mg) is lower than the 2-3 mg recommended to be safe and adequate (*Schoenemann HM et al. Consequences of severe copper deficiency are independent of dietary carbohydrate in young pigs. Am J Clin Nutr 52:147-54, 1990*).

Observational Study: The mean dietary intakes of 37% of 270 US Navy Sea, Air, and Land trainees were below the Recommended Dietary Allowances or the Estimated Safe and Adequate Intake range. Dietary intake was unassociated with plasma concentration (*Singh A et al. Magnesium, zinc, and copper status of US Navy SEAL trainees. Am J Clin Nutr 49:695-700, 1989*).

Observational Study: 75% of the daily diets in the U.S. fail to contain the Recommended Dietary Allowance of 2-3 mg/d (*Klevay LM. Biol Trace Elem Res 5:245-55, 1983*).

Observational Study: Dietary copper levels were determined spectrophotometrically for 22 men and women eating self-selected diets. 81% were found to consume less than 2/3 the US RDA for copper, even though the ave. daily protein intake exceeded the RDA (*Holden JM et al. Zinc and copper in self-selected diets. J Am Diet Assoc 75:23-8, 1979*).

Observational Study: The mean daily level of copper intake in hospital diets in the US was 0.76 mg (*Klevay LM et al. Evidence of dietary copper and zinc deficiencies. JAMA 241:1916-18, 1979*).

See Also:

Wolf WR et al. Daily intake of zinc and copper from self selected diets. Fed Proc 36:1175, 1977

Pregnant women may be in negative copper balance unless supplemented.

Experimental and Observational Study: 24 women in their second trimester were found to ingest less than the US RDA of copper. Copper retention was -0.02 mg/day until they were supplemented with copper which raised copper retention to 0.89 mg/day (*Taper L et al. Am J Clin Nutr 41:1184-92, 1985*).

Vegetarians are especially susceptible to copper deficiency.

Observational Study: A gp. of 44 vegetarians had statistically significantly lower plasma copper levels than controls *(Kadrabova J et al. Selenium status, plasma zinc, copper, and magnesium in vegetarians. Biol Trace Elem Res 50:13-24, 1995).*

Essential Fatty Acids

Intake is often inadequate.

Observational Study: The fatty acid profiles of >500 adults from the Framingham Heart Study were analyzed. More than 20% had biochemical evidence of an omega-3 or an omega-6 fatty acid deficiency, with ≥ 5% having a severe deficiency *(Siguel EN. Essential and trans fatty acid metabolism in health and disease. Compr Ther 20:500-10, 1994).*

Folic acid

Causes of deficiency include malabsorption (such as in celiac disease), exclusive ingestion of foods that are boiled for a long time, infant nutrition limited to goat's milk or the use of anti-folate drugs *(Barthelemy H, Chouvet B, Cambazard F. Skin and mucosal manifestations in vitamin deficiency. J Am Acad Dermatol 15(4-6):1263-74, 1986).*

Intake is often inadequate.

Review Article: 37 studies of elderly subjects published 1980-93 were reviewed. In several studies, a substantial proportion of subjects had folate intakes 2/3 below the country-specific recommended levels *(van der Wielen RPJ, de Groot LCPGM, van Staveren WA. Dietary intake of water soluble vitamins in elderly people living in a Western society (1980-1993). Nutr Res 14(4):605-38, 1994).*

Observational Study: Analysis of dietary data taken from a survey of US adults aged 19-74 (NHANES II) found mean daily folate intake to be 242 ± 2.8 μg for all adults, compared to the US RDA of 400 μg/d *(Subar AF et al. Folate intake and food sources in the US population. Am J Clin Nutr 50:508-16, 1989).*

Deficiency is not uncommon.

Observational Study: The U.S. Second National Health and Nutrition Examination Survey (NHANES II) found that about 11% of the normal US population could have deficient levels of serum folate (<3 μg/l) *(Senti FR, Pilch SM. Analysis of folate data from the Second National Health and Nutrition Examination Survey. J Nutr 115:1398-1402, 1985).*

Often deficient in the elderly *(Baker H et al. Severe impairment of dietary folate utilization in the elderly. J Am Geriatr Soc 26(5):218-21, 1978)* even despite adequate food intake and daily oral supplementation *(Frank O et al. Superiority of periodic intramuscular vitamins over daily oral vitamins in maintaining normal vitamin titers in a geriatric population. Am J Clin Nutr 30:630, 1977).*

Observational Study: Fasting serum folate levels were evaluated in 455 nursing home residents. 29% were taking folate supplements and 6% were taking phenytoin, a folate antagonist. None who were taking a folate supplement was low in folic acid. 9/325 (3%) residents not taking a folate supplement had low serum levels (<2.5 ng/mL). 2 of the 9 were receiving phenytoin. 5 of the 9 were characterized by staff as eating well. Results suggest that supplementation with a multivitamin containing 400 µg/d folic acid should be considered in nursing home residents (*Drinka PJ, Langer KH, Voeks SK, Goodwin JS. Low serum folic acid levels in a nursing home population: a clinical experience. J Am Coll Nutr 12(2):186-9, 1993*).

Observational Study: In a study of 92 elderly Canadians residing in an extended-care facility, 22% were deficient in folic acid. 9.2% were high-risk for a deficiency of RBC folate, while 30.9% were high-risk for serum folate deficiency. The correlation between the two levels was significant. The only variable found to correlate with folate deficiency was the length of stay in the facility (*Infante-Rivard C et al. Folate deficiency among institutionalized elderly: Public health impact. J Am Geriatr Soc 34:211-14, 1986*).

Observational Study: In a study of 403 elderly Danes residing in their own homes, folacin intake (66 µg mean; range 20-200 µg) was low in 100% as compared to the Recommended Dietary Allowances (RDA), Joint Nordic Recommendations (NNR) and the Absolute Minimal Necessary Amounts (AMA) (*Elsborg L et al. The intake of vitamins and minerals by the elderly at home. Int J Vitam Nutr Res 53:321-9, 1983*).

Observational Study: Low serum folate was found in 5-10% of elderly Americans living at home, and 15-20% of those admitted to hospitals or institutions (*Rosenberg IH et al. Folate nutrition in the elderly. Am J Clin Nutr 36:1060, 1982*).

Review Article: The results of several studies indicate that approx. 30% of the elderly in Great Britain have abnormally low blood folate levels (*Runcie J. Folate deficiency in the elderly, in MI Botez, EH Reynolds, Eds. Folic Acid in Neurology, Psychiatry, and Internal Medicine. New York, Raven Press, 1979:493-9*).

Often reduced in <u>adolescent females</u>.

Observational Study: The folacin status of 103 adolescent females aged 12, 14, and 16 yrs. was evaluated. 11.7% and 47.6% had serum and RBC folate levels <3 ng/ml (6.8 nmol/l) and 140 ng/ml (317 nmol/l), respectively. Folacin status was unrelated to per capita income (*Clark AJ et al. Folacin status in adolescent females. Am J Clin Nutr 46:302-6, 1987*).

For <u>premenopausal women</u>, the RDA of 180 µg daily may be inadequate.

Experimental Study: 17 nonpregnant women aged 21-27 consumed 200, 300, or 400 µg folate daily for 70 days. An intake of 200 µg daily was not sufficient to maintain folate status, and the women in this gp. showed elevated homocysteine levels (*O'Keffe CA et al. controlled dietary folate affects folate status in nonpregnant women. J Nutr 125:2717-25, 1995*).

In <u>pregnancy</u>, folic acid is the only vitamin whose requirement doubles. Serum and RBC folate levels decline during pregnancy and some degree of megaloblastic change can be found in substantial minorities of women in late pregnancy (*Truswell AS. Nutrition for pregnancy. Br Med J July, 1985*).

May be deficient in the absence of a megaloblastic anemia.

> **Experimental Study:** 3/17 elderly pts. with low concentrations of serum vitamin B_{12} or RBC folate but normal blood counts had bone marrow suppression, and 2 of the 3 also had megaloblastic changes in the marrow, suggesting that the low concentrations of serum B_{12} or RBC folate found in about 1/4 of elderly pts. might indicate actual tissue deficiencies even when blood counts were normal (*Matthews J et al. Effect of therapy with vitamin B_{12} and folic acid on elderly patients with low concentrations of serum vitamin B_{12} or erythrocyte folate but normal blood counts. Acta Haematologica 79:84-7, 1988*).

Dietary deficiency can result in a defect in the ability of intestinal cells to absorb folate when the diet is corrected (*Elsborg L. Reversible malabsorption of folic acid in the elderly with nutritional folate deficiency. Acta Haematology 55:140-7, 1976*).

Iodine

Severe iodine deficiency is common in many countries (*Hetzel BS. Iodine-deficiency disorders. Lancet i:1386-7, 1988*).

> **Observational Study:** The reference iodine intake in Britain is 140 µg daily, an intake all but special gps. such as vegans and infants manage to obtain. Based on the most recent national dietary survey, the ave. British intake is around 173 µg daily (*Lee SM, Lewis J, Buss DH, et al. Iodine in British foods and diets. Br J Nutr 72:435-46, 1994*).

Iron

Deficiency is believed to be the most prevalent worldwide nutritional deficiency and the most frequent cause of anemia (*Bernat I. Iron deficiency, in Iron Metabolism. New York, Plenum Press, 1983:215-74; Stoskman JA. Iron deficiency anemia: Have we come far enough? JAMA 258:1645-4, 1987*). It affects more than a quarter of the world's population (*DeMaeyer E, Adiels-Tegman M. The prevalence of anaemia in the world. World Health Stat Quart 38:302-16, 1985*).

> **Observational Study:** 548 healthy Danes (48% of whom were male) were evaluated. Appprox. 21.5% of the women and 15.5% of the men took daily iron supplements. Men at all ages had higher serum ferritin concentrations. Iron deficiency (serum ferritin <16 µg) was seen in about 14.7% of the women and 1% of the men. Iron-deficiency anemia was found in about 10% of the women with the highest incidence at ages 16-19; it was not found in the men. In women, iron supplementation reduced the risk of both iron deficiency and iron deficiency anemia (*Milman N, Clausen J, Jordal R. Iron status in young Danish men and women - a population survey comprising of 548 individuals. Ann Hematol 70(4):215-21, 1995*).

> **Review Article:** 20% of premenopausal American women (aged 18-44) have low iron stores based on serum ferritin (<12 µg/L), while 2.3% have anemia (reduced hemoglobin) (*Cook JD, Skikne BS, Lynch SR, Reusser ME. Estimates of iron sufficiency in the U.S. population. Blood 68:726-31, 1986*).

Frequently deficient in <u>children</u>.

Observational Study: An American study of >1,000 children found that their intakes at all ages were low in iron (*Nicklas TA, Farris RP, Myers L, Gerenson GS. Dietary intakes of electrolytes, minerals and trace metals in children's' diets: The Bogalusa Heart Study. <u>J Advancement Med</u> 8(4):241-58, 1995*).

Observational Study: In a study of 47 normal, healthy 1-year-old Irish children, 10 had low serum ferritin (<10 µg/L) and 3 had hemoglobin levels <11 g/dL (*Freeman VE, Hoey NMV, Gibney MJ. An assessment of the iron status of a sample of normal, healthy, 1-year-old children. <u>Proc Nutr Soc</u> 52:333A, 1993*).

Review Article: Iron deficiency is the most common nutrient deficiency in American children (*Worthington-Roberts B. Suboptimal nutrition and behavior in children, in <u>Contemporary Developments in Nutrition</u>. St. Louis, MO, CV Mosby, 1981:524-62*).

Frequently deficient in <u>adolescents</u>.

Observational Study: The dietary intakes of 79 lacto-ovo-vegetarian (LOV), 16 semi-vegetarian (SV) and 29 omnivorous (OM) females aged 13-19 were evaluated. 29% LOV, 44% SV, and 17% OM had low iron stores (plasma ferritin <12 µg/L), while only 3% had anemia. Intakes of iron and ascorbic acid were associated with serum iron (p<0.04) and total iron binding capacity (negatively: p<0.02), respectively; thus suboptimal iron status was attributed to a low intake of poorly available iron in all dietary gps. (*Donovan UM, Gibson RS. Iron and zinc status of young women aged 14 to 19 years consuming vegetarian and omnivorous diets. <u>J Am Coll Nutr</u> 14(5):463-72, 1995*).

Observational Study: 20% of a gp. of 114 British girls aged 11-14 had hemoglobin levels below 120 µg/L, with higher rates of low hemoglobin found in those of Asian origin and in vegetarians. The step test, a simple test of physical performance, showed that girls with a low hemoglobin status had impaired physical performance (*Nelson M, Bakaliou F, Trivedi A. Iron-deficiency anaemia and physical performance in adolescent girls from different ethnic backgrounds. <u>Br J Nutr</u> 72:427-43, 1994*).

Observational Study: The iron status of 207 Swedish subjects (220 females; 207 males) ages 15-16 was assessed. Iron deficiency (serum ferritin <16 µg/L) was present in 40% of the females and 15% of the males. Low serum ferritin levels were significantly correlated with reductions in transferrin saturation and hemoglobin concentration, confirming that these subjects were iron-deficient (*Hallberg L, Hulten L, Lilndstedt G et al. Prevalence of iron deficiency in Swedish adolescents. <u>Pediatr Res</u> 34:680-7, 1993*).

Observational Study: In a study of British middle-class 13-14 year olds, low levels of serum ferritin were found in 11% of 35 boys and 21% of 35 girls (*Southon S, Bailey AL, Wright AJA, et al. Micronutrient undernutrition in British schoolchildren. <u>Pro Nutr Soc</u> 52:155-63, 1993*).

Observational Study: 40% of 148 British students aged 14-18 had serum ferritin levels <10 µg/l (*Armstrong PL. Iron deficiency in adolescents. <u>Br Med J</u> 298:499, 1989*).

Frequently deficient in <u>adolescent female athletes</u>.

Observational Study: 22 Swedish teenage girls involved in elite gymnastic training who showed signs of delayed pubertal development including growth rate were compared to 22 girls not participating in sport. There was no difference in food intake between the 2 groups. While all the reference gp. had normal serum iron levels, 1/3 of the gymnasts had low serum iron. None had low hemoglobin *(Lindholm C, Hagenfeldt K, Hagman U. A nutrition study in juvenile elite gymnasts. Acta Paediatr 84:273-7, 1995).*

Dietary need is known to be increased during <u>pregnancy</u> and increased iron absorption may not be adequate to make up for the extra demands if storage iron is low *(Wallenburg HCS et al. Effect of oral iron supplementation during pregnancy on maternal and fetal iron status. J Perinat Med 12(1):7-12, 1984).*

Magnesium

Dietary intake is often inadequate.

Note: Based on long-term metabolic balance studies, the ideal ratio of calcium to magnesium intake appears to be 2- or 2.5-to-1 (Mildred Seelig, M.D., Ph.D. - interviewed by Zucker M in Let's Live, April, 1996:36-8).

Observational Study: The magnesium intakes of 28 American college females were markedly below the RDA *(Meacham SL, Taper LK, Volpe SL. Effect of boron supplementation on blood and urinary calcium, magnesium, and phosphorus, and urinary boron in athletic and sedentary women. Am J Clin Nutr 61:341-5, 1995).*

Observational Study: The mean intake of magnesium in the US is 279 mg a day compared to the RDA of 400 mg *(National Center for Health Statistics, Dietary Intake of Vitamins, Minerals and Fiber of Persons Age 2 Months and Over in the U.S., Advance Data No. 258, November 14, 1994).*

Review Article: Among elderly Americans, there is decreased availability of magnesium in the food supply, lower magnesium intake and widespread use of supplementation *(Costello RB, Moser-Veillon PB. A review of magnesium intake in the elderly. A cause for concern? Magnes Res 5(1):61-7, 1992).*

Observational Study: The mean dietary intakes of 34% of 270 US Navy Sea, Air, and Land trainees were below the Recommended Dietary Allowances or the Estimated Safe and Adequate Intake range. Dietary intake was unassociated with plasma concentration *(Singh A et al. Magnesium, zinc, and copper status of US Navy SEAL trainees. Am J Clin Nutr 49:695-700, 1989).*

Observational Study: In a survey of over 27,000 Americans, only 25% had a dietary intake of magnesium that equaled or exceeded the RDA *(Wester PO. Magnesium. Am J Clin Nutr 45(5 Suppl):1305-12, 1987).*

Observational Study: 39% of the population studied had daily intakes of less than 70% of the RDA for magnesium *(Marier JR. Magnesium content of the food supply in the modern-day world. Magnesium 5:108, 1986).*

Observational Study: Daily magnesium intakes based on 3-day dietary records from the USDA's 1977-8 Nationwide Food Consumption Survey were below the Recommended Dietary Allowance for all age and sex classes, with the exception of children younger than 5 years. Magnesium consumption was particularly low among adolescent females, adult females, and elderly males; 75-85% of individuals in these gps. ingested less than the RDA *(Morgan KJ et al. Magnesium and calcium dietary intakes of the U.S. population. J Am Coll Nutr 4:195, 1985).*

Review Article: While the typical American diet provides only 1/2 - 2/3 of the RDA (400 mg), it raises the magnesium requirement to 500-800 mg due to its high content of certain nutritional factors *(Seelig M. Magnesium Deficiency in the Pathogenesis of Disease. New York, Plenum Press, 1980).*

Pregnant women often have an inadequate intake.

Observational Study: The mean dietary intake of pregnant women in the US was 35-58% of the recommended dietary allowance of 450 mg. *(Franz KB. Magnesium intake during pregnancy. Magnesium 6:18-27, 1987).*

Frequently deficient in hospitalized patients, especially in those who are acutely medically ill.

Review Article: Magnesium deficiency and its clinical manifestations are common in pts. presenting to the emergency department. Since serum magnesium is the only readily available clinical test and may not be accurate in predicting intracellular magnesium, empirical magnesium therapy should be considered in high-risk pts. *(Reinhart RA. Magnesium deficiency: recognition and treatment in the emergency room setting. Am J Emerg Med 10(1):78-83, 1992).*

Observational Study: The frequency and prevalence of hypomagnesemia in the acute and chronic divisions of a medical center was studied. (The acute facility handles acute medical and all surgical cases, while the chronic facility handles primarily psychiatric cases.) In the acute population, the frequency was 41.4% (222/536 determinations) and the prevalence 26.1% (92/353 pts.) compared to 12.5% (50/399 determinations) and 3.5% (9/258 pts.), respectively, in the chronic population. In the acute care facility, the most common diagnoses associated with hypomagnesemia were coronary artery disease, malignancy, coronary artery bypass surgery, chronic obstructive pulmonary disease and alcoholism, while in the chronic care facility, alcoholism, liver disease and carcinoma were the most frequent diagnoses associated with hypomagnesemia *(Lum G. Hypomagnesemia in acute and chronic care patient populations. Am J Clin Pathol 97(6):827-30, 1992).*

Observational Study: Serum magnesium was measured "in 1033 serum specimens submitted for electrolyte analysis. Physician-initiated requests for magnesium measurements were received for 81 (7.4%) of these specimens. Serum magnesium abnormalities were identified in 546 of the 1033 specimens (hypomagnesemia [<0.74 mmol/L], 487); hypermagnesemia [>0.99 mmol/L], 59). Only 10% of the hypomagnesemic patients (48/487) and 13% of the hypermagnesemic patients (7/59) were identified by physician-initiated requests for this analyte. Fifty-three patients were both hypomagnesemic/hypokalemic and 30 patients were both hypomagnesemic/hyponatremic, but only 8 (15%) and 3 (10%), respectively, had physician-initiated requests for magnesium. Because magnesium abnormalities in significant numbers of patients are not being detected, we recommend routine measurement of this analyte when analyses of electrolytes are required for the care of patients" (Whang R, Ryder KW. Frequency of hypomagnesemia and hypermagnesemia. Requested vs routine. JAMA 263(22):3063-4, 1990).

Observational Study: In a coronary care unit, 7% of pts. were hypomagnesemic and 53% had low mononuclear cell magnesium (Ryzen E et al. Low blood mononuclear cell magnesium in intensive cardiac care unit patients. Am Heart J 111:475-80, 1986).

Observational Study: 65% of ICU pts. with serum creatinine concentrations of 1.1 mg/dl or less were hypomagnesemic. 1/3 of these also had hypocalcemia that was corrected with magnesium supplementation (Ryzen E et al. Magnesium deficiency in a medical ICU population. Crit Care Med 13:19-21, 1985).

Observational Study: Out of 102 consecutive pts. admitted to a medical ICU, 20% had hypomagnesemia (Reinhart R et al. Hypomagnesemia in patients entering the ICU. Crit Care Med 13(6):506, 1985).

Deficiency in the elderly, even when overtly healthy, may be common.

Observational Study: 36 healthy elderly subjects were compared with 53 healthy younger controls. With the exception of vitamin D in women, ave. energy and nutrient intakes were adequate. All subjects had serum magnesium levels within the reference range. Serum magnesium was significantly higher in the elderly subjects, while basal urinary magnesium excretion was significantly lower than that of the controls and 24-hour magnesium retention was greater. Since there was a negative correlation between magnesium retention and creatinine clearance, one could speculate that impaired renal function could contribute to increased magnesium retention; however, there was no evidence of delayed magnesium excretion among the elderly compared to the controls, since excretion the day after the magnesium load was increased to a similar extent. Magnesium retention was negatively correlated to basal urinary magnesium excretion and was positively correlated to serum magnesium. No correlation was found between magnesium retention and daily magnesium intake. Results suggest that apparently healthy elderly subjects, even with daily magnesium intake slightly above the Nordic recommendation, may have subclinical magnesium deficiency which is not detected by serum magnesium analysis (Gullestad L, Nes M, Rønneberg R, et al. Magnesium status in healthy free-living elderly Norwegians. J Am Coll Nutr 13(1):45-50, 1994).

Experimental Study: 14 apparently healthy elderly subjects, found to have lab evidence of marginal magnesium deficiency, randomly received 300 mmol (7.5 g) of magnesium as magnesium-lactate-citrate tabs, 3 mmol 3 times daily. 2 days later, there was evidence of improved magnesium status as assessed by increased baseline urinary magnesium excretion and decreased magnesium retention. However, serum magnesium significantly decreased, possibly due to improved renal function, since creatinine clearance increased while serum creatinine decreased. The improvement in lab chemistries following magnesium supplementation suggests that magnesium deficit "should be identified and supplementation began on liberal indications in elderly subjects" (Gullestad L, Nes M, Rønneberg R, et al. Magnesium status in healthy free-living elderly Norwegians. J Am Coll Nutr 13(1):45-50, 1994).

Observational Study: Low levels of both RBC magnesium and potassium were found in 20% of the subjects in a study of 381 unselected elderly men and women. Serum magnesium was low in 10% of the subjects *(Touitou Y, Godard JP, Ferment O, et al. Prevalence of magnesium and potassium deficiencies in the elderly. Clin Chem 33:518-23, 1987).*

Niacin

Approximately 33% of the US population in 1977-78 consumed less than the RDA for niacin and about 10% consumed less than 70% of the RDA *(Nutrition Monitoring in the United States: A Progress Report form the Joint Nutrition Monitoring Evaluation Committee. DHHS Publication No. (PHS)86-1255. Washington, DC: US Gov't Printing Office, 1986).*

Often deficient in the elderly, even despite adequate dietary intake and oral supplementation *(Frank O et al. Superiority of periodic intramuscular vitamins over daily oral vitamins in maintaining normal vitamin titers in a geriatric population. Am J Clin Nutr 30:630, 1977).*

> **Observational Study:** Deficient in 30% of institutionalized elderly Americans *(Baker H et al. Vitamin profiles in elderly persons living at home or in nursing homes, versus profiles in healthy subjects. J Am Geriatr Soc 27:444, 1979).*

Pantothenic Acid

Intake is frequently inadequate in the elderly.

> **Observational Study:** The ave. American nursing home resident surveyed consumed only 3.75 mg of pantothenic acid (unless supplemented with beverages and snacks), while the US RDA is 4-7 mg *(Walsh J H et al. Pantothenic acid content of a nursing home diet. Ann Nutr Metab 25:(3)178-81 1981).*

Potassium

Intake by children is frequently inadequate.

> **Observational Study:** An American study of >1,000 children found that their intakes at all ages were low in potassium *(Nicklas TA, Farris RP, Myers L, Gerenson GS. Dietary intakes of electrolytes, minerals and trace metals in childrens' diets: The Bogalusa Heart Study. J Advancement Med 8(4):241-58, 1995).*

Intake by the elderly is frequently inadequate.

> **Observational Study:** *Abdulla M et al. Dietary intake of potassium in the elderly. Letter. Lancet ii:562, 1975*

Occasionally deficient in the elderly.

> **Observational Study:** Low levels of both RBC magnesium and potassium were found in 20% of the subjects in a study of 381 unselected elderly men and women. Serum potassium was low in 2% of the subjects *(Touitou Y et al. Prevalence of magnesium and potassium deficiencies in the elderly. Clin Chem 33:518-23, 1987).*

Often deficient in <u>hospitalized patients</u>.

Observational Study: In a study of almost 3000 hospitalized American pts., approx. 20% had plasma potassium concentrations below 3.5 mEq/l (*Surawicz B et al. Clinical manifestations of hypopotassemia. Am J Med Sci 233:603, 1957*).

Riboflavin

Deficiency is primarily due to excessive carbohydrate and lipid intake with a relative protein deficiency. Chronic alcoholism and cirrhosis of the liver are also frequent causes (*Barthelemy H, Chouvet B, Cambazard F. Skin and mucosal manifestations in vitamin deficiency. J Am Acad Dermatol 15(4-6):1263-74, 1986*).

Intake by <u>the elderly</u> may be inadequate.

Observational Study: In a study of 403 elderly Danes residing in their own homes, riboflavin intake (2.3 mg mean; range 0.7-5.0 mg) was low in 10% as compared to the Recommended Dietary Allowances (RDA), in 4% as compared to the Joint Nordic Recommendations (NNR), and in 0.5% as compared to the Absolute Minimal Necessary Amounts (AMA) (*Elsborg L et al. The intake of vitamins and minerals by the elderly at home. Int J Vitam Nutr Res 53:321-9, 1983*).

Frequently marginally deficient in <u>the elderly</u>.

Observational Study: Riboflavin status in 19 hospitalized pts. ages 65-89 was compared to 10 healthy age-matched controls. Only one person in each gp. was deficient in vitamin B_2. The deficiency was not manifested clinically as a classic vitamin deficiency syndrome; thus biochemical assays are necessary for its detection (*Keatinge AM, Johnson AH, Collins PB, et al. Vitamin B_1, B_2, B_6 and C status in the elderly. Ir Med J 76(12):488-90, 1983*).

Observational Study: Marginal riboflavin deficiency was found in 30% of Britons over 65 years old (*Powers H, Thornham D. Br J Nutr 46:257, 1981*).

Frequently marginally deficient in <u>the poor</u>.

Observational Study: In a study of 210 low-socioeconomic-status adolescent Americans (ages 13-19), 26.6% of those not on supplements had abnormal RBC glutathione reductase activity (*Lopez R et al. Riboflavin deficiency in an adolescent population in New York City. Am J Clin Nutr 33:1283-6, 1980*).

Frequently marginally deficient in middle-class <u>schoolchildren</u>.

Observational Study: In a study of middle-class 13-14 year olds, the biochemical index of riboflavin status was low for around 30% of 35 girls and 19 boys (*Southon S, Bailey AL, Wright AJA, et al. Micronutrient undernutrition in British schoolchildren. Pro Nutr Soc 52:155-63, 1993*).

<u>Critically ill children</u> are frequently deficient.

Observational Study: Compared to tissue stores of healthy adults and children, approx. 3/80 children receiving intensive care and 1/6 children receiving chemotherapy were deficient in riboflavin. This deficiency was easily reversed with supplements (*Seear M, Lockitch G, Jacobson B, et al. Thiamin, riboflavin, and pyridoxine deficiencies in a population of critically ill children. J Pediatr 121:533-8, 1992*).

Selenium

Frequently inadequate in <u>Western diets</u>.

Review Article: In the early 1980's, it became evident that selenium intake in the Nordic countries was lower than the 'safe and adequate' intake of 50-200 μg proposed by the US National Academy of Sciences. In Finland, it averaged 20-30 μg, in Denmark 45 μg, in Sweden 30 μg, and in Norway 50-70 μg (*Tolonen M. Finnish studies on antioxidants with special reference to cancer, cardiovascular diseases and ageing. Int Clin Nutr Rev 9(2):68-75, 1989*).

Deficiency states have been demonstrated for inhabitants of regions where selenium supply is limited, in protein-energy malnutrition, and in pts. on total parenteral nutrition without selenium supplementation (*Neve J et al. Selenium deficiency. Clin Endocrinol Metab 14(3):629-56, 1985*).

It has been estimated that the typical selenium consumption in the United States is about 100 μg, while 250-300 μg daily can prevent most cancers (*Gerhard Schrauzer, professor of chemistry, U. of California, San Diego - 1981*).

<u>The elderly</u> are at greater risk for low plasma selenium levels.

Observational Study: 239 men and women were studied. Plasma selenium was found to decrease as a person aged. RBC selenium levels also decreased, but the results were not significant (*Berr C, Nicole A, Godin J, et al. Selenium and oxygen-metabolizing enzymes in elderly community residents: A pilot epidemiologic study. J Am Geriatr Soc 41:143-8, 1993*).

<u>Vegetarians</u> are especially susceptible to selenium deficiency.

Observational Study: A gp. of 44 vegetarians had lower levels of glutathione peroxidase, a selenium-dependent enzyme, than controls (*Kadrabova J et al. Selenium status, plasma zinc, copper, and magnesium in vegetarians. Biol Trace Elem Res 50:13-24, 1995*).

Thiamine

Intake is commonly below the Recommended Dietary Allowance.

Observational Study: 1039 French subjects aged 6-97 were studied. Most subjects had thiamine intakes below the French RDA (*Hercberg S, Preziosi P, Galan P, et al. Vitamin Status of a healthy French population: dietary intakes and biochemical markers. Int J Vitam Nutr Res 64(3):220-32, 1994*).

Deficiency is most frequently due to <u>chronic alcoholism</u> but can be due to <u>malabsorption</u> *(Barthelemy H, Chouvet B, Cambazard F. Skin and mucosal manifestations in vitamin deficiency. J Am Acad Dermatol 15(4-6):1263-74, 1986).*

<u>Children</u> are often deficient.

> **Observational Study:** In a study of British middle-class 13-14 year olds, the biochemical index of thiamine status was low for around 30% of 35 girls and 19 boys *(Southon S, Bailey AL, Wright AJA, et al. Micronutrient undernutrition in British schoolchildren. Proc Nutr Soc 52:155-63, 1993).*

> <u>Critically ill children</u> are frequently deficient.

>> **Observational Study:** Compared to tissue stores of healthy adults and children, 10/80 children receiving intensive care and 4/6 children receiving chemotherapy were thiamine-deficient. This deficiency was easily reversed with supplements *(Seear M, Lockitch G, Jacobson B, et al. Thiamin, riboflavin, and pyridoxine deficiencies in a population of critically ill children. J Pediatr 121:533-8, 1992).*

<u>The elderly</u> are often deficient *(Keatinge AMB et al. Irish Med J 76:488-90, 1983; Bowman BB, Rosenberg IH. Am J Clin Nutr 35:1142-51, 1982),* even when dietary intake appears to be adequate.

> **Observational Study:** Based on plasma thiamine levels, 43% of 30 consecutive American out-pts. aged 60-95 were at high risk for thiamine deficiency (< 2SD below the mean of gp. aged 20-60), and 13% were at moderate risk (< 10 ng/ml, the lower reference range of the younger gp.). Similarly, 27% were found to have red cell thiamine levels < 2 SD of the mean of the younger gp., while 33% had red cell thiamine levels < 138 ng/ml, the lower reference range of the younger group. Many of these pts. had symptoms associated with thiamine deficiency such as dizziness, heart problems, memory dysfunction and peripheral neuritis; however, 4 of these pts. also had deficient plasma vitamin B_{12} levels and one had a deficient folate level. The cause of their poor thiamine status was not ascertained *(Chen MF, Chen LT, Gold M, Boyce HW Jr. Plasma and erythrocyte thiamin concentrations in geriatric outpatients. J Am Coll Nutr 15(3):213-6, 1996).*

> **Observational Study:** Ave. daily thiamine intake of 60 free-living (30 male, 30 female) elderly Canadian subjects (≥65 yrs.) was above the recommended requirement (>0.4 mg/1000 Kcal) for each gender; however, almost half of the total study population had thiamine pyrophosphate effect >14%, suggesting thiamine deficiency. There was no correlation between thiamine intake and thiamine pyrophosphate effect, which raises questions about the reliability of dietary intake in assessing metabolic availability of thiamine in the elderly *(Nichols HK, Basu TK. Thiamin status of the elderly: dietary intake and thiamin pyrophosphate response. J Am Coll Nutr 13(1):57-61, 1994).*

> **Observational Study:** In a study of 98 free-living, healthy, middle-income Japanese over 60 yrs. of age, although mean dietary intake of thiamine was well above the RDA, about 10% of subjects consuming thiamine-fortified rice and 20-30% of subjects not consuming it were assessed on the basis of blood samples to have poor thiamine status in both July and December *(Itoh R et al. Nutritional status of thiamin, riboflavin and ascorbic acid in healthy elderly population in Japan. Nutr Rep Int 34(2):175-82, 1986).*

Elderly nursing home residents are often deficient.

Observational Study: Thiamine status was assessed by measuring dietary intake, red cell thiamine levels, and red cell transketolase activity. Thiamine status was found to be adequate in both young and elderly healthy individuals, but was low in elderly nursing home residents (*O'Rourke NP et al. Thiamine status of healthy and institutionalized elderly subjects: analysis of dietary intake and biochemical indices. Ageing 19:325-9, 1990*).

Elderly hospitalized patients are often deficient.

Observational Study: 36 consecutive non-demented, community-dwelling pts. admitted to an acute geriatric unit were studied. Based on the thiamine pyrophosphate effect, marginal thiamine deficiency was present in 31% and definite deficiency in 17%. Delirium occurred in 32% with normal thiamine and in 76% of thiamine-deficient patients. Results suggest that parenteral thiamine should be administered to all elderly pts. with delirium (*O'Keefe ST, Tormey WP, Glasgow R, Lavan JN. Thiamine deficiency in hospitalized elderly patients. Gerontology 40:18-24, 1994*).

Observational Study: Thiamine status in 19 hospitalized pts. ages 65-89 was compared to 10 healthy age-matched controls. Thiamine deficiency was common in both groups. This deficiency was not manifested clinically as a classic vitamin deficiency syndrome; thus biochemical assays are necessary for its detection (*Keatinge AM, Johnson AH, Collins PB, et al. Vitamin B_1, B_2, B_6 and C status in the elderly. Ir Med J 76(12):488-90, 1983*).

Vitamin A

Intake is frequently below the Recommended Dietary Allowance.

Observational Study: 1039 French subjects aged 6-97 were studied. Most subjects had vitamin A intakes below the French RDA (*Hercberg S, Preziosi P, Galan P, et al. Vitamin Status of a healthy French population: dietary intakes and biochemical markers. Int J Vitam Nutr Res 64(3):220-32, 1994*).

Review Article: In two major American nutrition surveys (NHANES I, 1971-74; USDA Nationwide Food Consumption Survey, 1977-78), vitamin A was found to be a problem nutrient, i.e., one in which ≥20% of the population surveyed was obtaining <70% of the Recommended Dietary Allowance. The data were confirmed more recently (NHANES II) (*Bendich A, Langseth L. Safety of vitamin A. Am J Clin Nutr 49:358-71, 1989*).

Intake may be inadequate among the elderly.

Observational Study: The mean vitamin A intake of 59 free-living healthy older persons (26 males, 33 females; ages 65-74) was found to meet the Canadian Recommended Intake (RNI) for both gender and season. However, probability analysis of dietary data revealed that, in summer and winter, 7 and 11% of males, and 8 and 14% of females, respectively, were at risk of deficiency. None exhibited biochemical evidence of vitamin A deficiency as determined by plasma levels of retinol and its transport proteins (*Basu TK, Donald EA,*

Hargreaves JA, et al. Seasonal variation of vitamin A (retinol) status in older men and women. J Am Coll Nutr 13(6):641-5, 1994).

Observational Study: In a study of 403 elderly Danes residing in their own homes, vitamin A intake (ave. 1500 µg; range 192-8700 µg) was low in 14% as compared to the Recommended Dietary Allowances (RDA) and the Joint Nordic Recommendations (NNR), and in 0.5% as compared to the Absolute Minimal Necessary Amounts (AMA) *(Elsborg L et al. The intake of vitamins and minerals by the elderly at home. Int J Vitam Nutr Res 53:321-9, 1983).*

Intake may be inadequate among low-income pregnant women.

Observational Study: 26% of 57 pregnant women in Iowa had a marginal vitamin A deficiency and another 9% had a definite deficiency. 50% of the Hispanic sub-gp. and 40% of the Afro-American sub-gp. had marginal deficiencies, suggesting that these were the highest risk gps. *(Duitsman PK, Cook LR, et al. Vitamin A inadequacy in socioeconomically disadvantaged pregnant Iowan women as assessed by the modified relative dose response (MRDR) test. Nutr Res 15(9):1263-76, 1995).*

It is estimated that 1 million people develop vitamin A deficiency each year *(Bauernfeind JC. The Safe Use Of Vitamin A: A Report of the International Vitamin A Consultative Group. Washington, DC: The Nutrition Foundation, 1980).*

Deficiency can result from a <u>deficient diet</u> or <u>malabsorption</u> due to a variety of causes *(Barthelemy H, Chouvet B, Cambazard F. Skin and mucosal manifestations in vitamin deficiency. J Am Acad Dermatol 15(4-6):1263-74, 1986).*

See Also:

Vitamin A Deficiency - a global disease. Nutr Rev 43:240-3, 1985

<u>Vitamin B$_6$</u>

Intake is frequently below the Recommended Dietary Allowance.

Observational Study: 1039 French subjects aged 6-97 were studied. Most subjects had vitamin B$_6$ intakes below the French RDA, and intakes were found to be related to the subjects' biological vitamin B$_6$ status *(Hercberg S, Preziosi P, Galan P, et al. Vitamin Status of a healthy French population: dietary intakes and biochemical markers. Int J Vitam Nutr Res 64(3):220-32, 1994).*

Review Article: Vitamin B$_6$ intake typically averages 50-75% below RDA levels *(Rall L, Meydani S. Vitamin B$_6$ and immune competence. Nutr Rev 51:217-25, 1993).*

Observational Study: Based on the Second National US Health and Nutrition Examination Survey (NHANES II) of 11,658 adults aged 19-74 yrs., 71% of males and 90% of females consumed less than the 1980 US RDA of vitamin B$_6$ *(Kant AK, Block G. Dietary vitamin B-6 intake and food sources in the US population: NHANES II, 1976-1980. Am J Clin Nutr 52:707-16, 1990).*

Observational Study: Based on data form the 1977-78 US Nationwide Food Consumption Survey, the ave. intake of vitamin B$_6$ by women aged 15-50, was 60% of the Recommended Dietary Allowance, with over 50% of all individuals consuming less than 70% of that level *(Pao EM, Mickle SJ. Problem nutrients in the United States. Food Tech 35:60-9, 1981).*

Marginally deficient in about 50% of <u>pregnant women</u>, and studies have shown that supplementation with 20 mg pyridoxine daily may be necessary to keep the laboratory measurements of vitamin B_6 (RBC glutamate-oxaloacetate transaminase) in the normal range *(Heller S et al. Vitamin B_6 status in pregnancy. Am J Clin Nutr 26(12):1339-48, 1973).*

<u>Middle-class schoolchildren</u> are often marginally deficient.

> **Observational Study:** In a study of middle-class 13-14 year olds, the biochemical index of vitamin B_6 status was low for 27% of 35 girls and 50% of 19 boys *(Southon S, Bailey AL, Wright AJA, et al. Micronutrient undernutrition in British schoolchildren. Proc Nutr Soc 52:155-63, 1993).*

<u>Children</u> often inadequate have an inadequate intake.

> **Observational Study:** In a study of children aged 2-10 in 4,000 households, vitamin B_6 intake was below the RDA in over 50% of the population *(Albertson AM, Tobelmann RC, Engstom A, Asp EH. Nutrient intakes of 2- to 10-year-old American children: 10-year trends. J Am Diet Assoc 92(12):1492-6, 1992).*

<u>The elderly</u> often have an inadequate intake.

> **Review Article:** 37 studies published 1980-93 were reviewed. Among the water-soluble vitamins, the intake of vitamin B_6 was most frequently below recommended levels *(van der Wielen RPJ, de Groot LCPGM, van Staveren WA. Dietary intake of water soluble vitamins in elderly people living in a Western society (1980-1993). Nutr Res 14(4):605-38, 1994).*

<u>The elderly</u> are often deficient, even despite adequate dietary intake and oral supplementation *(Frank O et al. Superiority of periodic intramuscular vitamins over daily oral vitamins in maintaining normal vitamin titers in a geriatric population. Am J Clin Nutr 30:630, 1977).*

> **Review Article:** Vitamin B_6 tissue stores often are low in seniors, partially as a result of reduced food consumption and altered vitamin metabolism. 1/3 elderly persons have plasma PLP (the main coenzyme form of vitamin B_6) levels of <30 nmol/L, indicating marginal vitamin B_6 status that can lead to a decline in immune response *(Rall L, Meydani S. Vitamin B_6 and immune competence. Nutr Rev 51:217-25, 1993).*

> **Observational Study:** In a study of 198 free-living, low-income, elderly persons (aged ≥60) in the U.S., vitamin B_6 status was low (PLP<32 nmol/L) in 32% and could be attributed to low dietary intakes and/or the presence of health problems reported to alter vitamin B_6 status *(Manore MM et al. Plasma pyridoxal 5^1-phosphate concentration and dietary B-6 intake in free-living, low-income elderly people. Am J Clin Nutr 50:339-45, 1989).*

> **Observational Study:** Deficient in elderly pts. as compared to healthy elderly controls *(Keatinge AMB et al. Vitamin B_1, B_2, B_6 and C status in the elderly. Ir Med J 76:488-90, 1983).*

> **Observational Study:** In a study of 403 elderly Danes residing in their own homes, pyridoxine intake was low in 83% as compared to the Recommended Dietary Allowances (RDA) and the Joint Nordic Recommendations (NNR), while only 1% took less than the

Absolute Minimal Necessary Amounts (AMA) which is 0.8 mg *(Elsborg L et al. The intake of vitamins and minerals by the elderly at home. Int J Vitam Nutr Res 53:321-9, 1983).*

Observational Study: Vitamin B_6 status in 19 hospitalized pts. ages 65-89 was compared to 10 healthy age-matched controls. Only the pts. were frequently deficient in vitamin B_6. This deficiency was not manifested clinically as the classic vitamin deficiency syndrome; thus biochemical assays are necessary for their detection *(Keatinge AM, Johnson AH, Collins PB, et al. Vitamin B_1, B_2, B_6 and C status in the elderly. Ir Med J 76(12):488-90, 1983).*

Observational Study: Compared to the US RDA, 55% of a gp. of elderly Americans were B_6-deficient *(Bowman BB, Rosenberg IH. Am J Clin Nutr 35:1142-51, 1982).*

Observational Study: Compared to the US RDA, 30% of institutionalized elderly Americans were B_6-deficient *(Baker H et al. Vitamin profiles in elderly persons living at home or in nursing homes, versus profiles in healthy subjects. J Am Geriatr Soc 27:444, 1979).*

Vitamin B$_{12}$

Deficiency is mainly due to malabsorption secondary to gastric disorders (ex. inadequate hydrochloric acid or intrinsic factor), intestinal disorders (ex. inadequate exocrine pancreatic secretion; complications of intestinal bypass surgery; *Bothriocephalus* infestation, malabsorption syndromes; alteration of the vitamin intrinsic factor complex fixation to the ileal wall) or congenital diseases *(Barthelemy H, Chouvet B, Cambazard F. Skin and mucosal manifestations in vitamin deficiency. J Am Acad Dermatol 15(4-6):1263-74, 1986).*

The elderly are often deficient, even despite adequate dietary intake and oral supplementation *(Frank O et al. Superiority of periodic intramuscular vitamins over daily oral vitamins in maintaining normal vitamin titers in a geriatric population. Am J Clin Nutr 30:630, 1977; Elsborg L et al. Serum vitamin B_{12} levels in the aged. Acta Med Scand 200:309-14, 1976).*

> *Note: Food cobalamin malabsorption occurs frequently in patients with unexplained low serum cobalamin levels (Carmel R et al. Food cobalamin malabsorption occurs frequently in patients with unexplained low serum cobalamin levels. Arch Intern Med 148(8):1715-9, 1988).*

Review Article: Cobalamin deficiency increases with age and has been found in a range of 3-42% of elderly people depending upon the population gp. studied or method used. As symptoms of cobalamin deficiency can be atypical, only 34% of elderly people with low serum cobalamin levels are diagnosed and treated *(Van Goor LP, Woiski MD, Lagaay AM, et al. Review: cobalamin deficiency and mental impairment in elderly people. Age Ageing 24:536-42, 1995).*

Review Article: The prevalence of vitamin B_{12} deficiency in the elderly (>60 yrs.) is estimated to be 5-8% *(Saltzman JR, Kemp JA, Bolner BB, et al. Effect of hypochlorhydria due to omeprazole treatment or atrophic gastritis on protein-bound vitamin B_{12} absorption. J Am Coll Nutr 13(6):584-91, 1994).*

Observational Study: 348 women and 200 men aged 67-96, all white, were evaluated. Serum cobalamin concentrations <258 pmol/L were found in 222 subjects (40.5%) compared with 17.9% of younger controls (p<0.001). Serum methylmalonic acid and total homocysteine concentrations were markedly elevated in association with these low cobalamin values in 11.3% and 5.7%, respectively, of the cohort, and both metabolites were increased in 3.8%, in association with lower RBC counts and higher mean cell volumes. 65 subjects (11.9%) had elevation of one or both metabolites and a reduced serum cobalamin concentration, findings strongly suggestive of cobalamin deficiency. Many elderly people with 'normal' serum vitamin concentrations are metabolically deficient in cobalamin or folate (*Lindenbaum J, Rosenberg IH, Wilson PWF, et al. Prevalence of cobalamin deficiency in the Framingham elderly population. Am J Clin Nutr 60:2-11, 1994*).

Observational Study: 809 elderly individuals (>65 yrs. old) were evaluated. 3.0% of the elderly assessed at a health fair and up to 5.1% of the elderly from retirement apartments had elevated levels of urinary methylmalonic acid, suggesting vitamin B_{12} deficiency. On follow-up, 18/35 had serum levels below 180 to 200 pg/mL, 12 were between 180-200 pg/mL and 250 pg/mL, and only 5 had normal serum levels (*Norman E, Morrison J. Screening elderly populations for cobalamin (vitamin B12) deficiency using the urinary methylmalonic acid assay by gas chromatography mass spectrometry. Am J Med 94:589-94, 1993*).

Observational Study: 14.5% of 152 out-pts. aged 65-99 were judged vitamin B_{12}-deficient (serum cobalamine levels <300 pg/L and elevated methylmalonic acid and/or homocysteine levels). Vitamin B_{12} significantly reduced or eliminated the elevated methylmalonic acid and/or homocysteine levels, demonstrating that serum B_{12} measurements alone will miss cases of B_{12} deficiency (*Pennypacker L, Allen R, Kelly J, et al. High prevalence of cobalamin deficiency in elderly outpatients. J Am Geriatr Soc 40:1197-1204, 1992*).

Observational Study: 100 male and female outpatients aged 65-93 were assessed. 36% had unacceptably low serum cobalamin levels (299 pg/mL or lower); 16% had serum cobalamin levels of 200 pg/mL or lower, and 21% had levels between 201 and 299. Many of the pts. showed no overt symptoms of vitamin B_{12} deficiency, despite low serum levels, while other pts. showed signs of peripheral neuropathy, macrocytic anemia, or type A gastritis. Based on these results, it is recommended that all persons aged 65-years and older be routinely screened for vitamin B_{12} deficiency. In addition to serum cobalamin level, tests for serum methylmalonic acid and total homocysteine levels should be conducted on pts. with serum cobalamin levels below 300 pg/mL, since low cobalamin levels are associated with alterations in these parameters and might help in the diagnosis of unexplained neuropsychiatric disorders (*Yao Y, Yao S, et al. Prevalence of vitamin B12 deficiency among geriatric outpatients. J Fam Pract 35:524-8, 1992*).

Observational Study: Serum samples were obtained from 152 hospital out-pts. aged 65-99. Vitamin B_{12} levels were low in 8.5% of pts. and were moderately low in 16.5%. Marked elevations of methylmalonic acid and homocysteine, vitamin B_{12} metabolites, were seen in 62% of those with very low serum B_{12} levels and in 56% of those with moderately low serum B_{12} levels (*Pennypacker C et al. High prevalence of cobalamin (CBL, vitamin B-12) deficiency in elderly outpatients. J Am Gerontol Soc 8:A9, 1990*).

People following a total vegetarian (vegan) diet may have reduced serum levels.

Observational Study: 2 mo. after 10 volunteers changed from a lacto-ovo-vegetarian diet to a total vegetarian diet, mean serum B_{12} level dropped 35% (p<0.0005) (*Crane MG, Sample C, Patchett S, Register UD. Vitamin B12 studies in total vegetarians (vegans). J Nutr Med 4:419-30, 1994*).

Deficiency is common following gastric surgery.

Observational Study: 19 of 61 (31%) gastric surgery pts. vs. 2% of 107 controls were found to have elevated methylmalonic acid, evidence of a vitamin B_{12} deficiency, and 63% of these 19 pts. had elevated total homocysteine (*Sumner A et al. Elevated methylmalonic acid and total homocysteine levels show high prevalence of vitamin B12 deficiency after gastric surgery. Ann Intern Med 124(5):469-75, 1996*).

May be deficient in the absence of a megaloblastic anemia and despite normal serum levels.

Review Article: In the elderly, a selected decline of transcobalamin II, a physiological transport protein, would result in higher serum cobalamin levels but lower intracellular levels, while most low serum cobalamin levels are due to gastric dysfunction in which protein-bound cobalamin is not digested. The latter condition can be corrected with oral administration of crystal cobalamin concentrate. Intracellular cobalamin deficiency is diagnosed by elevated serum methylmalonic acid and homocysteine levels. These tests should be performed on pts. who have hematological, neuropsychiatric or gastrointestinal disorders suggestive of cobalamin deficiency even though their serum cobalamin levels are >221 pmol/L (*Yulin Y et al. Decline of serum cobalamin levels with increasing age among geriatric outpatients. Arch Fam Med 3:918-22, 1994*).

Observational Study: In a gp. of pts. aged 57-98 attending a medical out-patient clinic, serum vitamin B_{12} levels were <200 pg/ml in 22 (7.8%) and <15 pg/ml in 15 pts. (5.3%). Only 47.8% of these vitamin B_{12}-deficient pts. had some hematological abnormality; 18% were anemic, 35.6% were leukopenic, and 31.8% had mean cell volumes >95 fl. Neurologic disorders were present in 40.9% and dementia in 72.7% of these patients (*Timiras M. Vitamin B_{12} deficiency in geriatric clinic patients. J Am Geriatr Soc 3898:A47, 1990*).

Observational Study: Only 45/70 (64%) consecutively diagnosed pts. with pernicious anemia had very low cobalamin levels (<74 pmol/L or <100 mg/L). Anemia was absent in 13 (19%), and macrocytosis was absent in 23 (33%); such absence was particularly common when cobalamin levels were only slightly or moderately low (74-184 pmol/L). In 9 pts., coexisting iron deficiency was responsible for the absence of macrocytosis. Of 10 pts. with neither anemia nor macrocytosis, neurological disturbance was prominent in 6, including 4 whose only noticeable abnormality was cerebral (*Carmel R. Pernicious anemia. The expected findings of very low serum cobalamin levels, anemia and macrocytosis are often lacking. Arch Intern Med 148(8):1712-14, 1988*).

Observational Study: 3/17 elderly pts. with low concentrations of serum vitamin B_{12} or red cell folate but normal blood counts had bone marrow suppression, and 2 of the 3 also had megaloblastic changes in the marrow, suggesting that the low concentrations of serum B_{12} or red cell folate found in about 1/4 of elderly pts. might indicate actual tissue deficiencies even when blood counts were normal (*Matthews J et al. Effect of therapy with vitamin B_{12} and folic acid on elderly patients with low concentrations of serum vitamin B_{12} or erythrocyte folate but not normal blood counts. Acta Haematologica 79:84-7, 1988*).

If deficient, supplementation may be beneficial.

Experimental Study: 14 hospital out-pts. aged 65-99 with marked elevations of methylmalonic acid and homocysteine, vitamin B_{12} metabolites, received vitamin B_{12} therapy. At the end of 8 wks., all 14 pts. had normal B_{12} metabolite levels (*Pennypacker C et al.*

High prevalence of cobalamin (CBL, vitamin B-12) deficiency in elderly outpatients. J Am Gerontol Soc 8:A9, 1990).

Experimental Study: 19 pts. aged 57-98 attending a medical out-patient clinic who had serum vitamin B_{12} levels <200 pg/ml were supplemented with vitamin B_{12}. 52.6% benefited. Hematological abnormalities were corrected in 5/7; neurologic abnormalities were corrected in 3/7; and mental status improved in 2/11 pts. with dementia (*Timiras M. Vitamin B_{12} deficiency in geriatric clinic patients. J Am Geriatr Soc 3898:A47, 1990*).

Vitamin C

Intake is commonly below the Recommended Dietary Allowance.

Observational Study: 1039 French subjects aged 6-97 were studied. Most subjects had vitamin C intakes below the French RDA, and intakes were found to be related to the subjects' biological vitamin C status (*Hercberg S, Preziosi P, Galan P, et al. Vitamin Status of a healthy French population: dietary intakes and biochemical markers. Int J Vitam Nutr Res 64(3):220-32, 1994*).

Observational Study: The Dutch RDAs are based on the goal of tissue vitamin C saturation. In a survey of 5898 subjects, most population gps. studied had a median vitamin C intake below the RDA. The lowest intake (median as percentage of RDA) was seen among boys (78%) and girls (75%) aged 13-15. Frank vitamin C deficiency is unlikely for most of the nonsmoking independently living population, but many of the Dutch population may not have tissue vitamin C saturation (*Löwik MR et al. Assessment of the adequacy of vitamin C intake in the Netherlands. Abstract. J Am Coll Nutr 10(5):544, 1991*).

Women frequently have an intake well below the Recommended Dietary Allowance.

Observational Study: In the 1985 (U.S.) National Food Consumption Survey, 20-50% of women received less than 70% of the RDA of 60 mg daily (*U.S. Department of Agriculture. National Food Consumption Survey, 1985*).

The healthy elderly occasionally have an inadequate intake.

Observational Study: In a study of 403 elderly Danes residing in their own homes, ascorbic acid intake averaged 64 mg with a range of 9-400 mg. This is adequate compared to the recommended daily intakes in England, Canada, the U.S. and Japan, but low compared to the recommended daily intakes in Holland, West Germany and the USSR. Based on the Joint Nordic Recommendations (NNR) of 60 mg, 24% did not receive enough vitamin C (*Elsborg L et al. The intake of vitamins and minerals by the elderly at home. Int J Vitam Nutr Res 53:321-9, 1983*).

The <u>chronically sick elderly</u> often have an inadequate intake.

Review Article: 37 studies published 1980-93 were reviewed. While vitamin C intakes were generally adequate in free-living elderly subjects, they tended to be low in institutionalized elderly *(van der Wielen RPJ, de Groot LCPGM, van Staveren WA. Dietary intake of water soluble vitamins in elderly people living in a Western society (1980-1993). Nutr Res 14(4):605-38, 1994).*

Observational Study: The mean dietary vitamin C intake of Dutch women living in nursing homes was 59% lower than for women living independently *(Lowik MRH, Hulshof K, Schneijder P, et al. Vitamin C status in elderly women: A comparison between women living in a nursing home and women living independently. J Am Diet Assoc 93:167-72, 1993).*

Observational and Experimental Study: Chronically sick elderly American women had low intakes and low blood concentrations of vitamin C. Small dietary supplements of vitamin C increased its concentrations in plasma and leukocytes to those found in both the active elderly and the young, confirming that low concentrations among the institutionalized and chronically sick elderly are primarily due to poor intake *(Newton HM et al. The cause and correction of low blood vitamin C concentrations in the elderly. Am J Clin Nutr 42(4):656-9, 1985).*

<u>Acutely hospitalized patients</u> are commonly deficient.

Observational Study: Within 72 hrs. of admission, fasting blood samples from 271 pts. at the Harborview Medical Center, Seattle, Washington were evaluated for vitamin C levels. 41% had low levels and 23% had deficient levels *(Baker B. Vitamin C deficiency common in hospitalized. Fam Pract News March 15, 1995:25).*

> *Note: Records from this study were kept separate from the medical chart. It was observed that vitamin C levels were not evaluated by the patients' physicians, and the vitamin C-deficient patients failed to receive adequate vitamin C to replenish their depleted stores (Baker B. Vitamin C deficiency common in hospitalized. Fam Pract News March 15, 1995:25).*

The <u>healthy elderly</u> may have low blood levels.

Experimental Study: Healthy elderly men needed 100-150 mg/d to reach plasma levels of 1 mg/dL, while elderly women required only 75-80 mg/d to maintain these levels. At an intake of 60 mg/d, the mean plasma ascorbate concentration for men was 0.5 mg/dL, as compared to 0.9 mg/dL for women. At this intake, about half of the men had plasma concentrations <0.4 mg/dL, which is considered a moderate risk for the development of a vitamin C deficiency and may indicate reduced body ascorbate stores *(Garry PJ, Goodwin JS, Hunt WC, Gilbert BA. Nutritional status in an healthy elderly population: vitamin C. Am J Clin Nutr 36(2):332-9, 1982; VanderJagt DJ, Garry PJ, Bhagavan HN. Ascorbic acid intake and plasma levels in healthy elderly people. Am J Clin Nutr 46(2):290-4, 1987).*

The <u>hospitalized elderly</u> may have low blood levels.

Observational Study: Ascorbic acid status in 19 hospitalized pts. ages 65-89 was compared to 10 healthy age-matched controls. Ascorbic acid deficiency was common in both groups. This deficiency was not manifested clinically as the classic vitamin deficiency syndrome; thus biochemical assays are necessary for its detection (*Keatinge AM, Johnson AH, Collins PB, et al. Vitamin B$_1$, B$_2$, B$_6$ and C status in the elderly. Ir Med J 76(12):488-90, 1983*).

The <u>chronically sick elderly</u> may have low blood levels.

> **Observational Study:** Dutch women living in nursing homes often had marginal blood levels of vitamin C (<23 mmol/L); sometimes these levels were low enough to be categorized as clinical scurvy (<11 mmol/L) (*Lowik MRH, Hulshof K, Schneijder P, et al. Vitamin C status in elderly women: A comparison between women living in a nursing home and women living independently. J Am Diet Assoc 93:167-72, 1993*).

Other groups at high risk for vitamin C deficiency are men who live alone, individuals who avoid 'acid'-containing foods due to dyspepsia or reflux esophagitis, food fadists, patients undergoing peritoneal dialysis and hemodialysis, and alcoholics (*Reuler JB et al. Adult scurvy. JAMA 253(6):805-7, 1985*).

Vitamin D

Lack of sunshine (ultraviolet light is necessary for endogenous vitamin D production) can cause vitamin D deficiency.

> **Observational Study:** Vitamin D levels of 23 older people were measured every 3 mo. for 16 months. In July, their levels were normal. By November, levels had dropped 19%. By February, levels had dropped 65% to a range where 9 had levels consistent with the development of disease. The May measurement was 62% below the initial measurement, which was equaled again in the next July measurement (*Lawson DE et al. Relative contributions of diet and sunlight to vitamin D state in the elderly. Br Med J ii:303-5, August 4, 1979*).

<u>The elderly</u> commonly have an intake below the US Recommended Daily Allowance (200 IU) and serum levels are often low.

> **Review Article:** Vitamin D deficiency may now be more common among older people than in infants and is related to age-related skin changes, renal function, gut absorption and sunlight exposure, with as much as a 40% reduction in vitamin D absorption in the gut as compared to younger individuals (*Gloth FM III. Vitamin D deficiency in older people. J Am Geriatric Soc 45:822-8, 1995*).

> **Observational Study:** 116 American subjects ≥aged 65 confined indoors for at least 6 mo. were compared to a healthy ambulatory group. All subjects were free of diseases or medications that might interfere with their vitamin D status. Results suggest that, despite a relatively high degree of vitamin supplementation in the US, homebound elderly persons are likely to suffer from vitamin D deficiency (*Gloth FM III. Vitamin D deficiency in homebound elderly persons. JAMA 274(21):1683-6, 1995*).

> **Observational Study:** Wintertime serum 25-hydroxyvitamin D concentrations were measured in 824 elderly people from 11 European countries. 36% of men and 47% of women had concentrations below 30 nmol/L. Users of vitamin D supplements and/or sunlamps had higher concentrations (median 54 nmol/L) than non users (median 31

nmol/L). Surprisingly, the lowest concentrations were seen in southern European countries. "These findings show that free-living elderly Europeans are at substantial risk of inadequate vitamin D status during winter and that dietary enrichment or supplementation with vitamin D should be seriously considered during this season" (van der Wielen RPJ, Löwik MRH, van den Berg H, et al. Serum vitamin D concentrations among elderly people in Europe. Lancet 346:207-10, 1995).

> *Note: 30 nmol/L was used as the minimal desirable concentration as lower levels are associated with secondary hyperparathyroidism, increased bone turnover, and decreased bone-mass density at the hip* (van der Wielen RPJ, Löwik MRH, van den Berg H, et al. Serum vitamin D concentrations among elderly people in Europe. Lancet 346:207-10, 1995).

Observational Study: In a cross sectional survey of 109 nursing home residents, the ave. vitamin D intake was 379 IU/d, with 16% having an intake below the RDA. Of the subjects taking supplements of 400 IU/d, none had serum calcidiol (25-hydroxyvitamin D3) levels below 15 ng/mL. However, of those with vitamin D intakes of 200-400 IU/d, 46% had serum calcidiol levels below 15 ng/mL and 14% had levels below 10 ng/mL (Dowd K, Clemens T, Kelsey J, et al. Exogenous calciferol (vitamin D) and vitamin D endocrine status among elderly nursing home residents in the New York City area. J Am Geriatr Soc 41:414-21, 1993).

Observational Study: In a study of 403 elderly Danes residing in their own homes, vitamin D intake (2.4 µg mean; range 1-26 µg) was low in 62% as compared to the Recommended Dietary Allowances (RDA) and Joint Nordic Recommendations (NNR) (Elsborg L et al. The intake of vitamins and minerals by the elderly at home. Int J Vitam Nutr Res 53:321-9, 1983).

Observational Study: In a 5-yr. prospective study, calcidiol was measured in 166 American women and 138 men, all healthy and active and with a mean age of 72. Although 25% took 400 IU daily as a supplement, the majority were consuming less than 100 IU daily. The ave. serum vitamin D level was 15.5 ng/ml compared to 29.1 ng/ml in a younger control gp., and 15% had a serum vitamin D below 8 ng/ml. Vitamin D levels were lower in women than in men. There was an inverse relationship between total serum alkaline phosphatase and serum vitamin D, suggesting chronic bone loss as a result of vitamin D deficiency (Omdahl JL et al. Nutritional status in a healthy elderly population: vitamin D. Am J Clin Nutr 36:1225-33, 1982).

See Also:

> Editorial: Vitamin D supplementation in the elderly. Lancet i:306-7, 1987

> Parfitt AM et al. Vitamin D and bone health in the elderly. Am J Clin Nutr 36(5 Suppl):1014-31, 1982

Vitamin E

Intake is frequently below the Recommended Dietary Allowance.

Observational Study: 1039 French subjects aged 6-97 were studied. Most subjects had vitamin E intakes below the French RDA, and intakes were found to be related to the subjects' biological vitamin E status (*Hercberg S, Preziosi P, Galan P, et al. Vitamin Status of a healthy French population: dietary intakes and biochemical markers. Int J Vitam Nutr Res 64(3):220-32, 1994*).

Observational Study: Based on 24-hr. recall data from 11,658 adults interviewed in the US Second National Health and Nutrition Examination Survey (NHANES II), median intakes of vitamin E were considerably lower than the U.S. RDA for both men and women, although the mean intakes were close to the RDA (*Murphy SP et al. Vitamin E intakes and sources in the United States. Am J Clin Nutr 52:361-7, 1990*).

Observational Study: In the 1985 (U.S.) National Food Consumption Survey, 70% of women aged 19-50 received less than 100% of the RDA for vitamin E, while 41% received less than 70% (*U.S. Department of Agriculture. National Food Consumption Survey, 1985*).

The ratio of vitamin E to polyunsaturated fatty acids may be low.

Observational Study: Based on 24-hr. recall data from 11,658 adults interviewed in the US Second National Health and Nutrition Examination Survey (NHANES II), if a ratio of vitamin E to PUFAs of ≥0.4 is considered desirable, 23% of men and 15% of women had diets with low ratios (*Murphy SP et al. Vitamin E intakes and sources in the United States. Am J Clin Nutr 52:361-7, 1990*).

Vitamin K

Subclinical deficiency during <u>pregnancy</u> and in <u>the newborn</u> is common.

Observational Study: 46 normal mother-infant pairs were studied at term. 13 infants (28%) and 7 mothers (15%) were found to be vitamin K-deficient as judged by PIKVA (protein induced by vitamin K absence) status, and maternal PIKVA status correlated with infant status (p<0.03) (*Block CA et al. Mother-infant prothrombin precursor status at birth. J Pediatr Gastroenterol Nutr 3(1):101-3, 1984*).

<u>Postmenopausal women</u> are at risk for subclinical deficiency (*Ferland G. Subclinical vitamin K deficiency: recent development. Nutr Rep 12(1), January, 1994*).

Zinc

Commonly inadequate in the Western diet (*Prasad AS. Role of zinc in human health. Contemp Nutr 16(5), 1991*).

Observational Study: The mean dietary intakes of 44% of 270 US Navy Sea, Air, and Land trainees were below the Recommended Dietary Allowances or the Estimated Safe and Adequate Intake range. Dietary intake was unassociated with plasma concentration (*Singh A et al. Magnesium, zinc, and copper status of US Navy SEAL trainees. Am J Clin Nutr 49:695-700, 1989*).

Observational Study: In a study of 403 elderly Danes residing in their own homes, zinc intake (ave. 10 mg; range 4-26 mg) was low in 87% as compared to the Recommended Dietary Allowances (RDA) and the Joint Nordic Recommendations (NNR) (*Elsborg L et al. The intake of vitamins and minerals by the elderly at home. Int J Vitam Nutr Res 53:321-9, 1983*).

Observational Study: Dietary zinc levels were determined spectrophotometrically for 22 American men and women eating self-selected diets. 68% were found to consume less than 2/3 the RDA for zinc, even though the ave. daily protein intake exceeded the RDA *(Holden JM et al. Zinc and copper in self-selected diets. J Am Diet Assoc 75:23, 1979).*

Children and adolescents are especially susceptible to zinc deficiency due to their increased requirements for growth and development *(Sandstead HH. Zinc nutrition in the United States. Am J Clin Nutr 26(11):1251-60, 1973).*

Vegetarians are especially susceptible to zinc deficiency.

Observational Study: A gp. of 44 vegetarians had statistically significantly lower plasma zinc levels than controls *(Kadrabova J et al. Selenium status, plasma zinc, copper, and magnesium in vegetarians. Biol Trace Elem Res 50:13-24, 1995).*

Intake by children is often inadequate.

Observational Study: An American study of >1,000 children found that their intakes at all ages were low in potassium *(Nicklas TA, Farris RP, Myers L, Gerenson GS. Dietary intakes of electrolytes, minerals and trace metals in childrens' diets: The Bogalusa Heart Study. J Advancement Med 8(4):241-58, 1995).*

Observational Study: In a study of children aged 2-10 in 4,000 households, zinc intake was below the RDA in over 50% of the population *(Albertson AM, Tobelmann RC, Engstom A, Asp EH. Nutrient intakes of 2- to 10-year-old American children: 10-year trends. J Am Diet Assoc 92(12):1492-6, 1992).*

Intake by adolescents is often inadequate.

Observational Study: The dietary intakes of 79 lacto-ovo-vegetarian (LOV), 16 semi-vegetarian (SV) and 29 omnivorous (OM) females aged 13-19 were evaluated. 24% LOV, 33% SV, and 18% OM had low serum zinc (<10.71 µmol/L) and 14% LOV, 14% SV, and 17% OM had hair zinc <1.68 µmol/g. Phytate to zinc molar ratios were negative associated with serum zinc (p<0.04). Suboptimal zinc status was attributed to a low intake of poorly available zinc in all dietary gps. *(Donovan UM, Gibson RS. Iron and zinc status of young women aged 14 to 19 years consuming vegetarian and omnivorous diets. J Am Coll Nutr 14(5):463-72, 1995).*

Zinc nutriture is often inadequate during pregnancy.

Observational Study: Pregnant women ingested only about 2/3 of the Recommended Dietary Allowance of zinc *(Hambridge KM et al. Zinc nutritional status during pregnancy: A longitudinal study. Am J Clin Nutr 37:429-42, 1983).*

Observational Study: Plasma zinc declined about 30% during pregnancy, while WBC and hair zinc also declined *(Truswell AS. Nutrition for pregnancy. Br Med J July, 1985).*

The elderly are especially susceptible to zinc deficiency due to:
1. lower zinc consumption than younger individuals.
2. poor bioavailability of their dietary zinc.
3. the presence of certain disease states.

4. the use of various medications which affect zinc nutriture.
(Greger JL. Prevalence and significance of zinc deficiency in the elderly. Geriatr Med Today 3(1):24-30, 1984; Hutton CW, Hayes-Davis RB. Assessment of the zinc nutritional status of selected elderly subjects. J Am Diet Assoc 82(2):148-53, 1983).

Review Article: The mean intake of zinc in the elderly (aged 50-80) has been reported to be 9 mg daily, only 69% of the RDA. Zinc deficiency is common in the elderly and defined as a plasma zinc concentration of < 15 µmol/L *(Heyneman CA. Zinc deficiency and taste disorders. Ann Pharmacotherapy 30:186-7, 1996).*

Negative Observational Study: 53 healthy elderly Swiss subjects (mean age 77) consumed an ave. of 62% of the US RDA daily (9.2 mg); yet there was no evidence, based on mean serum zinc, zinc depletion, and zinc in leukocyte subfractions, of poor zinc status. Supplementation increased serum and urine zinc, which only means that it was absorbed *(Swanson CA et al. Zinc status of healthy elderly adults: Response to supplementation. Am J Clin Nutr 48:343-9, 1988).*

Observational Study: In a study of 100 elderly subjects aged 60-89 yrs., zinc ingestion was below the RDA in more than 90% *(Bogden JD et al. Zinc and immunocompetence in the elderly: Baseline data on zinc nutriture and immunity in unsupplemented subjects. Am J Clin Nutr 46(1):101-9, 1987).*

Observational Study: The ave. elderly American nursing home resident surveyed was found to consume only one-half of the US RDA for zinc *(Hutton CW et al. Assessment of the zinc nutritional status of selected elderly subjects. J Am Diet Assoc 82(2):148-53, 1983).*

Severe zinc deficiency can occur with total parenteral nutrition unless supplementation is given *(Goldwasser B, Werbin N, Stadler J, Wiznitzer T. Zinc deficiency during intravenous hyperalimentation. Isr J Med Sci 17(12):1155-7, 1981).*

Hospital diets may be inadequate in zinc.

Observational Study: Dietary registration was undertaken in 56 consecutive pts. admitted to a department of general medicine ward for an ave. of 10.2 days. Only 1/56 (1.8%) received zinc in the quantity recommended for healthy adults *(Stellfeld M, Gyldendorf B. [Dietary investigation in a internal medical ward: The energy, protein and zinc intakes of 56 pts. during hospitalization.] Ugeskr Laeger 150(25):1537-40, 1988).*

Observational Study: The mean daily level of zinc intake in hospital diets in the U.S. was 9.4 mg compared to the 13 mg thought to be required daily by adults *(Klevay LM et al. Evidence of dietary copper and zinc deficiencies. JAMA 241:1916-18, 1979).*

Chapter Three

BIOAVAILABILITY OF NUTRITIONAL SUPPLEMENTS

GENERAL INFORMATION

Effect of Food on Supplement Absorption

"Most vitamins and minerals are better absorbed if taken with a meal" *(Harrison A. Supplements in perspective. Editorial. Nutr Rep 12(10):74, 1994; Whitney E, Rolfes S. Understanding Nutrition. St. Paul/Minneapolis, West Publishing Co., 1993:321).*

Quality

"Very often, [supplement tablets] are made so hard and are so insoluble that they pass through the system with hardly any disintegration at all. I have tested various nutritional supplements made by different companies using the official methods for the disintegration of pharmaceutical tablets. Some of these products have proven to be slow dissolving or almost totally insoluble, even when tested for several days, in an apparatus which simulates the human stomach" *(Zimmerman, PW. HealthWatch: are your tablets dissolving? Townsend Letter for Doctors, April, 1988:145).*

"In light of the standard formulation procedures used by some manufacturers of nutritional supplements, many vitamins and minerals may be defective" *(Shangraw RF. Factors to consider in the selection of a calcium supplement. Pub Health Rep Suppl. October, 1987:46-50).*

Supplements vs. Food Sources of Nutrients

If the goal is to increase nutriture of a specific nutrient, provision of a dietary supplement may sometimes be more feasible than attempting to increase the dietary intake of that nutrient from food sources.

Example: Folic Acid

Experimental Controlled Study: 41 women randomly received either a folic acid supplement (400 µg/d), folic-acid-fortified foods (an additional 400 µg/d), dietary folate (an additional 400 µg/d), dietary advice on increasing folate intake, or served as controls. After 3 mo., red cell folate concentrations increased significantly in the gps. taking folic acid supplements or food fortified with folic acid ($p < 0.01$ for both gps.). By contrast, although aggressive intervention with dietary folate or dietary advice significantly increased intake of food folate ($p < 0.001$ and $p < 0.05$, respectively), there was no significant change in folate status *(Cuskelly GJ, McNulty H, Scott JM. Effect of increasing dietary folate on red-cell folate: implications for prevention of neural tube defects. Lancet 347:657-9, 1996).*

See Also:

Gregory JF. The bioavailability of folate, in LB Bailey, Ed. <u>Folate in Health and Disease</u>. New York, Marcel Dekker, 1995:195-235

Supplement Formulation

- Compounding

WARNING: In multivitamin/multimineral preparations, <u>vitamin B$_{12}$</u> (cyanocobalamin), through an interaction with the combination of <u>thiamine</u>, <u>vitamin C</u> and <u>copper</u>, may be converted into inactive analogs which may fail to stimulate or even inhibit cobalamin-dependent enzymes, suggesting that vitamins and minerals should be provided separately *(Kondo H, Mitchell JB, Kolhouse FJ, et al. Presence and formation of cobalamin analogs in multivitamin-mineral pills. <u>J Clin Invest</u> 70(4):889-98, 1982).*

"The pharmaceutical literature is replete with formulation factors that can influence the dissolution and absorption of a drug preparation, assuming that the purity and potency of the active component is known. The issue then becomes the potential interactions between the active ingredients and the excipients, which make up the formulation. . . . Many of the potential pharmaceutical interactions involving binding, complexation, dissolution, or solubility interactions may affect absorption rate. These problems can be detected and screened out if in vitro dissolution and release assays are conducted on batches of drug produced. . . . These quality control procedures are implicit to the Good Manufacturing Practice process and adhered to by all generic and pioneer drug manufacturers *(Riviere JE. Influence on compounding on bioavailability. <u>J Am Vet Med Assoc</u> 205(2):226-31, 1994).*

- Dissolution Time

Supplements that dissolve the most rapidly have the highest physiological bioavailability because nutrients have a much more limited and defined region of absorption in the intestinal tract than is often the case with drugs *(Bland J. Nutrient bioavailability and fast acting formulas. <u>Int Clin Nutr Rev</u> 5(1):25-9, 1985; Chapman DG, Crisalfio R. The relation between in vitro disintegration time of coated tablets and physiological availability. <u>J Am Pharm Assoc</u> 65:374, 1956; Morrison AB, Chapman DG, Campbell JA. Further studies on the relation between in vitro disintegration time of tablets and urinary excretion rates of riboflavin. <u>J Am Pharm Assoc</u> 68:634, 1959).*

<u>Magnesium stearate</u>, a lubricant added to many supplements, may reduce bioavailability by increasing dissolution time. (It is possible that <u>calcium stearate</u> and <u>stearic acid</u> have the same effect.)

In vitro Experimental Study: A drug, ketorolac tromethamine, was mixed with crospovidone and lactose and the powder was compared with a mixture of the same ingredients plus magnesium stearate. When mixing time was 10 min., the percent dissolution for the powder after 20 min. in solution was reduced from 80-90% without magnesium stearate to 25% with the stearate. When mixing time was 28 min., the percent dissolution of the powder containing magnesium stearate after both 20 and 35 min. in solution was reduced to 20%. It was found that interactions between the magnesium stearate and both the drug and crospovidone appeared to cause the magnesium stearate to flake; these flakes adhered to the drug-crospovidone agglomerates, causing a reduction in the drug dissolution rate (*Chowhan ZT, Chi L-H. Drug-excipient interactions resulting from powder mixing, II: possible mechanism of interaction with crospovidone and its effect on in vitro dissolution. Pharm Tech, April, 1985, pp. 28-41*).

In vitro Experimental Study: Prolonged mixing of magnesium stearate with a powder containing a water-soluble drug, lactose and corn starch resulted in agglomeration of the starch grains, flaking of the magnesium stearate, and increased adhesion of magnesium stearate to starch grain agglomerates and drug particles. These interactions appeared to be responsible for a decrease in the rate of drug dissolution from uncompacted, hand-filled, hard gelatin capsules (*Chowhan ZT, Chi L-H. Drug-excipient interactions resulting from powder mixing. I. possible mechanism of interaction with starch and its effect on drug dissolution. Pharm Technol 9(3):84-97, 1985*).

- Emulsification

In contrast to water-soluble nutrients, nutrients that are fat-soluble must first be emulsified by bile; then they are absorbed, predominantly in the lymph. Formulations that improve emulsification and lymphatic uptake may thus enhance their bioavailability (*Azizi E, Szeinberg A. Abetalipoproteinaemia treated with oral vitamins A and E and medium chain triglycerides. Acta Paediatr Scand 67:797, 1978; Bland J. Nutrient bioavailability and fast acting formulas. Int Clin Nutr Rev 5(1):25-9, 1985*).

- Gelatin Capsules, Hard

Generally made from a mixture of animal gelatins of bovine and porcine origin plus additives.

Except for fragments from the capsule shell, they should disintegrate within 45 minutes in the USP standardized test procedure.

- Gelatin Capsules, Soft

Typically composed of ≈50% gelatin, ≈30% glycerin and water along with additives.

Except for fragments from the capsule shell, they should disintegrate within 45 minutes in the USP standardized test procedure.

While they dissolve reasonably soon, these capsules leave an oily, pasty capsule-shaped mass that does not dissolve or disperse readily (*Miller OH. Bio-availability of common vitamin-mineral products. J Appl Nutr 27(2-3):52-9, 1975*).

Soft gelatin capsules are somewhat permeable to oxygen; thus it is possible for their contents to become partially oxidized after encapsulation. Both the plasticizer content of the capsules and their storage conditions affect their permeability to oxygen (*Shukla VKS, Perkins EG. The presence of oxidative polymeric materials in encapsulated fish oils. Lipids 26:23-6, 1991*).

Note: *The addition of vitamin E, an anti-oxidant, to the contents may prevent oxidation.*

- Microencapsulation

Formulation of a mineral salt in a microencapsulated multiple-unit dosage form neither guarantees wide dispersion in the stomach nor the absence of a high local concentration *(Graham DY, Smith JL, Bouvet AA. What happens to tablets and capsules in the stomach: endoscopic comparison of disintegration and dispersion characteristics of two microencapsulated potassium formulations. J Pharm Sci 79(5):420-4, 1990).*

- Mineral Chelation

In order to chelate a mineral, a molecule (ligand) must contain at least two atoms capable of donating a pair of electrons to the mineral. These donating atoms must be located within the molecule so that they permit the formation of a ring (chelate ring) *(Mellor D. Historical background and fundamental concepts, in F Dwyer, D Mellor, Eds. Chelating Agents and Metal Chelates. New York, Academic Press, 1964:17).*

"The bioavailability and metabolism of chelates differ depending on the properties of the ligand that forms the chelate -- some are helpful, while others are not and may even be destructive" *(Jeppsen RB. Biochemistry and physiology of Albion® metal amino acid chelates as proofs of chelation. Albion Laboratories, Inc. , International Conference on Human Nutrition, Salt Lake City, UT, January 1995).*

Amino Acid Chelates

Di- and tri-peptides are actively absorbed through the intestinal wall *(Matthews DM. Protein Absorption. New York, Wiley-Liss, 1991:245-7; Roberts PR, Zaloga GP. Dietary bioactive peptides. New Horiz 2(2):237-43, 1994).* Chelates that are produced by combining mineral salts with amino acids are intended to take advantage of this mechanism *(Ashmead HD, Graff DJ. Ashmead HH. Intestinal Absorption Of Metal Ions And Chelates. Springfield, IL, Charles C. Thomas, 1985).*

However, mineral supplements labeled as amino acid chelates may not be true chelates, especially if they are formed from metal salts and either hydrolyzed protein or amino acids derived from hydrolyzed protein. Since the products of protein hydrolyzation have a wide range of molecular weights, there is no assurance of the nature of the chelates or the percentage of the metal that has been chelated *(Bailer JC. Chemistry. Orlando, Academic Press, 1984:144-6; Committee for Product and Label Integrity, National Nutritional Foods Association, USA, NNFA Newsletter, 1992).* If a mineral supplement contains true amino acid chelates, the label should list the name of the amino acid to which the mineral is chelated.

Note: Albion Laboratories, Inc., Clearfield, Utah produces patented mineral chelates that meet strict standards to ensure chelation and bioavailability.

- Prolonged-Release Formulations

"Data on which to base an evaluation of effectiveness are inadequate or unavailable for the prolonged-release forms of many drugs. . . . In some instances, a pharmaceutical manufacturer develops a prolonged-release product solely to permit extension and/or retention of a competitive position in the marketplace while providing no significant advantage to the patient" (*Drug response variation and dosing information. AMA Drug Evaluations Subscription. American Medical Association, Fall, 1993*).

Book: The older studies of phenylpropanolamine (immediate-release) found an ave. wt. loss of 0.62 lb/wk, while the newer studies, which used time-release phenylpropanolamine, found an ave. wt. loss of only 0.31 lb/wk (*Hobbs LS. The New Diet Pills. Irvine, CA, Pragmatic Press, 1995*).

- Tablet Coatings

Enteric Coating

"Enteric-coated tablets are most apt to be poorly absorbed because of the water-proofing characteristics of part of the coating" (*Miller OH. Bio-availability of common vitamin-mineral products. J Appl Nutr 27(2-3):52-9, 1975*).

See Also:

> *Alvarez WC. Do enteric coatings of pills do what they are supposed to do? Gastroenterology 9:219-21, 1947*

Film Coating

Like uncoated tablets, they should disintegrate within 30 minutes in the USP standardized test procedure.

Film-coated tablets disintegrate and dissolve readily and are well absorbed (*Miller OH. Bio-availability of common vitamin-mineral products. J Appl Nutr 27(2-3):52-9, 1975*).

"Some manufacturers actually use shellac, which is known to be insoluble in an acidic medium, in their tablet coatings" (*Shangraw RF. Factors to consider in the selection of a calcium supplement. Pub Health Rep Suppl, October, 1987:46-50*).

> *Note: "Pharmaceutical glaze" usually refers to shellac, while "vegetable protein coating" is a corn protein.*

Sugar Coating

Should disintegrate within 45 minutes in the USP standardized test procedure.

"Sugar coated tablets are most apt to be poorly absorbed because of the water-proofing characteristics of part of the coating. . . . Patients should be instructed to bite sugar-coated vitamin tablets so as to crack any overly-resistant coating, prior to swallowing them" (*Miller OH. Bio-availability of common vitamin-mineral products. J Appl Nutr 27(2-3):52-9, 1975*).

NUTRIENTS

Amino Acids and Protein Hydrolysates

Not uncommonly, manufacturers mislabel the amino acid content of their products. In protein hydrolysates, high quality protein may not be used, or the levels of free amino acids may be low.

> **Observational Study:** 8 protein products sold in Canada were analyzed. 6 were labeled as amino acid products derived from protein hydrolysates, while 2 claimed to be mixtures of crystalline amino acids. In the 'protein hydrolysates', the levels of free amino acids were very low (<1-9% of total amino acids), although the labels of 4 of these products implied total hydrolysis or digestion to free amino acids. 2 products only contained lysine and large amts. of ammonia as ammonium salts; one was labeled as pure free amino acids, while the other as containing up to 100% pharmaceutical grade free crystalline amino acids. Based on amino acid composition, 4 products contained a protein source other than the high quality protein listed on the labels (casein, lactalbumin, egg albumin), possibly gelatin, a nutritionally incomplete protein. There were also notable differences between the label claims for individual amino acid contents and the actual findings (*Sarwar G et al. J Can Diet Assoc 53:159-63, 1992*).

Beta-Carotene

> **Note:** *Beta-carotene supplements may be therapeutically equivalent to vitamin A (retinyl palmitate) for the alleviation of vitamin A deficiency, at least in the formulation currently recommended by the World Health Organization (Carlier C, Coste J, Etchepare M, et al. A randomised controlled trial to test equivalence between retinyl palmitate and beta carotene for vitamin A deficiency. BMJ 307:1106-10, 1993). However, beta-carotene supplementation may fail to increase plasma retinoid concentrations in non-vitamin A-deficient subjects, suggesting that there may be little tissue metabolism of beta-carotene to retinoids (Johnson EJ, Suter PM, Sahyoun N, et al. Relation between β-carotene intake and plasma and adipose tissue concentrations of carotenoids and retinoids. Am J Clin Nutr 62:598-603, 1995).*

Efficient absorption of fat-soluble nutrients depends upon the presence of adequate bile, pancreatic enzymes and bicarbonate as well as a normal small intestine (*Gallo-Torres HE. Obligatory role of bile for the intestinal absorption of vitamin E. Lipids 5:379, 1970*).

Since dietary fats generally promote absorption of fat-soluble substances, fat-soluble beta-carotene supplements should be taken with a meal. Taking the supplement in portions several times a day will usually increase its utilization (*Vitamin E Fact Book. VERIS (Vitamin E Research & Information Service, 5325 S. 9th Ave., LaGrange, IL 60525, 1994*).

- Natural vs. Synthetic

Natural beta-carotene supplements contain 9-*cis* beta-carotene which is not present in synthetic beta-carotene.   It may be more biologically effective than synthetic (all-*trans*) beta-carotene.

Experimental Study: Male subjects were given a basal diet supplemented with 40 mg daily of synthetic beta-carotene (Hoffman-La Roche) or dry *Dunaliella bardawil* powder (an algae containing about equal amts. of the all-*trans* and 9-*cis* isomers) for 14 days. The preferential serum absorption of all-*trans* beta-carotene over 9-*cis* beta-carotene, in parallel with the appearance of a high concentration of oxidized dienic products in the all-*trans* gp. compared to a low concentration in the gp. receiving the natural isomer mixture, suggests that 9-*cis*-beta-carotene acts as an *in vivo* lipophilic antioxidant more efficiently than does all-t*rans* beta-carotene (*Ben-Amotz A, Levy Y. Bioavailability of a natural isomer mixture compared with synthetic all-trans β-carotene in human serum. Am J Clin Nutr 63:729-34, 1996*).

Experimental Placebo-controlled Study: 28 pts. with histologically-confirmed premalignant gastric mucosal lesions received natural beta-carotene (a mixture of 51% all-*trans* and 34% of 9-*cis* beta-carotene) 30 mg/day, synthetic beta-carotene 95% all-*trans* beta-carotene) 30 mg/day or placebo. After 180 days, although plasma levels of both preparations increased, only natural beta-carotene demonstrated significant effectiveness against inflammation of gastric tissue and gastric dysplasia (p<0.05), suggesting that 9-*cis* beta-carotene protects gastric tissue more effectively than all-*trans* beta-carotene (*Yeum K-J, Zhu S, Xiao S, et al. β-carotene intervention trial in premalignant gastric lesions. Abstract. J Am Coll Nutr 14(5):536, 1995*).

- Oil-soluble vs. Water-soluble

Emusol® beta-carotene (Bioglan, Ca) ('micellized' beta-carotene), and perhaps other water-soluble forms of beta-carotene, may be better absorbed than oil-soluble beta-carotene.

Note: Fat-soluble beta-carotene is about one-fifth as well absorbed as water-soluble beta-carotene (Gissen AS. Carotene confusion: choosing a carotenoid supplement. Vitamin Research Products Newsletter, December, 1993).

Note: Oil-filled, gelatin capsules usually contain the fat-soluble, less well absorbed form of beta-carotene, while the dry beadlets are usually the better absorbed, water-soluble form. Capsules can be tested by placing them in water. If they dissolve to form orange to red water, they are water-soluble; if they dissolve to become orange oil floating on top of the water, they are fat-soluble (Gissen AS. Carotene confusion. Vitamin Research Products Newsletter (VRP, Inc. 3579 Hwy. 50 East, Carson City, NV 89701, December, 1993).

Note: Supplements containing carotenoids or carotenes should be very orange to red in color. If they are not, they are either very low in potency or are badly oxidized, as the oxidation products of most carotenoids are colorless (*Gissen AS. Carotene confusion. <u>Vitamin Research Products Newsletter</u> (VRP, Inc. 3579 Hwy. 50 East, Carson City, NV 89701), December, 1993*).

Experimental Study: 6 normal subjects randomly received 25,000 retinol equivalents of beta-carotene either as an oil or in micellized form. The micellized form was absorbed much faster and, at 2 hrs., doubled the plasma beta-carotene level, an increase that was 5 times that of the oil. At 6 hrs., the plasma level resulting from ingestion of micellized beta-carotene was unchanged, while that from ingestion of the oil had increased to 2/3 that of micellized beta-carotene (*Bland J - summarized in Rutolo DA Jr. Nutrition delivery systems II: micellization and fat soluble nutrients. <u>Int Clin Nutr Rev</u> 9(4):206-12, 1989*).

Calcium

"The task for individuals to meet calcium requirements on a continuing daily basis [without the use of calcium supplements] is a formidable challenge" (*NIH Consensus Development Panel on Optimal Calcium Intake. Optimal calcium intake. <u>JAMA</u> 272(24):1942-8, 1994*).

Retention is not necessarily enhanced by supplementation.

Experimental Study: The ingestion of milk or calcium supplements may not increase calcium retention in healthy young men due to depression of calcium absorption in the gut and fractional tubular absorption in the kidneys; whether the same is true for healthy young women is uncertain (*Lewis NM et al. Calcium supplements and milk: effects on acid-base balance and on retention of calcium, magnesium, and phosphorus. <u>Am J Clin Nutr</u> 49:527-33, 1989*).

Experimental Study: "Our data suggest that many women may respond to calcium supplementation by increasing urinary calcium excretion moderately; however, a significant number may exhibit hypercalciuria or no response to calcium supplementation. Therefore, monitoring urinary calcium levels in response to short-term supplementation might be a quick way to assess which women should be evaluated further because calcium supplementation may induce hypercalciuria and related problems" (*Storey ML et al. Urinary calcium and magnesium excretion by women in response to short-term calcium supplementation. <u>Nutr Res</u> 8:617-24, 1988*).

Absorption of calcium supplements is most efficient in individual doses of 500 mg or less (*Levenson DI, Bockman RS. A review of calcium preparations. <u>Nutr Rev</u> 52(7):221-32, 1994; NIH Consensus Development Panel on Optimal Calcium Intake. Optimal calcium intake. <u>JAMA</u> 272(24):1942-8, 1994*).

Absorption may be enhanced by concurrent supplementation with <u>vitamin D</u>.

Experimental Placebo-controlled Study: The addition of vitamin D 600 IU to a 1000 mg of a preparation of calcium carbonate resulted in increased calcium absorption followed by increased urinary calcium excretion (*Mortensen L, Charles P. Bioavailability of calcium supplements and the effect of vitamin D: comparisons between milk, calcium carbonate, and calcium carbonate and vitamin D. <u>Am J Clin Nutr</u> 63:354-7, 1996*).

- Absorption from Different Sources

Over 5 times better absorbed from <u>milk</u> than from <u>spinach</u> (mean of 27.6% vs. 5.1%), since the calcium in spinach is bound to oxalate (*Heaney RP et al. Calcium absorbability from spinach. <u>Am J Clin Nutr</u> 47:707-9, 1988*).

Some people may utilize calcium from dairy products more adequately than calcium from supplements (*Recker RR, Bammi A, Barger-Lux J, Heaney RP. Calcium absorbability from milk products, and imitation milk, and calcium carbonate. <u>Am J Clin Nutr</u> 47:93-5, 1988*).

Experimental Controlled Study: 24 male and 51 female normotensive adults aged 19-25 randomly received either 1000 mg elemental calcium daily as highly bioavailable calcium carbonate tablets (Os-Cal, Marion Labs, Kansas City) or dietary calcium supplementation (24 fluid oz of skim, 2% or whole milk containing about 1000 mg elemental calcium), or served as controls for 6 weeks. While baseline dietary calcium intakes were below the RDA, total calcium intakes during the study were above the RDA. Serum ionic calcium levels increased significantly ($p<0.05$) for the dietary calcium-supplemented gp. but not for the calcium tablet-supplemented gp. (*Knight KB, Keith RE. Effects of oral calcium supplementation via calcium carbonate versus diet on blood pressure and serum calcium in young, normotensive adults. <u>J Optimal Nutr</u> 3(4):152-8, 1994*).

- When To Provide Oral Supplementation

Absorption of supplemental calcium is about 10% higher when it is coingested with food (*Heaney RP. Optimal calcium intake. Letter. <u>JAMA</u> 274(13):1012, 1995*). Even though food may contain oxalates, phytates and other antiabsorbers (*Levenson DI, Bockman RS. A review of calcium preparations. <u>Nutr Rev</u> 52(7):221-32, 1994*), they are irrelevant as they are already fully complexed with the calcium in the food source (*Heaney RP. Optimal calcium intake. Letter. <u>JAMA</u> 274(13):1012, 1995*).

Note: Calcium supplements taken with food may interfere with the absorption of iron and possibly other nutrients (NIH Consensus Development Panel on Optimal Calcium Intake. Optimal calcium intake. <u>JAMA</u> 272(24):1942-8, 1994).

Unless hydrochloric acid production is reduced, supplementation may be most effective when given in the evening.

Experimental Study: 18 premenopausal women received calcium citrate (1000 mg of elemental calcium) for 14 days. When given at 11 p.m. vs. 8 a.m., supplementation reversed the night time increase in parathyroid hormone, slowed the circadian increase in bone resorption and reduced overall daily bone resorption (*Blumsohn A et al. The effect of calcium supplementation on the circadian rhythm of bone resorption. <u>J Clin Endocrinol Metab</u> 79(3):730-5, 1994*).

Experimental Study: In a previous study, calcium carbonate 2 g daily over 2 yrs. failed to affect urinary hydroxyproline excretion, a reliable indicator of calcium resorption from bone. In the present study, 15 post-menopausal women with osteoporosis but normal calcium absorption received 1 g calcium (5.23 g calcium lactate gluconate and 0.8 g calcium carbonate) at 2100 hr daily.   Urinary hydroxyproline decreased, indicating a significant decrease in bone resorption (*Horowitz M et al. Biochemical effects of calcium supplementation in postmenopausal osteoporosis. Eur J Clin Nutr 42:775-8, 1988*).

- Forms and Formulations

For some calcium salts, such as <u>calcium carbonate</u>, <u>tribasic calcium phosphate</u> and <u>calcium sulfate</u>, dissolution is impaired in the presence of reduced levels of stomach acid, a common finding among postmenopausal females and elderly males.   Other salts are relatively pH independent; these are mostly those with low calcium loads (low percentages of calcium by weight) - such as <u>calcium lactate</u>, <u>calcium citrate</u> and <u>calcium gluconate</u> (*Carr CJ, Shangraw RF. Nutritional and pharmaceutical aspects of calcium supplementation. Am Pharm NS27(2):49-57, 1987*). For example, among achlorhydric subjects, calcium citrate is ten times as well absorbed as is calcium carbonate (*Recker RR. Calcium absorption and achlorhydria. N Engl J Med 313(2):70-3, 1985*).

> *Note: However, in the presence of reduced levels of stomach acid, if calcium carbonate is taken with meals, its absorption is unimpaired* (*Bilezikian JF. Optimal calcium intake. Letter. JAMA 274(13):1012-13, 1995*).

<u>Calcium Chelazome</u>® (Albion Labs, Utah, USA), an amino acid chelate, may be more highly absorbable than other calcium formulations.

> **Experimental Study:** Calcium Chelazome®, given without food, was absorbed at a rate that was 82% greater than calcium citrate, 87% greater than calcium carbonate, and 165% greater than calcium as hydroxyapatite (*Heaney RP, Recker RR, Weaver CM. Absorbability of calcium sources; the limited role of solubility. Calcif Tissue Int 46(5):300-4, 1990*).

Calcium present within whole bone extract (<u>microcrystalline hydroxyapatite compound</u>) is generally better absorbed than simple calcium salts.   Moreover, in contrast to calcium carbonate and calcium gluconate, it does not produce carbon dioxide in the stomach (which may cause symptoms of gas) or interfere with digestion (*Dixon AS. Editorial. Non-hormonal treatment of osteoporosis. Br Med J [Clin Res] 286:999-1000, 1983*).

> *Note: MCHC is prepared from bovine bone by a process that leaves intact and in their natural ratios both the organic and inorganic constituents of normal bone with preservation of the organic protein matrix* (*Durance RA, Parsons V, Atkins CJ. Treatment of osteoporotic patients: a trial of calcium supplements (MCHC) and ashed bone. Clin Trials J 3:67-74, 1973; Epstein O, Kato Y, Dick R, Sherlock S. Vitamin D, hydroxyapatite, and calcium gluconate in treatment of cortical bone thinning in postmenopausal women with primary biliary cirrhosis. Am J Clin Nutr 36:426-30, 1982*). *It contains calcium phosphate (as hydroxyapatite microcrystals) with a 2:1 calcium to phosphorus ratio, fluorine, (presumably as fluorapatite), other minerals (including magnesium, zinc, strontium, silicon and iron), collagen, protein, peptides, amino acids, and glycosaminoglycans* (*Windsor ACM, Miscra DP, Loudon JM, Staddon CE. The effect of whole-bone extract on ^{47}Ca absorption in the elderly. Age Ageing 2:230-4, 1973*).

Note: MCHC 800 mg tablets provide 178 mg calcium and 83 mg phosphorus. Each gram of powder contains 829 mg, providing 176 mg calcium and 82 mg phosphorus.

Note: In animal studies, MCHC has been shown to present no hematological, biochemical or morphological signs of toxicity and, in human use, no significant adverse effects have been reported (Kohn R, in Osteoporosis. A Multi-Disciplinary Problem. Royal Society of Medicine International Congress & Symposium Series No. 55, 1983:165-7).

Experimental Controlled Study: 53 post-menopausal women with seriously impaired calcium absorption and accelerated bone loss due to primary biliary cirrhosis received either vitamin D$_2$ 100,000 IU IM monthly alone, or vitamin D$_2$ along with 1000 mg of either calcium gluconate or hydroxyapatite. After 14 mo., the control gp. showed significant loss of cortical bone, the calcium gluconate gp. showed no change in bone status, and the hydroxyapatite gp. showed a significant increase in bone thickness *(Epstein O et al. Vitamin D, hydroxyapatite, and calcium gluconate in treatment of cortical bone thinning in postmenopausal women with primary biliary cirrhosis. Am J Clin Nutr 36:426-30, 1982).*

Experimental Controlled Study: 64 randomly selected postmenopausal women with primary biliary cirrhosis received either MCHC or calcium gluconate while a control gp. received no calcium supplementation. All received vitamin D. After 1 yr., the control gp. lost a significant amt. of cortical bone, the calcium gluconate gp. was unchanged, and the MCHC gp. had a gain in cortical bone of 6.1% *(Nilsen KH, Jayson MI, Dixon AS. Microcrystalline hydroxyapatite compound in corticosteroid treated rheumatoid patients: a controlled study. Br Med J ii:1124, 1978).*

Experimental Study: 15 elderly osteoporotic pts. received whole-bone extract (MCHC powder) and calcium gluconate separated by an interval of 2 weeks. At both 1/2 hr. and 2 hrs. absorption of ^{47}Ca tracer was significantly greater with MCHC than with calcium gluconate *(Windsor ACM, Miscra DP, Loudon JM, Staddon CE. The effect of whole-bone extract on ^{47}Ca absorption in the elderly. Age Ageing 2:230-4, 1973).*

Experimental Study: Using ^{47}Ca as a tracer, MCHC was better absorbed in osteoporotic pts. than calcium gluconate. It was concluded that the calcium to phosphorus ratio in MCHC was crucial in determining absorption *(Parsons V, Veall NB, Butterfield WJ. The clinical use of orally administered ^{47}Ca for the investigation of intestinal calcium absorption. Calcif Tissue Res 2(1):83-92, 1968).*

Experimental Study: Whole bone extract was nearly twice as effective as calcium gluconate in promoting absorption of a calcium tracer (^{47}Ca) over a 2-hr. period in fasting pts. with osteoporosis *(McCance RA et al. Biochem J 36:686-91, 1942).*

Calcium citrate may be more bioavailable than many other calcium salts *(Harvey JA, Kenny P, Poindexter J, Pak CYC. Superior calcium absorption from calcium citrate than calcium carbonate using external forearm counting. J Am Coll Nutr 9(6):583-7, 1990; Nicar MJ, Pak CY. Calcium bioavailability from calcium carbonate and calcium citrate. J Clin Endocrinol Metab 61(2):391-3, 1985; Schutte SA, Knowles JB. Intestinal absorption of Ca(H₂PO₄)₂ and Ca citrate compared by two methods. Am J Clin Nutr 47(5):884-8, 1988; Wabner CL, Pak CYC. Modification by food of the calcium absorbability and physicochemical effects of calcium citrate. J Am Coll Nutr 11(5):548-52, 1992).*

> **WARNING:** Calcium citrate increases absorption of dietary aluminum *(Coburn JW et al. Am J Kidney Dis 17(6):708-11, 1991; Nolan CR et al. Aluminum and lead absorption from dietary sources in women ingesting calcium citrate. South Med J 87(9):894-8, 1994; Nestel AW et al. Effect of calcium supplement preparation containing small amounts of citrate on the absorption of aluminum in normal subjects and in renal failure patients. Nephron 68:197-201, 1994).*

> *Note: Alkali citrate may <u>inhibit</u> calcium absorption, perhaps due to complexation of calcium by citrate (Rumenapf G, Schwille PO. The influence of oral alkali citrate on intestinal calcium absorption in healthy man. Clin Science 73:117-21, 1987).*

Experimental Study: At dosages from 200-2000 mg, calcium absorption from calcium citrate was superior to that from calcium carbonate. In fact, using an oral calcium load, calcium absorption following a 500 mg load of calcium as calcium citrate was higher than after a 2000 mg load of calcium from carbonate. Results suggest that physicians cannot compensate for deficient calcium absorption by simply prescribing larger doses of calcium carbonate *(Harvey JA, Zobitz MM, Pak CYC. Dose dependency of calcium absorption: a comparison of calcium carbonate and calcium citrate. J Bone Min Res 3(3):253-8, 1988).*

Negative Experimental Study: Calcium absorption from carbonate, acetate, lactate, gluconate, and citrate salts of calcium, and from whole milk, was similar in fasting healthy subjects following a 500 mg dose *(Sheikh MS, Santa Ana CA, Nicar MJ, et al. Gastrointestinal absorption of calcium from milk and calcium salts. N Engl J Med 317(9):532-6, 1987).*

In contrast to calcium carbonate, calcium citrate is well absorbed in the presence of gastric hypoacidity.

Experimental Study: 9 normals and 11 achlorhydric fasting subjects were studied. While fractional calcium absorption from calcium carbonate and calcium citrate was similar in normochlorhydric subjects, achlorhydric subjects absorbed an ave. of 10 times as much calcium from calcium citrate as calcium carbonate *(Recker RR. Calcium absorption and achlorhydria. N Engl J Med 313(2):70-3, 1985).*

Experimental Study: 12 normals received 1500 mg calcium daily as either calcium carbonate or as monocalcium citrate. Monocalcium citrate was well absorbed regardless of gastric acid production. By contrast, subjects taking calcium carbonate who had higher levels of gastric acid excreted more urinary calcium than those with lower levels, suggesting that higher levels of gastric acid are needed to optimize calcium carbonate absorption *(Hunt JN, Johnson C. Relation between gastric secretion of acid and urinary excretion of calcium after oral supplements of calcium. Dig Dis Sci 28(5):417-21, 1983).*

<u>Calcium citrate-malate</u>, like calcium citrate, may be more bioavailable than calcium carbonate. It may even be superior to calcium citrate as it has about 6 times the solubility

of either calcium citrate or calcium malate (*Smith KT, Heaney RP, Flora L, Hinders SM. Calcium absorption from a new calcium delivery system (CCM).* Calcif Tissue Int *41:351-2, 1987*).

Experimental Double-blind Study: 301 healthy postmenopausal women, half of whom had a calcium intake lower than 400 mg/d and half an intake of 400-650 mg/d randomly received calcium carbonate or calcium citrate malate (500 mg Ca/d) or placebo for 2 years. Among women with the lower calcium intake who had been postmenopausal for 6 yrs. or more, calcium citrate malate significantly prevented bone loss (p<0.05) at the femoral neck, radius and spine, while calcium carbonate maintained bone density only at the femoral neck and radius. Among the women who had been postmenopausal for 6 yrs. or more and who had the higher calcium intake, those in all 3 treatment gps. maintained bone density at the hip and radius and lost bone from the spine (*Dawson-Hughes B, Dallal GE, Krall EA, et al. A controlled trial of the effect of calcium supplementation on bone density in postmenopausal women.* N Engl J Med *323:878-83, 1990*).

Experimental Double-blind Crossover Study: 12 healthy adolescents (6 males, 6 females) received a calcium supplement in the form of calcium carbonate or calcium citric and malic acids ingested with a standard breakfast and given in random order in a crossover design. Relative to calcium carbonate, calcium-citrate-malate had an increased fractional absorption (p<0.03) (*Miller JZ, Smith DL, Flora L, et al. Calcium absorption from calcium carbonate and a new form of calcium (CCM) in healthy male and female adolescents.* Am J Clin Nutr *48:1291-4, 1988*).

Calcium absorption from <u>milk</u>, <u>oyster shell</u> and <u>dolomite</u> appears to be similar as does calcium absorption from <u>calcium carbonate</u>, <u>calcium lactate</u>, and <u>calcium gluconate</u> (*Kohls KJ, Kies C. Calcium bioavailability: a comparison of several different commercially available calcium supplements.* J Appl Nutr *44(3&4):50-61, 1992; Spencer H, Norris S. Intestinal absorption of calcium from different sources. Abstract.* J Am Coll Nutr *13(5):534, 1994*).

Experimental Placebo-controlled Study: Absorption of calcium from a calcium carbonate preparation was at least equal to calcium absorption from milk (*Mortensen L, Charles P. Bioavailability of calcium supplements and the effect of vitamin D: comparisons between milk, calcium carbonate, and calcium carbonate and vitamin D.* Am J Clin Nutr *63:354-7, 1996*).

Experimental Study: Calcium absorption from carbonate, lactate, and gluconate salts was similar in fasting healthy subjects following a 500 mg dose (*Sheikh MS, Santa Ana CA, Nicar MJ, et al. Gastrointestinal absorption of calcium from milk and calcium salts.* N Engl J Med *317(9):532-6, 1987*).

<u>Calcium phosphate</u> is commonly used in Europe. It appears to have comparable absorbability to calcium carbonate (*Levenson DI, Bockman RS. A review of calcium preparations.* Nutr Rev *52(7):221-32, 1994*).

Some brands of calcium carbonate fail to be properly absorbed due to excessive disintegration and dissolution times (*Carr CJ, Shangraw RF. Nutritional and pharmaceutical aspects of calcium supplementation.* Am Pharm *NS27(2):49-57, 1987; Kobrin SM, Goldstein SJ, Shangraw RF, Raja RM. Variable efficacy of calcium carbonate tablets.* Am J Kidney Dis *14(6):461-5, 1989*), especially tablets that are over-compressed to achieve a smaller size or formulated without starch *(Carr CJ, Shangraw RF. Nutritional and pharmaceutical aspects of calcium supplementation. Am Pharm NS27(2):49-57, 1987).*

Clinical Observations: Either a name-brand or a chewable calcium carbonate supplement is more likely to be well absorbed, and liquids are generally no better absorbed than tablets *(Robert P Heaney, professor of medicine, Osteoporosis Research Center, Creighton U., Omaha, Nebraska - interviewed in Doheny K. Mythbusters. Los Angeles Times April 18, 1995).*

Laboratory Study: 1/3 of 31 calcium tablets took over 45 min. to dissolve and thus were ineffective *(Health Letter, June, 1987).*

The availability of calcium from calcium carbonate tablets for absorption can be easily determined at home *(Whiting SJ, Pluhator MM. Comparison of in vitro and in vivo tests for determination of availability of calcium from calcium carbonate tablets. J Am Coll Nutr 11(5):553-60, 1992):*

"Place one tablet in 6 ounces of vinegar at room temperature. Stir the vinegar every 2 to 3 minutes. At the end of 30 minutes, the tablet should have disintegrated (not dissolved) into fine particles" *(Kobrin SM, Goldstein SJ, Shangraw RF, Raja RM. Variable efficacy of calcium carbonate tablets. Am J Kidney Dis 14(6):461-5, 1989).*

See Also:

Review Article: *Levenson D, Bockman R. A review of calcium preparations. Nutr Rev 52(7):221-32, 1994*

Carnitine

L-carnitine supplementation has been shown to be bioavailable regardless of the customary level of dietary carnitine *(Rebouche CJ, Chenard CA. Metabolic fate of dietary carnitine in human adults. J Nutr 121(4):539-46, 1991).*

Carnitine supplements are often poorly manufactured.

Observational Study: 12 American brands of carnitine were evaluated. Most were poorly manufactured, and 2 contained little or no carnitine *(Duke U., 1992 - reported in Nutrition Action Newsletter, March, 1995).*

Cartilage extract

Bioavailability studies of shark cartilage components are lacking. Newer products produced by enzymatic digestion claim to have at least a 10% greater protein content than available 100% pure products. However, no comparative laboratory data exist to show a benefit for them over existing pure shark cartilage. "Assays of the biologic effects (modulation of angiogenesis) of all shark cartilage brands should be made available and such activity should be shown to be present consistently in products that are promoted on the basis of a putative anti-angiogenic effect" *(Holt S. Shark cartilage and nutriceutical update. Altern Compliment Therap 11-12/95:414-16).*

Choline

Phosphatidyl choline consumed as a nutritional supplement is more bioavailable than phosphatidyl choline in foods (*Zeisel S, Growdon JH, Wurtman RJ, et al. Lecithin therapy in neurologic diseases: plasma choline responses to ingested lecithin. Neurology 30:1226-9, 1980*).

The amount of phosphatidyl choline required to increase plasma choline levels depends upon its purity. With an 80% pure phosphatidyl choline preparation, 5 to 7 gms are needed to increase plasma choline significantly. In most studies, enough phosphatidyl choline has been given to at least double plasma choline levels, but in individual diseases, this may be either too much or too little (*Growdon JH. An overview of phosphatidylcholine, in I Hanin and GB Ansell, Eds. Lecithin. New York, Plenum Publishing Company, 1987*).

- Lecithin as a Source of Phosphatidyl Choline

Commercial lecithin usually contains only 10-20% phosphatidyl choline, much larger quantities of unknown phospholipids, and possible impurities (*Growdon JH. An overview of phosphatidylcholine, in I Hanin and GB Ansell, Eds. Lecithin. New York, Plenum Publishing Company, 1987*). While consumption of 9 gms of phosphatidyl choline will double blood choline levels within 2 hours (*Lopez G-C, Berry IR. Plasma choline levels in humans after oral administration of highly purified phosphatidylcholine (PC) in capsules, in RJ Wurtman et al, Eds. Alzheimer's Disease: Advances in Basic Research and Therapies. Proc 4th Mtg Int Study Gp on the Pharmacology of Memory Disorders Assoc with Aging, Zurich, Switzerland, 1987*), blood choline levels are unlikely to increase at all if the same amount of commercial lecithin is ingested as most of the free choline is destroyed by intestinal bacteria (*Lecithin and its uses. Advanced Nutritional Technology, Inc., P. O. Box 3225, Elizabeth, NJ 07207, 1986*).

- Choline chloride vs. Phosphatidyl choline

Compared to choline chloride, phosphatidyl choline, which is a natural dietary constituent, can raise human serum choline levels 3 times as much at an equivalent dose, and the rise persists 3 times as long (12 hrs. vs. 4 hrs.) (*Wurtman RJ, Hirsch MJ, Growdon JH. Lecithin consumption raises serum free choline levels. Lancet ii:68-9, 1977*).

Chondroitin sulfate

Manufacturers use one of two grades. The lower grade is very crude and consists of barely refined trachea powder containing perhaps 30-40% chondroitin sulfates in a poorly absorbable form. The higher grade, which is much more expensive, varies from 80-100% in purity and is highly absorbable (*Luke Bucci, Ph.D. - interviewed in Anderson GD. Glycosaminoglycans: Interview with Luke Bucci, Part II. Dynamic Chiropractic July 17, 1995*).

Chromium

Note: Chromium supplementation is only beneficial if chromium is deficient; however, since there are no reliable tests for chromium status, the only way to detect a deficiency is to begin supplementation and monitor the effects on glucose tolerance (Mertz W. Chromium in human nutrition: A review. J Nutr 123:626-33, 1993).

- Forms and Formulations

"Chromium is available for dietary supplementation as either inorganic or organic complexes. <u>Chromium chloride</u> is the main inorganic form, whereas three organic (that is, carbon-containing) forms are currently found in the marketplace: <u>chromium nicotinate</u>, <u>chromium picolinate</u>, and <u>GTF extracted from Brewer's yeast</u>. In addition, laboratory studies in animals have employed <u>chromium acetate</u> as well as <u>chromium citrate</u>, both of which have shown effective biological activity" (*Leibovitz B. Chromium wars: As I see it. <u>Muscular Development</u> 26(12):23,76,78, 1989*).

"Inorganic <u>chromium chloride</u> is poorly absorbed (estimates range from 1 to 3%), while <u>GTF-chromium</u> is the most active . . . (10-25% absorbable). The uptake of other organic chromium compounds is thought to be better than chromium chloride, but worse than GTF chromium. . . . In spite of the poor absorption of inorganic chromium, numerous studies have documented that chromium chloride is effective in both humans and animals" (*Leibovitz B. Chromium wars: As I see it. <u>Muscular Development</u> 26(12):23,76,78, 1989*).

<u>Brewer's yeast</u> is the richest known source of glucose tolerance factor. However, it typically contains only 2 µg of chromium per gram of yeast; furthermore, less than half of the chromium present is in the biologically active GTF form (*Toepfer E et al. Chromium in foods in relation to biological activity. <u>J Agr Food Chem</u> 21(1):69-73, 1973*).

Much higher amounts of chromium are present in <u>yeast-bound chromium products</u> ('<u>high chromium yeast</u>'; '<u>GTF chromium</u>'). These products consist of biologically synthesized GTF which is produced by introducing an inorganic salt such as chromium chloride to live yeast cultures, resulting in the conversion of about 25% of the chromium into GTF. These products are marketed in tablets containing 100-200 µg chromium. They must be distinguished from <u>chromium-fortified yeast-based products</u> that, although often labeled as GTF chromium, consist of little more than a crude mixture of Brewer's yeast and an inorganic chromium salt (*Choosing a chromium supplement. Product brochure. InterHealth Company, Concord, CA 1990*).

> **Experimental Study:** Using as the criterion the maximum decrease in fasting blood glucose level produced in 6 men and 1 woman aged 22-42 by the administration of a single dose of 100 µg chromium in various forms, high chromium yeast and Cr^{+++}-EDTA complex were more active than either inorganic Cr^{+++} (chromic chloride) or conventional brewer's yeast (*Vinson JA, Hsiao KH. Comparative effect of various forms of chromium on serum glucose: An assay for biologically active chromium. <u>Nutr Rep Int</u> 32:1-7, 1985*).
>
> > *Note: Such differences may not apply to chronic daily administration, where serum chromium builds up to a rather constant plateau* (*Flodin NW. <u>Pharmacology of Micronutrients</u>. New York, Alan R. Liss, Inc., 1988*).

While its exact composition remains unknown, GTF is believed to consist of chromium linked to niacin along with amino acids that appear to help stabilize the complex (*Anderson RA, Mertz W. Glucose tolerance factor: an essential dietary agent. <u>Trends Biochem Sci</u> 2:277-9, 1979; Mertz W. Effects and metabolism of glucose tolerance factor. <u>Nutr Rev</u> 33:129, 1975*), although there is some evidence that

GTF from brewer's yeast need not contain chromium (*Haylock SJ, Buckley PD, Blackwell LF. The relationship of chromium to the glucose-tolerance factor. II. J Inorg Biochem 19:105-17, 1983; Hwang DL, Lev-Ran A, Papoian T, Beech WK. Insulin-like activity of chromium-binding fractions from brewer's yeast. J Inorg Biochem 30:219-25, 1987*). Studies have found that the addition of 100 mg/d of nicotinic acid to 200 μg of chromium chloride synergistically increases glucose tolerance, decreases fasting glucose (*Urberg M, Zemel MB. Evidence for synergism between chromium and nicotinic acid in the control of glucose tolerance in elderly humans. Metabolism 36(9):896-9, 1987*) and decreases serum cholesterol (*Urberg M, Benyi J, John R. Hypocholesterolemic effects of nicotinic acid and chromium supplementation. J Fam Pract 27(6):603-6, 1988*).

Amino acid-chelated chromium is made of predigested protein (usually from soy or milk) bound to chromium. While better absorbed than inorganic chromium, it does not exhibit GTF activity (*Choosing a chromium supplement. Product brochure. InterHealth Company, Concord, CA 1990*).

Coenzyme Q_{10}

Degrades rapidly when exposed to light (*Gissen AS. Coenzyme Q: The ubiquitous quinone. Vitamin Research Products Newsletter (VRP, Inc. 3579 Hwy. 50 East, Carson City, NV 89701, November, 1993*).

Efficient absorption of fat-soluble nutrients depends upon the presence of adequate bile, pancreatic enzymes and bicarbonate as well as a normal small intestine (*Gallo-Torres HE. Obligatory role of bile for the intestinal absorption of vitamin E. Lipids 5:379, 1970*).

- When to Provide Oral Supplementation

Since dietary fats generally promote absorption of fat-soluble substances, fat-soluble coenzyme Q_{10} supplements should be taken with a meal. Taking the supplement in portions several times a day will usually increase its utilization (*Vitamin E Fact Book. VERIS (Vitamin E Research & Information Service, 5325 S. 9th Ave., LaGrange, IL 60525, 1994*).

- Formulations

A soft gelatin capsule of CoQ_{10} in soy bean oil has superior bioavailability to a hard capsule containing the powder mixed with an inert substance. Additives to the soft gelatin capsule, instead of improving absorption, may decrease it (*Weis M, Mortensen SA, Romer Rassing M, et al. Bioavailability of four oral coenzyme Q_{10} formulation in healthy volunteers. Paper presented at the International Symposium on Coenzyme Q, Stockholm, Sweden, November 1993; Fred Crane, professor of biology, Purdue U. and discoverer of coenzyme Q_{10} - interviewed in Nutrition Action Newsletter, March, 1995*).

Copper

Bioavailability of copper from human milk is high, whereas it is lower from cow's milk and infant formula (*Lönnerdal B. Bioavailability of copper. Am J Clin Nutr 63:821S-9S, 1996*).

Copper gluconate may *not* be bioavailable.

Experimental Double-blind Study: 7 volunteers received 10 mg copper daily as copper gluconate or placebo. After 12 wks., supplemented subjects had no change in the level of copper in the serum, urine or hair (*Pratt WB, Omdahl JL, Sorenson JR. Lack of effect of copper gluconate supplementation. Am J Clin Nutr 42(4):681-2, 1985*).

L-Cysteine

Readily oxidizes to insoluble cystine, a cause of kidney stones and tissue damage (*Higashi T et al. Sulfur Amino Acids: Biochemical and Clinical Aspects. New York, Alan R. Liss, 1983:419-34*); thus N-acetylcysteine may be a more bioavailable source (*see 'N-acetylcysteine' below*).

Because it is hygroscopic and corrosive, the label should indicate the expiration date (*Labeling Standard for Amino Acid Products, National Nutritional Food Association, 150 E. Paularino Ave., Suite 285, Costa Mesa, CA 92626*).

Folic Acid

Unstable in acid conditions. Decomposed by sunlight.

In the elderly, a good diet and a daily 'multivitamin' may fail to maintain adequate folate nutriture, and intramuscular injections may be necessary.

> **Experimental Study:** 228 ambulatory residents of a nursing home, mean age 87, who had not undergone major surgical procedures, ate a 'good' diet, and received at least one multivitamin pill daily for 3-5 of the preceding months, were compared to 204 healthy volunteers aged 20-50. 88/228 (39%) showed deficits of up to 5 of the B complex vitamins, one of which was folic acid. Oral vitamin supplementation was stopped and a single IM injection of multivitamins was given. After 3 mo., these deficits were no longer detectable in the blood of 89-100% of the previously vitamin-deficient pts. (*Baker H, Frank O, Jaslow SP. Oral versus intramuscular vitamin supplementation for hypovitaminosis in the elderly. J Am Geriatr Soc 28(1):42-5, 1980*).

- When to Provide Oral Supplementation

A water-soluble vitamin, folic acid is absorbed with or without food although food, by slowing the rate of absorption, may increase the length of time that blood levels are increased and thereby reduce its eventual excretion. A similar improvement in absorption can be achieved by dividing the total dosage into several portions and taking them throughout the day (*Yung S, Mayersohn M, Robinson JB. Ascorbic acid absorption in man: influence of divided dose and food. Life Sci 28(22):2505-11, 1981*).

- Folinic Acid

Folinic acid (5-formyltetrahydrofolate; leucovorin; citrovorum factor) bypasses several steps in the conversion of dietary folic acid to 5-methyltetrahydrofolate and avoids the usual process of biliary secretion and reabsorption (*Whitehead VM, Pratt R, Viallet A, Cooper BA. Intestinal conversion of folinic acid to 5-methyltetrahydrofolate in man. Br J Haematol 22:63-72, 1972*). Absorption kinetic studies of orally administered folinic acid (20 mg) have found a bioavailability of 92-98% (*McGuire BW, Sia LL, Haynes JD, et al. Absorption kinetic studies of orally administered leucovorin calcium NCI Monogr 5:47-56, 1987; McGuire BW, Sia LL, Leese PT, et al. Pharmacokinetics of leucovorin calcium after intravenous, intramuscular, and oral administration. Clin Pharm 7:52-8, 1988*).

Folinic acid metabolism, in contrast to the metabolism of dietary or supplemental folic acid, bypasses the reductase enzymes which are among the most commonly reported defects in congenital folate malabsorption (*Irons M, Levy HL, O'Flynn ME, et al. Folinic acid therapy in treatment of dihydropteridine reductase deficiency. J Pediatr 110:61-7, 1987; Poncz M, Colman N, Herbert V, et al. Therapy of congenital folate malabsorption. J Pediatr 98:76-9, 1981; Steinschneider M, Sherbany A, Pavlakis S, et al. Congenital folate malabsorption: Reversible clinical and neurophysiologic abnormalities. Neurology 40:1315, 1990*).

Folinic acid is more readily transported into the central nervous system than folic acid (*Levitt M, Nixon PF, Pincus JH, Bertino JR. Transport characteristics of folate in cerebrospinal fluid; a study utilizing doubly labeled 5-methyltetrahydrofolate and 5-formyltetrahydrofolate. J Clin Invest 50:1301-8, 1971; Poncz M, Colman N, Herbert V, et al. Therapy of congenital folate malabsorption. J Pediatr 98:76-9, 1981*).

In inflammatory bowel disease, folinic acid is more bioavailable than folic acid.

> *Note: Folic acid is absorbed in the small intestines; thus folinic acid may only be more bioavailable in inflammatory disease of the small intestines.*

Experimental Study: Pts. with inflammatory bowel disease and folate deficiency received 15 mg or either folic or folinic acid. After 1 mo., red cell folate, an indicator of folate body stores, was significantly higher in those receiving folinic acid than those taking folic acid (p<0.01) (*Pironi L, Cornia GL, Ursitti MA, et al. Evaluation of oral administration of folic and folinic acid to prevent folate deficiency in patients with inflammatory bowel disease treated with salicylazosulfapyridine. Int J Pharm Res 8:143-8, 1988*).

Glutathione

The systemic availability of oral glutathione is uncertain and may be idiosyncratic (*Smith CV. Will glutathione become a hot new supplement? Nutr Report 11(11), November, 1993*).

> *Note: In mice and rats, hepatic gamma-glutamyltransferase activity is an order of magnitude lower; thus, in contrast to humans, their plasma glutathione levels can be boosted fairly easily by oral supplementation and the results of studies of oral glutathione supplementation performed on these animals should not be extrapolated to humans (Witschi A, Reddy S, Stofer B, Lauterburg BH. The systemic availability of oral glutathione. Eur J Clin Pharmacol 43(6):667-9, 1992).*

In a study of 7 healthy volunteers, a dose of about 3 g (0.15 mmol/kg body wt.) failed to increase plasma concentrations of glutathione, cysteine or glutamate after 4.5 hours. Even though 3 subjects had at least a transient increase in plasma levels, and one of them had a less than two-fold rise that lasted 4 hours, the researchers concluded that "because of its hydrolysis by intestinal and hepatic gamma-glutamyltransferase, dietary glutathione is not a major determinant of circulating glutathione" (*Witschi A, Reddy S, Stofer B, Lauterburg BH. The systemic availability of oral glutathione. Eur J Clin Pharmacol 43(6):667-9, 1992*).

Other investigators found that an oral dose of 1.25 g (15 mg/kg) increased plasma glutathione levels 1.5 to 10 fold in 4 out of 5 subjects with the maximal level at 1 hour, while equivalent amounts of the 3 amino acid constituents of glutathione failed to increase plasma glutathione levels, indicating that this increase was due to glutathione absorption *(Jones DP et al. Oral administration of glutathione (GSH) increases plasma GSH concentration in humans. Abstract. FASEB J 3(4):A1250, 1989).*

Even without detectable elevations in systemic glutathione concentrations, oral supplementation could theoretically be beneficial, since it has been shown to increase intestinal glutathione content, at least in rats, and thus could support intestinal detoxification of dietary lipid peroxides *(Aw TY, Williams MW. Intestinal absorption and lymphatic transport of peroxidized lipids in rats: effect of exogenous GSH. Am J Physiol 263(5 Pt 1):G665-72, 1992).*

Iron

If deficient, oral supplementation is preferred *(Fairbanks VF, Bentler E. Iron deficiency, in Hematology. McGraw Hill, 1983:466-89).*

There is no significant absorptive advantage in giving iron less often than once daily *(Cook JV, Reddy MB. Efficacy of weekly compared with daily iron supplementation. Am J Clin Nutr 62:117-20, 1995).*

Supplements are best absorbed when taken away from meals.

Case Report: Supplemental iron given to a healthy fasting subject increased plasma iron levels by 100%, while the same dose given during or after a meal produced hardly any elevation of plasma iron *(Martinez-Torres C, Layrisse M. Nutritional factors in iron deficiency: Food iron absorption. Clin Haematol 2(2):339-52, 1973).*

- Forms

Ferrous iron is 1 1/2 to 15 times better absorbed than ferric iron *(Hahn PF et al. The relative absorption and utilization of ferrous and ferric iron in anemia as determined with the radioactive isotope. Am J Physiol 143:191, 1945; Moore CV et al. Absorption of ferrous and ferric radioactive iron by human subjects and dogs. J Clin Invest 23:755, 1944).*

Heme iron (found in meat) is much better absorbed than iron in plant foodstuffs (non-heme iron) *(Hallberg L, Rossander L. Effect of soy protein on nonheme iron absorption in man. Am J Clin Nutr 36:514, 1982).*

Experimental Placebo-controlled Study: Premenopausal non-pregnant women with low serum ferritin levels received either 9 or 27 mg of an iron supplement comprising 11% heme and 89% inorganic iron or placebo for 6 months. While the 9 mg dose failed to correct iron stores, the 27 mg supplement corrected both mild anemia and storage iron depletion. This compares to the 1-200 mg daily of inorganic iron that is usually prescribed to increase iron stores, a dosage that frequently causes GI symptoms *(Fogelholm M, Suominen M, Rita H. Effects of low-dose iron supplementation in women with low serum ferritin concentrations. Eur J Clin Nutr 48:753-6, 1994).*

Ferrous sulfate is the most frequently utilized iron supplement.

Compared to ferrous sulfate, ferrous iron amino acid chelate (glycine-iron-glycine; Ferrochel™, Albion Labs, Clearfield, Utah) is more bioavailable.

Experimental Double-blind Study: 100 adolescents aged 10-19 with a hemoglobin of <12 g/dL received one of two enteric-coated supplements of ferrous iron, commercial ferrous sulfate 120 mg or a water-soluble preparation in which the iron 30 mg, 60 mg or 120 mg) was chelated with glycine and then stabilized. In addition, all gps. received 250 µg folic acid. After 4 wks., all treatments raised hemoglobin levels 2.4-2.9 g/dL. Ferritin increases from both 120 mg iron sources and the 60 mg of iron chelate were significant. Gastric distress with the 120 mg dosage of the amino acid chelate was far less than from ferrous sulfate (*Pineda O, Ashmead HD, Perez JM, Lemus CP. Effectiveness of iron amino acid chelate on the treatment of iron deficiency anemia in adolescents. J Appl Nutr 46(1&2), 1994*).

Compared to ferrous sulfate, ferrous fumarate has similar bioavailability, while ferrous succinate, ferrous saccharate and ferric pyrophosphate are less bioavailable.

Experimental Study: In adult volunteers, compared to ferrous sulfate, the absorption of ferrous fumarate was similar, ferrous succcinate was 92%, ferrous saccharate (10%Fe) was 74%, and ferric pyrophosphate was only 39% (*Hurrell RF, Furniss DE, Burri J, et al. Iron fortification of infant cereals: a proposal for the use of ferrous fumarate or ferrous succinate. Am J Clin Nutr 49(6):1274-82, 1989*).

Compared to ferrous sulfate, ferritin and iron chondroitinsulfuric acid complex have similar bioavailability.

Experimental Study: 69 pregnant women, anemic and non-anemic received ferrous sulfate, iron chondroitinsulfuric acid complex, ferritin alone, or ferritin along with folinic acid and cobamamide. After 50 days, based on hematological findings (Hb, RCC, Ht, CV, iron, and transferrrin IBC), the 4 products demonstrated similar efficacy in maintaining anemic conditions under control. Only ferrous sulfate caused side effects (*Fochi F, Ciampini M, Caccarelli G. Efficacy of iron therapy: a comparative evaluation of four iron preparations administered to anaemic pregnant women. J Int Med Res 13(1):1-11, 1985*).

- Formulations

The bioavailability of enteric-coated ferrous sulfate tablets, as compared to film-coated tablets and an oral solution, is considerably lower; thus these products should not be considered interchangeable (*Walker SE, Paton TW, Cowan DH, et al. Bioavailability of iron in oral ferrous sulfate preparation in healthy volunteers. Can Med Assoc J 141(6):543-7, 1989*).

Controlled-release iron preparations reduce gastric irritation and are equally as bioavailable as conventional supplements (*Krzysko K, Bokowski W, Wichlinski LM. Biopharmaceutical evaluation of ferrous salts in form of oral long-acting tablets. Pol J Pharmacol Pharm 36(1):73-7, 1984| Ricketts CR. Iron bioavailability from controlled-release and conventional iron supplements. J Appl Nutr 45(1):13-19, 1993*).

Lactobacillus acidophilus

Beneficial microorganisms should generally be taken with food *(Khem Shahani, professor of Food Science Technology, U. of Nebraska)*.

Many lactobacillus products on the market are of inferior quality, contaminated, or do not contain *Lactobacillus acidophilus*, the acidophilus species found to be effective.

> **In vitro Study:** 16 non-prescription lactobacillus products were compared. All contained lactobacilli; however, only 4/16 (25%) contained *Lactobacillus acidophilus*. At least one contaminant was detected in 11/16 (69%) of the products: *Enterococcus faecium* (n=10), *Colstridium sporogenes* (n=1), *Streptococcus mitis* (n=1), and *Pseudomonas species* (n=1). Recently, lactobacillus species that produce hydrogen peroxide have been associated with normal vaginal flora; 10/16 (62%) products were found to produce hydrogen peroxide *(Hughes VL, Hillier SL. Microbiologic characteristics of Lactobacillus products used for colonization of the vagina. Obstet Gynecol 75(2):244-8, 1990)*.

Lecithin   See '**Choline**' above.

Magnesium

In the stomach, dietary magnesium combines with hydrochloric acid to form magnesium chloride which is then absorbed in the small intestine, particularly in the proximal portions *(Classen HG. Magnesium and potassium deprivation and supplementation in animals and man: aspects in view of intestinal absorption. Magnesium 3:257-64, 1984)*.

Oral supplementation may restore magnesium depots in patients with magnesium deficiency within six weeks.

> **Experimental Double-blind Study:** 40 elderly pts. with suspected magnesium deficiency randomly received oral magnesium citrate/lactate 5 mmol 3 times daily or placebo for 6 wks., while another gp. of 23 pts. received 30 mmol of magnesium sulfate IV daily for 7 days. Controls consisted of 30 pts. without known predisposition to magnesium deficiency and 27 young, healthy subjects. Based on IV magnesium-loading tests, magnesium retention after 6 wks. of oral supplementation, but not after placebo, was comparable to that observed after 7 days of parenteral administration and to that in both control gps. *(Gullestad L, Oystein DL, Birkeland K, et al. Oral versus intravenous magnesium supplementation in patients with magnesium deficiency. Magnes Trace Elem 10(1):11-16, 1991-2)*.

- When to Provide Oral Supplementation

Magnesium supplements may be more bioavailable when taken with meals.

> *Note: The absorption of magnesium decreases rapidly at doses above about 200 mg when taken with meals (Fine KD, Santa Ana CA, Porter JL, Fordtran JS. Intestinal absorption of magnesium from food and supplements. J Clin Invest 88:(2)396-402, 1991)*.

Experimental Study: 7 normal subjects and 4 pts. with recurrent calcium oxalate nephrolithiasis were studied. When magnesium citrate or magnesium oxide were administered with meals, versus when they were administered on an empty stomach, urinary magnesium showed larger increases *(Lindberg J, Harvey J, Pak CY. Effect of magnesium citrate and magnesium oxide on the crystallization of calcium salts in urine: changes produced by food-magnesium interaction. J Urol 143(2):248-51, 1990).*

- Formulations

Intestinal absorption appears to be the same from various preparations so long as magnesium is free and in its ionized form when it reaches the absorptive area *(Leonhard S, Smith E, Martens H, et al. Transport of magnesium across an isolated preparation of sheep rumen: A comparison of magnesium chloride, magnesium aspartate, magnesium pidolate, and Mg-EDTA. Magnes Trace Elem 9(5):265-71, 1990).*

Magnesium chloride is the recommended form of magnesium for oral supplementation according to the Consensus Panel of the American Diabetes Association *(Magnesium supplementation in the treatment of diabetes. American Diabetes Association. Diabetes Care 15(8):1065-7, 1992).* It is considerably more soluble than most magnesium salts (ex. magnesium oxide, carbonate, citrate, hydroxide or sulfate) *(Lange NA. Handbook of Chemistry, Edition 10. San Francisco, McGraw-Hill, 1967:282-5; Lowenthal DT. Clinical pharmacology of magnesium chloride, in TD Giles, MS Seelig, Eds. The Role of Magnesium Chloride Therapy in Clinical Practice. Clifton NJ, Oxford Health Care, 1988)* and does not require stomach acid for solubility *(Laban E, Charbon GA. Magnesium and cardiac arrhythmias: Nutrient or drug? J Am Coll Nutr 5:521-32, 1986).*

Moreover, chloride is a particularly suitable anion for a magnesium salt. Many of the conditions that predispose patients to magnesium deficiency (e.g. diuretic therapy; congestive heart failure) often precipitate metabolic alkalosis. Metabolic alkalosis can worsen after supplementation with other magnesium salts as 50-70% of the magnesium chloride formed in the stomach is lost via the feces before it can be absorbed; thus only compounds containing both magnesium and chloride (such as magnesium chloride or magnesium aspartate hydrochloride) can correct a magnesium deficiency while not provoking or aggravating metabolic alkalosis in high risk patients *(Classen HG. Magnesium and potassium deprivation and supplementation in animals and man: aspects in view of intestinal absorption. Magnesium 3:257-64, 1984; Schimatschek HT, Classen HG, Thoni H, Haubold W. [Acid-base changes in rats kept on highly magnesium enriched diets using different magnesium compounds.] Magnesium Bull 9:161-76, 1987).* In addition, chloride has a positive effect on magnesium absorption and distribution *(Classen HG, Marquardt P, Spaeth M, et al. Improvement by chlorine of the intestinal absorption of inorganic and organic Mg compounds and their protective effect against adrenergic cardiopathy. Rec Adv Stud Cardiac Struct Metab 6:111-19, 1975).*

> *Note: Because magnesium chloride is hygroscopic (moisture-retaining), magnesium chloride tablets must be enteric coated to protect their integrity (Seelig M. Cardiovascular consequences of magnesium deficiency and loss: Pathogenesis, prevalence and manifestations - magnesium and chloride loss in refractory potassium repletion. Am J Cardiol 63(14):4G-21G, 1989). However, enteric coating may reduce magnesium bioavailability:*

Experimental Study: "Magnesium absorption from a commercially available enteric-coated magnesium chloride tablet was much less than from magnesium acetate, suggesting that enteric coating can impair magnesium bioavailability" *(Fine KD, Santa Ana CA, Porter JL, Fordtran JS. Intestinal absorption of magnesium from food and supplements. J Clin Invest 88:(2)396-402, 1991).*

Note: The bioavailability of magnesium chloride solution appears similar to that of slow-release magnesium chloride tablets (White J, Massey L, Gales SK, et al. Blood and urinary magnesium kinetics after oral magnesium supplements. Clin Ther 14(5):678-87, 1992).

Case Report: A pt. who abused magnesium cathartics developed a hypochloremic/hypokalemic alkalosis which was thought to be due to gastric conversion of magnesium oxide to magnesium chloride and fecal excretion of endogenous chloride *(Urakabe S, Nakata K, Ando A, et al. Hypokalemia and metabolic alkalosis resulting from overuse of magnesium oxide. Jpn Circ J 39:1135-7, 1975).*

Case Reports: Alkalosis was worsened when buffered potassium rather than potassium chloride was provided *(Kassirer JP, Barkman PM, Lawrenz DR, Schwartz WB. The critical role of chloride in the correction of hypokalemic alkalosis in man. Am J Med 38:172-90, 1965).*

Several magnesium salts appear to be adequately bioavailable, although comparisons between them are rare:

Magnesium acetate is as bioavailable as magnesium from almonds, a magnesium-rich natural source *(Fine KD, Santa Ana CA, Porter JL, Fordtran JS. Intestinal absorption of magnesium from food and supplements. J Clin Invest 88:(2)396-402, 1991).*

Magnesium citrate is highly soluble, even in water, and provides bioavailable magnesium; it is superior in both solubility and bioavailability to magnesium oxide *(Lindberg JS, Zobitz MM, Poindexter JR, Pak CYC. Magnesium bioavailability from magnesium citrate and magnesium oxide. J Am Coll Nutr 9(1):48-55, 1990).*

Tablets containing magnesium citrate/lactate with or without magnesium hydroxide, magnesium hydroxide tablets alone and magnesium chloride solution alone were all equally bioavailable *(Bohmer T, Roseth A, Holm H, et al. Bioavailability of oral magnesium supplementation in female students evaluated from elimination of magnesium in 24-hour urine. Magnes Trace Elem 9(5):272-8, 1990).*

In an animal study, magnesium lactate tolerance and bioavailability compared favorably to that of enteric-coated magnesium chloride, even in conditions of reduced gastric acidity *(Robins TL, Imondi AR, Murphy PE, et al. Magnesium lactate bioavailability in dogs is not impaired by decreased gastric acidity. Abstract. J Am Coll Nutr 8(5):462, 1989).*

Magnesium aspartate has excellent absorption *(Mühlbauer B, Schwenk M, Coram WM, et al. Magnesium-L-aspartate-HCl and magnesium-oxide: bioavailability in healthy volunteers. Eur J Clin Pharmacol 40(4):437-8, 1991)* and is well-tolerated *(Hallberg D. Magnesium problems in gastroenterology. Acta Med Scand Suppl 661:19-20, 1982; Nyhlin H, Dyckner T, Ek B, Wester PO. Magnesium in Crohn's disease. Acta Med Scand Suppl 661:21-5, 1982).*

Magnesium gluconate appears to be as bioavailable as magnesium chloride (*White J, Massey L, Gales SK, et al. Blood and urinary magnesium kinetics after oral magnesium supplements. Clin Ther 14(5):678-87, 1992*).

Magnesium oxide is insoluble in water; thus its bioavailability may be poor in patients with decreased gastric acidity (*Lindberg JS, Zobitz MM, Poindexter JR, Pak CYC. Magnesium bioavailability from magnesium citrate and magnesium oxide. J Am Coll Nutr 9(1):48-55, 1990*) and other magnesium salts may be preferable.

> **Experimental Study:** In a parallel gp. design, 3 gps. of 8 healthy volunteers received one of two formulations of magnesium-L-aspartate HCL (Magnesiocard® tablets or granules, Verla-Pharm, Germany) or magnesium oxide (Magnetrans® forte capsules, Fresenius, Germany). Magnesium oxide showed significantly lower absorption than magnesium-L-aspartate HCL (*Mühlbauer B, Schwenk M, Coram WM, et al. Magnesium-L-aspartate-HCl and magnesium-oxide: bioavailability in healthy volunteers. Eur J Clin Pharmacol 40(4):437-8, 1991*).

The bioavailability of magnesium hydroxide appears similar to that of magnesium oxide (*Davenport GM, Boling JA, Gay N. Bioavailability of magnesium in beef cattle fed magnesium oxide or magnesium hydroxide. J Anim Sci 68(11):3765-72, 1990*).

N-Acetylcysteine

Rapidly absorbed following oral administration (*Bonanomi L, Gazzaniga A. Toxicological, pharmacokinetic and metabolic studies on acetylcysteine. Eur J Respir Dis 61 (Suppl):45-51, 1980*).

Niacin

In the elderly, a good diet and a daily 'multivitamin' may fail to maintain adequate niacin nutriture, and intramuscular injections may be necessary.

> **Experimental Study:** 228 ambulatory residents of a nursing home, mean age 87, who had not undergone major surgical procedures, ate a 'good' diet, and received at least one multivitamin pill daily for 3-5 of the preceding months, were compared to 204 healthy volunteers aged 20-50. 88/228 (39%) showed deficits of up to 5 of the B complex vitamins, one of which was niacin. Oral vitamin supplementation was stopped and a single IM injection of multivitamins was given. After 3 mo., these deficits were no longer detectable in the blood of 89-100% of the previously vitamin-deficient pts. (*Baker H, Frank O, Jaslow SP. Oral versus intramuscular vitamin supplementation for hypovitaminosis in the elderly. J Am Geriatr Soc 28(1):42-5, 1980*).

- When to Provide Oral Supplementation

A water-soluble vitamin, niacin is absorbed with or without food although food, by slowing the rate of absorption, may increase the length of time that blood levels are increased and thereby reduce its eventual excretion. A similar improvement in absorption can be achieved by dividing the total dosage into several portions and taking them throughout the day (*Yung S, Mayersohn M, Robinson JB. Ascorbic acid absorption in man: influence of divided dose and food. Life Sci 28(22):2505-11, 1981*).

- Formulation

Inositol hexanicotinate is a niacin ester that consists of six niacin molecules surrounding a single molecule of inositol. While rapidly absorbed as the intact ester, it has a slow rate of metabolism, thus producing the therapeutic advantages of a sustained-release preparation of niacin and inositol but with less side effects than those of sustained-release niacin (*Welsh AL, Ede M. Inositol hexanicotinate for improved nicotinic acid therapy. Int Record Med 174:9-15, 1961*).

Omega-3 Fatty Acids

Fish oils are commonly used as a source of omega-3 fatty acid supplements. Because they are highly unsaturated, they are easily oxidized.

Observational Study: 5/6 samples of soft gelatin-encapsulated fish oils, although they contained the antioxidant vitamin E (164-7,965 ppm), showed 1-10% dimeric triacylglycerols and one contained 6.3% trimeric triacylglycerols and 3.1% oligomeric triacylglycerols, thermal oxidation products which may have formed during high-temperature deodorization or as a result of auto-oxidation prior to encapsulation. Also soft gelatin capsules are somewhat permeable to oxygen which would allow some oxidation of the oil after encapsulation (*Shukla VKS, Perkins EG. The presence of oxidative polymeric materials in encapsulated fish oils. Lipids 26:23-6, 1991*).

- Enteric Coating

As the rate of absorption of the component omega-3 fatty acids in fish oil is high when they are administered in the form of an enteric-coated preparation (Purepa, Tillotts Pharma, Ziefen, Switzerland), the dose needed to achieve the incorporation of fish-oil fatty acids into phospholipids membranes is one-third of that used previously (*Belluzzi A, Brignola C, Campieri M, et al. Effects of new fish oil derivative on fatty acid phospholipid-membrane pattern in a group of Crohn's disease patients. Dig Dis Sci 39:2589-94, 1994*).

Omega-6 Fatty Acids

Common commercial sources of gamma-linolenic acid:

Evening primrose seed oil:	7-8% GLA
Black current seed oil:	15-17% GLA
Borage seed oil:	22-24% GLA

- Borage vs. Evening Primrose Oil

Evening primrose oil and borage oil are equivalent sources of tissue gamma-linolenic acid (GLA) and dihomogammalinolenic acid (DGLA) concentrations when equivalent dosages of gamma-linolenic acid are provided (*Raederstorff D, Moser U. Borage or primrose oil added to standardized diets are equivalent sources for gamma-linolenic acid in rats. Lipids 27(12):1018-23, 1992*). However, there is evidence that, due to differences in its composition, borage oil is an inferior source of GLA.

Review Article: Evening primrose oil (EPO) contains 8-9% GLA almost entirely in the form of dilinoleoyl-monogammalinolenyl glycerol (DLMG), a triglyceride which comprises glycerol with one molecule of GLA and two molecules of linoleic acid attached to it. Scotia pharmaceuticals has isolated DLMG from EPO and shown that the oil's biological activity is almost entirely explained by its DLMG content: in biological tests in which sunflower oil is inactive but EPO is active, the addition of the right level of DLMG makes sunflower oil as active as EPO. Compared to EPO, borage oil is much more complex, with the GLA spread among many more triglycerides, and fatty acids other than GLA or linoleic acid present in these triglycerides. These other fatty acids also have biological effects, and may interfere with the absorption of GLA or with its metabolism once absorbed *(Horrobin DF. Guest editorial. Natural ≠ safe. Pharmaceutical Technology Europe, December, 1994).*

Animal Experimental Study: Either 1% evening primrose oil (EPO) or 1% borage oil was added to the diet of diabetic rats. While EPO produced a near complete correction of nerve conduction, borage oil, despite a higher GLA content, produced only a 25% correction. Increasing the amt. of borage oil in the diet to 3% resulted in even less improvement, suggesting that some ingredient in the oil may be actively toxic *(Dines KC, Cotter MA, Cameron NE. Effects of dietary supplementation with oils containing γ-linolenic acid on nerve function in diabetic rats. Presentation to The Physiological Society Meeting, Aberdeen, UK, September 14-16, 1994).*

Experimental Study: Normal male volunteers were administered borage oil. In contrast to the effect of evening primrose oil which inhibits platelet aggregation and reduces thromboxane levels, platelet aggregation and the formation of thromboxane A_2 (a strong pro-aggregatory agent) increased *(Barre DE, Holum BJ, Chapkin RS. Effect of borage oil supplementation on human platelet aggregation, thromboxane B_2, prostaglandin E_1 and E_2 formation. Nutr Res 13:739-51, 1993).*

Animal Experimental Study: As compared to corn oil, both borage oil and evening primrose oil (EPO) increased the level of PGE_1 in mice. However, while EPO more than doubled the amt. of PGI_2 (a powerful anti-platelet aggregating agent) as compared to corn oil, borage oil halved it *(Fan YY, Chapkin RS. Mouse peritoneal macrophage prostaglandin E_1 synthesis is altered by dietary gamma-linolenic acid. J Nutr 1600-06, 1992).*

Pancreatic Enzymes

Note: *"Pancreatic enzyme products are not pharmaceutical equivalents, are not tested one against the other, and cannot be expected to behave identically"* *(Rheinstein PH. Regulatory status of pancreatic enzyme products. JAMA 263(18):2491-2, 1990).*

- When to Provide Oral Supplementation

Pancreatic enzymes are best taken with meals (*DeMagno EP, Malagelada JR, Go WL, Moertel CG. Fate of orally ingested enzymes in pancreatic insufficiency. N Engl J Med 296(23):1318-22, 1977; Pap V, Varro V. Replacement therapy in pancreatic insufficiency with a new pancreatin preparation respecting the physiological ratio of lipase/trypsin activity. Hepato-gastroenterol 35:83-6, 1988*).

- Formulations

Pancreatin granules may be more bioavailable than enteric-coated pancreatin tablets.

> *Note: Pancreatin is a commercially prepared and dried pancreatic compound that contains digestive enzymes standardized for amylase, trypsin and lipase, usually of porcine or bovine origin.*

Experimental Study: 12 pts. with chronic pancreatitis received the manufacturers' recommended doses of pancreatin in two different formulations. There was a significantly greater improvement in fat absorption following administration of the non-enteric-coated enzymes than following administration of the enteric-coated ones ($p<0.001$) (*Marotta F, O'Keefe SJD, Marks IN, et al. Pancreatic enzyme replacement therapy: importance of gastric acid secretion, H2-antagonists, and enteric coating. Dig Dis Sci 3493):456-61, 1989*).

Experimental Study: In a study of both pancreatic insufficient and healthy subjects, intestinal enzyme activity did not markedly increase in either gp. following administration of pancreatin tablets, but amylase, lipase, phospholipase and trypsin were significantly increased following administration of pure pancreatin granules (*Schneider MU, Knoll-Ruzicka ML, Domshke S, et al. Pancreatic enzyme replacement therapy: comparative effects of conventional and enteric-coated microspheric pancreatin and acid-stable fungal enzyme preparations on steatorrhoea in chronic pancreatitis. Hepato-gastroenterol 32:97-102, 1985*).

Review Article: Pts. with clinically documented hypo- or hyperchlorhydria will benefit from enteric-coated pancreatin microspheres. "In all other patients, this preparation is no better than cheap pancreatin" (*DeMagno EP. Controversies in the treatment of exocrine pancreatic insufficiency. Dig Dis Sci 27(6):481-4, 1982*).

Observational Study: 16 commercially available pancreatic extracts were assayed. Lipase activity *in vitro* correlated with potency *in vivo* in decreasing steatorrhea for both tablets and capsules. Enteric-coated tablets were found to be less effective (*Graham DY. Enzyme replacement therapy of exocrine pancreatic insufficiency in man. Relation between in vitro enzyme activities and in vivo potency in commercial pancreatic extracts. N Engl J Med 296:1314-17, 1977*).

Phosphatidylcholine   See '<u>Choline</u>' above.

Potassium

- Formulations

Bioavailability of various potassium preparations tested is excellent and appears to be similar.

> *Note: Correction of a potassium deficit should be via oral or nasogastric administration, if possible. Parenteral administration should be limited to the intravenous route, as subcutaneous and intramuscular injections present many hazards (Snively WD Jr, Sweeney MJ. Fluid Balance Handbook for Practitioners. Springfield, IL, Charles C. Thomas, 1956).*

Potassium Chloride

> **WARNING:** Potassium chloride is irritating to the gastric and intestinal mucosa, and enteric-coated potassium chloride may cause ulceration and stenosis of the small intestine *(Snively WD Jr, Westerman RL. The clinician views potassium deficit. Minn Med June, 1965, pp. 713-19)*. Formulation of the salt in a microencapsulated multiple-unit dosage form neither guarantees wide dispersion in the stomach nor the absence of a high local concentration *(Graham DY, Smith JL, Bouvet AA. What happens to tablets and capsules in the stomach: endoscopic comparison of disintegration and dispersion characteristics of two microencapsulated potassium formulations. J Pharm Sci 79(5):420-4, 1990).*

Experimental Single-blind Crossover Study: 10 healthy volunteers received potassium chloride solution (PS) and potassium chloride wax-matrix tablets (WMT) and a new microencapsulated potassium chloride tablet (MET). Results based on urinary potassium excretion showed that all 3 formulas have excellent bioavailability, indicating that potassium absorption in the stomach (from the solution) is similar to that in more distal portions of the gut (from the slow-release tablets). The slow-release characteristic of both MET and WMT were confirmed. No side effects were reported with any of the formulations *(Caplain H, Dahan R, Pamphile R, Thebault JJ. A single blind normal volunteer bioavailability study of a new microencapsulated potassium chloride tablet compared to reference potassium formulations. Eur J Drug Metab Pharmacokinet 16(3):241-4, 1991).*

Experimental Study: 10 healthy subjects received a standard sustained-release preparation of potassium chloride embedded in a wax material, formulations containing 20% hydrogenated vegetable oil and hydroxypropyl methylcellulose and an enteric-coated potassium chloride tablet. Mean recoveries in 24-hr. urine potassium levels were similar, and there was no significant difference in the time to reach maximal excretion rates among the 3 sustained release tablets.   No adverse effects were reported *(Senel S, Capan Y, Dalkara T, et al. Formulation, bioavailability, and pharmacokinetics of sustained-release potassium chloride tablets. Pharm Res 8(10):1313-17, 1991).*

Experimental Crossover Study: 28 healthy male volunteers received 40 meq doses of a suspension containing microencapsulated potassium chloride, a microencapsulated potassium chloride capsule and a potassium chloride solution. The pattern of excretion of the solution indicated rapid absorption and elimination. The potassium from the suspension and the capsules was excreted more slowly and over a longer period, indicating that the potassium content from these formulas was not being dumped. The extent of absorption was similar in all 3 products (*Melikian AP, Cheng LK, Wright GJ, et al. Bioavailability of potassium from three dosage forms: suspension, capsule, and solution. J Clin Pharmacol 28(11):1046-50, 1988*).

Experimental Study: 13 volunteers on a low potassium diet received a single dose of 32 mmol potassium either in the form of a controlled-release multiple-unit tablet (Kalinorm) and a single-unit tablet (Slow-K), either with or without water loading. Irrespective of procedure, the two products had the same bioavailability based on urinary potassium excretion (*Bechgaard H, Shephard NW. Bioavailability of potassium from controlled-release tablets with and without water loading. Eur J Clin Pharmacol 21(2):143-7, 1981*).

Experimental Study: Based on urinary potassium excretion in 10 healthy volunteers, a sustained-release potassium chloride tablet was as bioavailable as a non-sustained release potassium chloride tablet (*Muller A, Thoma M Renker H. [Biological availability of potassium from a sustained release preparation.] Schweiz Med Wochenschr 106(1):27-30, 1976*).

Potassium Citrate

> **WARNING:** Potassium citrate mixture BP, because of its alkalizing action, is used to relieve the discomfort of cystitis. However, even when renal function is normal, severe hyperkalemia may occur (*Elizabeth JE, Carter NJ. Potassium citrate mixture: soothing but not harmless? Br Med J 295:993, 1987*).

Experimental Placebo-controlled Study: After stabilization on a constant metabolic diet, subjects took a single dose of placebo, slow-release potassium citrate (60 meq) or rapid-release potassium citrate liquid (60 meq). Timed urine specimens were analyzed for potassium, citrate and pH. Similar biochemical findings were observed, with the onset and decline of changes being slightly more rapid for the liquid than the tablet preparation (*Harvey JA, Zobitz MM, Pak CY. Bioavailability of citrate from two different preparations of potassium citrate. J Clin Pharmacol 29(4):338-41, 1989*).

Potassium Tartrate

Experimental Study: The bioavailability of potassium from a potassium tartrate tablet was evaluated in 20 normal subjects. The formulation was found to be highly bioavailable (*Whiting SJ, Gorecki DK, Jones D. In vitro and in vivo assessment of the bioavailability of potassium from a potassium tartrate tablet. Biopharm Drug Dispos 12(3):207-13, 1991*).

Phosphatidylserine

A comparison of bovine brain cortex and soy-derived phosphatidylserine (in regard to their effects on mouse brain) found the latter, which lacks certain long-chain fatty acids, to be inactive (*Toffano G, Leon A, Benvegnu D, et al. Effect of brain cortex phospholipids on catechol-amine content of mouse brain. Pharmacol Res Commun 8(6):581-90, 1976*).

Quercetin

Absorption of orally administered quercetin is uncertain, although newer evidence suggests that it may be bioavailable (*Hollman PCH et al. Absorption of dietary quercetin glycosides and quercetin in healthy ileostomy volunteers. Am J Clin Nutr 62:1276-82, 1995*).

Riboflavin

Destroyed under alkaline conditions. Light at acid and neutral pH converts riboflavin to lumichrome; at alkaline pH, light converts it to lumiflavin, a riboflavin-antagonist.

- When to Provide Oral Supplementation

A water-soluble vitamin, riboflavin is absorbed with or without food - although food, by slowing the rate of absorption, may increase the length of time that blood levels are increased and thereby reduce its eventual excretion. A similar improvement in absorption can be achieved by dividing the total dosage into several portions and taking them throughout the day (*Yung S, Mayersohn M, Robinson JB. Ascorbic acid absorption in man: influence of divided dose and food. Life Sci 28(22):2505-11, 1981*).

- Supplements vs. Food Sources

In the presence of ethanol, riboflavin supplements are better absorbed than are dietary sources of riboflavin (flavin mononucleotide and flavin adenine dinucleotide) (*Pinto J, Huang YP, Rivlin RS. Mechanisms underlying the differential effects of ethanol on the bioavailability of riboflavin and flavin adenine dinucleotide. J Clin Invest 79(5):1343-8, 1987*).

S-Adenosylmethionine

While unstable in acid, it is efficiently absorbed when administered in enteric-coated tablets and taken up intact by various tissues, including hepatocytes (*Stramentinoli G. Pharmacologic aspects of S-adenosylmethionine. Am J Med 84(suppl 5A):35-42, 1987*).

Selenium

- Organic versus Inorganic

1. Organic selenium (L-selenomethionine) is rapidly and completely absorbed, while inorganic selenium (selenite and selenate) is less well absorbed and retained (*Swanson CA et al. Human [^{74}Se]selenomethionine metabolism: a kinetic model. Am J Clin Nutr 54:917-26, 1991*).

Experimental Double-blind Study: 33 New Zealand women aged 18-23 received selenium 200 µg as selenium-enriched yeast (selenomethionine) or brewer's yeast mixed with selenate, or placebo. Selenomethionine was more effective in raising blood selenium concentrations than selenate (*Thomson CD, Robinson MF, Butler JA, Whanger PD. Long-term supplementation with selenate and selenomethionine: selenium and* *glutathione peroxidase (EC 1.11.1.9) in blood components of New Zealand women. Br J Nutr 69(2):577-88, 1993).*

Animal Experimental Study: 60 weanling male rats were fed Torula yeast-based diets containing 0.5, 1.5 or 2.5 parts per million of selenium as either L-selenomethionine or sodium selenate. After 4 wks., selenium retention was greater in every tissue when selenomethionine was fed in comparison to selenate. Hair and nail selenium levels reflect both liver and muscle selenium pools when selenomethionine is the source of selenium. When selenate is fed, however, hair and nails accumulate selenium while muscle selenium levels remain relatively unchanged *(Salbe AD, Levander OA. Hair and nails as indicators of selenium status in rats fed elevated dietary levels of selenium as L-selenomethionine (SeMet) or sodium selenate (Na_2SeO_4). Fed Proc 46(4), March 5, 1987).*

Experimental Study: Blood selenium of volunteers given organic selenium increased more in relation to dose than did blood selenium of volunteers given sodium selenate *(Jaakkola K et al. Selenium levels in whole blood of Finnish volunteers before and during organic and inorganic selenium supplementation. Scand J Clin Lab Invest 43(6):473-6, 1983).*

2. Inorganic selenium, in contrast to organic selenium, has been found to be nearly ineffective in various *in vitro* experiments against selenium deficiency in several species, starting with the study of Schwartz and Fultz *(J Biol Chem 233:245-51, 1958)* and reconfirmed repeatedly *(Schrauzer GN. Benefits of nutritional selenium. Report of presentation from the Fourth International Symposium on Selenium in Biology and Medicine, Tubingen U., W. Germany, July, 1988. Anabolism 7(4):5, 1988).*

3. Inorganic selenium causes a rapid rise in serum selenium with an early plateau and a sharp decline in blood levels upon discontinuation, while selenomethionine causes a slow but progressive rise in serum selenium with a very slow decline in blood levels following discontinuation due, presumably, to selenomethionine body stores. Therefore, selenium toxicity is more likely to be caused by prolonged use of excessive doses of selenomethionine *(Levander OA, Alfthan G, Arvilommi H, et al. Bioavailability of selenium to Finnish men as assessed by platelet glutathione peroxidase activity and other blood parameters. Am J Clin Nutr 37(6):887-97, 1983).*

4. The body may treat selenomethionine as methionine and incorporate much of it into tissue protein, thus making it less available than inorganic selenate for incorporation into tissue glutathione peroxidase *(Thomson CD, Robinson MF, Butler JA, Whanger PD. Long-term supplementation with selenate and selenomethionine: selenium and glutathione peroxidase (EC 1.11.1.9) in blood components of New Zealand women. Br J Nutr 69(2):577-88, 1993).*

Experimental Double-blind Study: 33 women aged 18-23 consumed 200 μg/d of selenium as either selenium-enriched yeast (selenomethionine) or brewer's yeast mixed with selenate, or placebo. After 32 wks., selenate was more effective in raising glutathione peroxidase levels in platelets, while both were equally effective in raising glutathione peroxidase activities in whole blood, erythrocytes and plasma *(Thomson C, Robinson M, Butler J, et al. Long-term supplementation with selenate and selenomethionine: selenium and glutathione peroxidase (C 1.11.1.9) in blood components of New Zealand women. Br J Nutr 69:577-88, 1993).*

Experimental Double-blind Study: 3 gps. of 11 women each received, for 32 wks., yeast tablets with no added selenium or 200 µg selenium daily either as selenate or as selenium-enriched yeast (selenomethionine). Supplementation with selenomethionine increased selenium content in plasma and RBCs to a greater extent than supplementation with selenate. The percentage of selenium associated with glutathione peroxidase was greater in RBCs and plasma of women taking selenate than of those taking selenomethionine. Blood selenium concentrations correlated better with glutathione peroxidase activity in women taking selenate, possibly because the accumulation of selenium in the hemoglobin of women taking selenomethionine (*Butler JA, Thomson CD, Whanger PD, Robinson MF. Selenium distribution in blood fractions in New Zealand women taking organic or inorganic selenium. Am J Clin Nutr 53:748-54, 1991*).

5. Inorganic selenium may be more effective than organic selenium in animal models of cancer (*Greeder GA, Milner JA. Factors influencing the inhibitory effect of selenium on mice inoculated with Ehrlich ascites tumor cells. Science 209:825-7, 1980; Griffin AC, Jacobs MM. Effect of selenium on azo dye hepatocarcinogenesis. Cancer Lett 3:177-81, 1977; Milner JA, Greeder GA, Poirer KA. Selenium and transplantable tumors, in JE Spallholz et al, Eds. Selenium in Biology and Medicine. Westport, CT, AVI Publishing Co., 1981:146-59; Thompson HJ. Selenium as an anticarcinogen. J Agric Food Chem 32:422-5, 1984*).

- Forms of Organic Selenium

1. Ingestion of selenomethionine (which is plant-derived) will produce higher blood and tissue selenium levels than ingestion of selenocysteine (which is animal-derived) as animals treat selenomethionine as methionine. They thus incorporate it into proteins in place of methionine and, when catabolized, it becomes nutritionally available for incorporation into glutathione peroxidase. Selenocysteine, by contrast, is only incorporated into selenoproteins such as glutathione peroxidase and is excreted once the enzyme reaches control levels. Thus selenium levels merely reflect differences in the plant and animal components of the diet (*Burk RF. Letter. JAMA 262(6):775, 1989*).

2. Selenomethionine may be more bioavailable than selenium-enriched yeast.

> *Note: About half of the selenium in selenium-enriched yeast is in the form of protein-bound selenomethionine; however it also contains other selenium compounds that have not yet been identified (Myers G, Wang CS, Novelli R, et al. Selenium yeast studies, in JE Spallholz, JL Martin, HE Ganther, Eds. Selenium in Biology and Medicine. Westport, CT, AVI Publishing Co., 1981:531-4).*

Experimental Controlled Study: 31 lactating women and 22 nonlactating women randomly received selenomethionine (2.7 µmol Se), selenium-enriched yeast (2.9 µmol Se) or no selenium. Plasma selenium declined in unsupplemented lactating women but not in nonlactating women. Selenomethionine increased plasma selenium in both lactating and nonlactating women whereas selenium-enriched yeast increased plasma selenium only in nonlactating women. Milk selenium declined markedly for 20 wks. after parturition in unsupplemented women. Selenomethionine significantly increased milk selenium concentrations whereas selenium-enriched yeast prevented a decline (*McGuire MK, Burgert SL, Milner JA,* *et al. Selenium status of lactating women is affected by the form of selenium consumed. Am J Clin Nutr 58:649-52, 1993).*

- Forms of Inorganic Selenium

Selenite has been shown to interact with glutathione in the presence of oxygen to generate free radicals. Since glutathione is found in all cells, this form of selenium may be unsuitable for human use *(Schrauzer GN. Benefits of nutritional selenium. Report of presentation from the Fourth International Symposium on Selenium in Biology and Medicine, Tubingen U., W. Germany, July, 1988. Anabolism 7(4):5, 1988).*

Sodium selenite should not be taken concurrently with vitamin C, as it is reduced by vitamin C *in vitro* to the ineffective elemental selenium, a reaction which is the basis for the analytical measurement of selenium *(Newberry & Christian, JOAC 48:322, 1965).*

> **Experimental Study:** In healthy subjects, absorption of 1 mg selenium as sodium selenite 2 hrs. given with breakfast or juice was measured by fecal and urinary excretion. When ascorbic acid 1 g was added to the selenium supplement and both were consumed 2 hrs. before a meal, absorption was significantly reduced. Ascorbic acid reduces selenite to elemental selenium which is poorly absorbed *(Robinson MF, Thomas CD, Huemmer PK. Effect of a megadose of ascorbic acid, a meal and orange juice on the absorption of selenium as sodium selenite. N Z Med J 98:627-9, 1985).*

Thiamine

Unstable in alkali conditions.

In the elderly, a good diet and a daily 'multivitamin' may fail to maintain adequate thiamine nutriture, and intramuscular injections may be necessary.

> **Experimental Study:** 228 ambulatory residents of a nursing home, mean age 87, who had not undergone major surgical procedures, ate a 'good' diet, and received at least one multivitamin pill daily for 3-5 of the preceding months, were compared to 204 healthy volunteers aged 20-50. 88/228 (39%) showed deficits of up to 5 of the B complex vitamins, one of which was thiamine. Oral vitamin supplementation was stopped and a single IM injection of multivitamins was given. After 3 mo., these deficits were no longer detectable in the blood of 89-100% of the previously vitamin-deficient pts. *(Baker H, Frank O, Jaslow SP. Oral versus intramuscular vitamin supplementation for hypovitaminosis in the elderly. J Am Geriatr Soc 28(1):42-5, 1980).*

- When to Provide Oral Supplementation

A water-soluble vitamin, thiamine is absorbed with or without food although food, by slowing the rate of absorption, may increase the length of time that blood levels are increased and thereby reduce its eventual excretion. A similar improvement in absorption can be achieved by dividing the total dosage into several portions and taking them throughout the day *(Yung S, Mayersohn M, Robinson JB. Ascorbic acid absorption in man: influence of divided dose and food. Life Sci 28(22):2505-11, 1981).*

- Forms and Formulations

Thiamine hydrochloride is the most common commercially available form.

Thiamine mononitrate is often found in multivitamin preparations and is preferred over the hydrochloride in food enrichment because of its greater stability in processing and storage (*Flodin NW. Pharmacology of Micronutrients. New York, Alan R. Liss, Inc., 1988*).

Thiamine administered as lipophilic benfotiamine is substantially more bioavailable than water-soluble thiamine mononitrate (*Bitsch R, Wolf M, Moller J, et al. Bioavailability assessment of the lipophilic benfotiamine as compared to a water-soluble thiamin derivative. Ann Nutr Metab 35(5):292-6, 1991*).

Allithiamine is formed in garlic bulbs and other plants of the allium species by the conjugation of allicin with thiamine. In Japan, a number of allithiamine derivatives have been synthesized, such as thiamine propyl disulfide whose biologic activity was found to be significantly greater than thiamine hydrochloride (*Fujiwara M. Absorption, excretion and fate of thiamine and its derivatives in (the) human body, in M Shimazono, E Katsura, Eds. Beriberi and Thiamine. Edition 2. Tokyo, Igaku Shoin, 1965:179-213*). More recently, a synthetic, thiamine tetrahydrofurfuryl disulfide (Takeda Chemical Industries, Osaka), has almost completely replaced the earlier compounds as it appears to have the same biologic activity but does not leave the patient with the pungent odor of garlic and no toxic effects have been observed (*Lonsdale D. A Nutritionist's Guide to the Clinical Use of Vitamin B-1. Tacoma, WA, Life Sciences Press, 1987:64-70*).

See Also:

> Lonsdale D. Allithiamine and its synthetic derivatives: a review. *J Nutr Med* 2:305-11, 1991

> Lonsdale D. Thiamine and its fat soluble derivatives as therapeutic agents. *Int Clin Nutr Rev* 7(3):114-25, 1987

> Sakuma A et al. Clinical effects of TTFD tablets on so-called neuralgia. *Jap J Clin Exp Med* 52:2890-301, 1975

> Pincus JH, Cooper JR, Itokawa Y, et al. Subacute necrotizing encephalomyelopathy: effect of thiamine and thiamine propyl disulfide. *Arch Neurol* 24:511-17, 1971

> Thomson AD, Frank O, Baker H, et al. Thiamine propyl disulfide: absorption and utilization. *Ann Intern Med* 74:529-34, 1971

Vanadium

Bis(maltolato)oxovanadium, an organic vanadium complex, may be more readily absorbed than inorganic vanadium salts (such as vanadyl sulfate) (*Yuen VG, Orvig C, McNeill JH. Comparison of the glucose-lowering properties of vanadyl sulfate and bis(maltolto)oxovanadium(IV) following acute and chronic administration. Can J Physiol*

Pharmacol 73(1):55-64, 1995; Yuen VG, Orvig C, McNeill JH. Glucose-lowering effects of a new organic vanadium complex, bis(maltolto)oxovanadium(IV). _Can J Physiol Pharmacol_ 71(3-4):263-9, 1993).

Vitamin A

Unstable in acid conditions.

Beta-carotene may be therapeutically equivalent to vitamin A (retinyl palmitate) for the alleviation of vitamin A deficiency in the formulation currently recommended by the World Health Organization (Carlier C, Coste J, Etchepare M, et al. A randomised controlled trial to test equivalence between retinyl palmitate and beta carotene for vitamin A deficiency. _BMJ_ 307:1106-10, 1993).

Efficient absorption of fat-soluble vitamins depends upon the presence of adequate bile, pancreatic enzymes and bicarbonate as well as a normal small intestine (Gallo-Torres HE. Obligatory role of bile for the intestinal absorption of vitamin E. _Lipids_ 5:379, 1970).

- When to Provide Oral Supplementation

Since dietary fats generally promote absorption of oil-soluble substances, vitamin A supplements should be taken with a meal. Taking the supplement in portions several times a day will usually increase its utilization (_Vitamin E Fact Book_. VERIS (Vitamin E Research & Information Service, 5325 S. 9th Ave., LaGrange, IL 60525, 1994).

- Formulations

Patients with pancreatic disease absorb water-miscible preparations adequately, but oil-soluble preparations poorly, while patients with intestinal disease or resection absorb all oral preparations poorly, whether oil-soluble or water-miscible (Johnson EJ, Krasinski SD, Howard LJ, et al. Evaluation of vitamin A absorption by using oil-soluble and water-miscible vitamin A preparations in normal adults and in patients with gastrointestinal disease. _Am J Clin Nutr_ 55(4):857-64, 1992).

Emusol® A (Bioglan, CA) ('micellized A'), may be more bioavailable than emulsified A which, in turn, may be more bioavailable than the oil.

Experimental Study: 50,000 IU or retinol activity from vitamin A palmitate from an oil, emulsified A or micellized A were compared in a study of 8 normal subjects. 8 hrs. after ingestion, micellized A produced plasma levels 4.7 times those of the oil form, while emulsified A produced plasma levels double that of the oil form (Internal studies. Bioglan Laboratories - summarized in Rutolo DA Jr. Nutrient delivery systems II. Micellization and fat soluble nutrients. _Int Clin Nutr Rev_ 9(4):206-12, 1989).

Bioavailability of injectable preparations varies greatly.

Case Reports: 6 women, 4 with primary biliary cirrhosis and 2 with idiopathic chronic cholestatic liver disease, who were receiving monthly IM injections of vitamin A reported unusually severe local pain immediately after the injection followed by local erythema and swelling lasting 1-3 wks. and then followed by peeling of the overlying skin. Inquiries showed the formulation had been changed from an oil base to a water base, and polyoxyl 40 hydrogenated castor oil (Cremophor RH) had been added as a solubilizer. Data supplied by Roche when the product was licensed showed that the bioavailability of the new product was roughly 50% compared to about 1% for the old preparation (*McCormick PA, Hughes JE, Burroughs AK, McIntyre N. Reformulation of injectable vitamin A: potential problems. BMJ 301:924, 1990*).

Vitamin B₆

In the elderly, a good diet and a daily 'multivitamin' may fail to maintain adequate vitamin B₆ nutriture, and intramuscular injections may be necessary.

> **Experimental Study:** 228 ambulatory residents of a nursing home, mean age 87, who had not undergone major surgical procedures, ate a 'good' diet, and received at least one multivitamin pill daily for 3-5 of the preceding months, were compared to 204 healthy volunteers aged 20-50. 88/228 (39%) showed deficits of up to 5 of the B complex vitamins, one of which was vitamin B₆. Oral vitamin supplementation was stopped and a single IM injection of multivitamins was given. After 3 mo., these deficits were no longer detectable in the blood of 89-100% of the previously vitamin-deficient pts. (*Baker H, Frank O, Jaslow SP. Oral versus intramuscular vitamin supplementation for hypovitaminosis in the elderly. J Am Geriatr Soc 28(1):42-5, 1980*).

- When to Provide Oral Supplementation

A water-soluble vitamin, vitamin B₆ is absorbed with or without food although food, by slowing the rate of absorption, may increase the length of time that blood levels are increased and thereby reduce its eventual excretion. A similar improvement in absorption can be achieved by dividing the total dosage into several portions and taking them throughout the day (*Yung S, Mayersohn M, Robinson JB. Ascorbic acid absorption in man: influence of divided dose and food. Life Sci 28(22):2505-11, 1981*).

- Forms

For most patients, although pyridoxal-5-phosphate (P5P) is the biologically active form of vitamin B₆ and the predominant form of the vitamin in the plasma, pyridoxine appears to be preferable form of vitamin B₆ for oral administration, since orally administered P5P is largely split into pyridoxal and phosphate by intestinal phosphatases (*Friedrich W. Vitamin B₆, in W Friedrich, Ed. Vitamins. New York, Walter de Gruyter, 1988:543-618; Middleton HM. Intestinal hydrolysis of pyridoxal-5'-phosphate in vitro and in vivo in the rat. Gastroenterology 91:343-50, 1986*). Moreover, non-phosphorylated B₆ isomers are better able to cross the blood-brain barrier (*Soukes TL. Nutrients and cofactors required for monoamine synthesis in nervous tissue. Nutr Brain 3:265-99, 1979*) as well as other membrane barriers (*Friedrich W. Vitamin B₆, in W Friedrich, Ed. Vitamins. New York, Walter de Gruyter, 1988:543-618*).

P5P may be preferable to pyridoxine, however, when given to patients with a deficiency or inhibition of pyridoxal kinase, the phosphorylating enzyme required for the conversion of pyridoxine to its active form. This defect may be congenital, it may be acquired as the result of liver dysfunction or, since magnesium and/or zinc activate the enzyme, deficiencies of these minerals may cause its activity to be reduced.

WARNING: Phosphates interfere with the absorption of some minerals by forming insoluble salts; thus pyridoxal phosphate should be not be taken within 4 hours of a mineral supplement.

Clinical Observation: On the basis of a functional measure of vitamin B_6 (EGPT stimulation), when pts. had reduced levels of magnesium and/or zinc, normalization of the measure could be achieved with one-tenth the dosage of pyridoxal phosphate compared to the dosage of pyridoxine HCl (*Pangborn JB. Monograph on pyridoxal phosphate. Bionostics, Inc., P.O. Drawer 400, Lisle, IL 60532, Ca. 1990*).

Observational Study: All 41 pts. with alcoholic liver disease were deficient in pyridoxal-5-phosphate (*Majumdar SK et al. Blood vitamin status (B_1, B_2, B_6, folic acid and B_{12}) in patients with alcoholic liver disease. Int J Vitam Nutr Res 52(3):266-71, 1982*).

Experimental Study: Pyridoxal-5'-phosphate levels were significantly reduced in 22/31 pts. with decompensated cirrhosis or subacute hepatic necrosis. IV pyridoxine HCl increased plasma pyridoxal-5'-phosphate levels in only 1/3 of the pts., while all pts. responded to IM pyridoxal 5'-phosphate, although the response was significantly less than that found in normal controls. While impaired hepatic phosphorylation may be responsible for the difference, increased degradation of pyridoxal 5'-phosphate by the liver is a more likely cause (*Labadarios D, Rossouw JE, McConnell JB, et al. Vitamin B_6 deficiency in chronic liver disease - evidence for increased degradation of pyridoxal-5'-phosphate. Gut 18(1):23-7, 1977*).

Case Report: A 72 year-old woman with primary acquired sideroblastic anemia, otherwise in good health, failed to respond to oral supplementation with pyridoxine 100 mg twice daily along with folic acid 5 mg 3 times daily and ascorbic acid 200 mg twice daily, but showed a prompt and lasting response to IM pyridoxal-5-phosphate, initially 250 mg daily, and later reduced to a maintenance dosage of 250 mg daily (*Mason DY, Emerson PM. Primary acquired sideroblastic anaemia: response to treatment with pyridoxal-5-phosphate. Br Med J i:389-90, 1973*).

Note: Primary acquired sideroblastic anemia appears to be due to a defect in heme synthesis caused by a block in the conversion of pyridoxine to pyridoxal-5-phosphate, the active coenzyme form of the vitamin. Response to pyridoxine is almost always suboptimal and very large doses, often 100 times the normal nutritional requirement, may be necessary (Mason DY, Emerson PM. Primary acquired sideroblastic anaemia: response to treatment with pyridoxal-5-phosphate. Br Med J i:389-90, 1973).

Vitamin B_{12}

- When to Provide Oral Supplementation

A water-soluble vitamin, vitamin B_{12} is absorbed with or without food although food, by slowing the rate of absorption, may increase the length of time that blood levels are increased and thereby reduce its eventual excretion. A similar improvement in absorption can be achieved by dividing the total dosage into several portions and taking them throughout the day *(Yung S, Mayersohn M, Robinson JB. Ascorbic acid absorption in man: influence of divided dose and food. Life Sci 28(22):2505-11, 1981).*

- Causes Of Malabsorption

Due to the importance of intrinsic factor in promoting vitamin B_{12} absorption, conditions that reduce its production (such as atrophic gastritis or gastrectomy) will lead to B_{12} deficiency and pernicious anemia *(Hathcock JN, Troendle GJ. Oral cobalamin for treatment of pernicious anemia? Editorial. JAMA 265(1):96-7, 1991).*

Moreover, since the vitamin B_{12} complex with intrinsic factor is absorbed mainly in the distal small intestine, any process that disrupts the normal function of that area (such as ileitis, ileal resection, tropical sprue or celiac disease) may reduce B_{12} absorption. Also, bacterial overgrowth in that location (due, for example, to surgically-produced blind loops, strictures, anastomoses, or diverticulae) may metabolize ingested B_{12} to inactive analogs *(Vitamin B-12 analogues and intestinal bacteria. Nutr Rev 37:45-6, 1979).*

Exocrine pancreatic insufficiency frequently results in malabsorption of crystalline B_{12} as shown by the Schilling test; however food-derived B_{12} usually is adequately absorbed to prevent B_{12} deficiency *(Flodin NW. Pharmacology of Micronutrients. New York, Alan R. Liss, Inc., 1988).*

> *Note: Vitamin B_{12} from plant foods may not be bioavailable (Dagnelie PC, van Staveren WA, van den Berg H. Vitamin B-12 from algae appears not to be bioavailable. Am J Clin Nutr 53:695-7, 1991).*

- Forms

The human body contains 3 main cobalamins: hydroxocobalamin (or very closely related compounds), adenosylcobalamin (cobamamide; cobinamide; coenzyme B_{12}), and methylcobalamin *(Matthews DM, Linnell JC. Vitamin B_{12}: an area of darkness. Br Med J September 1, 1979, pp. 533-5).*

Cyanocobalamin is the most common pharmaceutical form of vitamin B_{12} although, in the body, it is present only in traces and is often undetectable, and its biochemical significance, if any, is uncertain *(Matthews DM, Linnell JC. Vitamin B_{12}: an area of darkness. Br Med J September 1, 1979, pp. 533-5).*

> *Note: Cyanocobalamin contains cyanide; thus there is some concern about possible cyanide toxicity when given repeatedly, although the cyanide dosage in 1000 μg of cyanocobalamin has been judged to be toxicologically insignificant (Hathcock JN, Troendle GJ. Oral cobalamin for treatment of pernicious anemia? Editorial. JAMA 265(1):96-7, 1991).*

Hydroxocobalamin is available for injection and may be preferable to cyanocobalamin for therapeutic use *(Matthews DM, Linnell JC. Vitamin B_{12}: an area of darkness. Br Med J September 1, 1979, pp. 533-5).*

> *Note: In several conditions (including Leber's optic atrophy and dominantly inherited optic atrophy), the percentage of plasma cyanocobalamin to total plasma*

cobalamins is greatly increased. Also, in <u>tobacco amblyopia</u>, cyanide intake is increased due to its content in tobacco smoke. Hydroxocobalamin is concerned with the detoxification of cyanide by conversion into cyanocobalamin, and all of these conditions may have a derangement in cyanide metabolism. It seems obvious that hydroxocobalamin is preferable to cyanocobalamin in these conditions. Not surprisingly, some of the optic neuropathies appear to respond to massive doses of hydroxocobalamin, and have been claimed to be adversely affected by administration of cyanocobalamin (Matthews DM, Linnell JC. Vitamin B_{12}: an area of darkness. <u>Br Med J</u> September 1, 1979, pp. 533-5). *Similarly, hydroxocobalamin has been found to be superior to cyanocobalamin for the treatment of tobacco amblyopia* (Chisholm JA, Bronte-Stewart J, Foulds WS. Hydroxocobalamin versus cyanocobalamin in treatment of amblyopia induced by tobacco. <u>Lancet</u> ii:450, 1967).

<u>Adenosylcobalamin</u> (coenzyme B_{12}; cobamamide; cobinamide) is the metabolically active form of vitamin B_{12}. In order to be activated, cyanocobalamin or hydroxocobalamin must be converted in the hepatic mitochondria into adenosylcobalamin (Fenton WA, Rosenberg LE. Mitochondrial metabolism of hydroxocobalamin: synthesis of adenosylcobalamin by intact rat liver mitochondria. <u>Arch Biochem Biophys</u> 189(2):441-7, 1978). It is better absorbed orally than cyanocobalamin and accumulated to a greater extent in the liver (Heinrich HC, Gabbe E. Metabolism of the vitamin B_{12} coenzyme in rats and man. <u>Ann N Y Acad Sci</u> 112:871, 1964). In certain circumstances, it may be more effective than either cyanocobalamin or hydroxocobalamin.

Animal Experimental Study: Among 3 cobalamins studied, the enzymatically active derivatives 5'-deoxy-adenosylcobalamin and methylcobalamin significantly increased the survival time of leukemic mice, while cyanocobalamin was inactive (Tsao CS, Myashita K. Influence of cobalamin on the survival of mice bearing ascites tumor. <u>Pathobiology</u> 61(2):104-8, 1993).

Negative Experimental Study: In a study of 11 pts. with methylmalonic aciduria, therapy with deoxyadenosylcobalamin offered no advantage over hydroxocobalamin (Chalmers RA, Bain MD, Mistry J, et al. Enzymologic studies on patients with methylmalonic aciduria: basis for a clinical trial of deoxyadenosylcobalamin in a hydroxocobalamin-unresponsive patient. <u>Pediatr Res</u> 30(6):560-3, 1991).

Case Report: A 7-month-old girl with hydroxocobalamin-resistant methylmalonic acidemia responded to adenosylcobalamin (Bhatt HR, Linnell JC, Barltrop D. Treatment of hydroxocobalamin-resistant methylmalonic acidaemia with adenosylcobalamin. Letter. <u>Lancet</u> ii:465, 1986).

Experimental Study: 2 gps. of pts. from the same hepatitis A epidemic received either coenzyme B_{12} or hydroxycobalamin. The gp. treated with coenzyme B_{12} demonstrated a more rapid return of serum aminotransferase levels to normal (Iwarson S, Lindberg J. Coenzyme-B12 therapy in acute viral hepatitis. <u>Scand J Infect Dis</u> 9(2):157-8, 1977).

- Routes Of Administration

The usual practice of giving vitamin B_{12} as an <u>intramuscular injection</u> has several drawbacks, as injections can be painful, difficult to provide for some patients and costly

(Lederle FA. Commentary. Oral cobalamin for pernicious anemia. Medicine's best kept secret? JAMA 265(1):94-5, 1991).
However, many clinicians believe that parenteral administration is far more bioavailable than the oral route, even for patients without B_{12} malabsorption.

Case Report: A healthy, 23 year-old fasting male received two 1000 μg tablets of B_{12} resin as cyanocobalamin orally, the same preparation sublingually, 10 μg hydroxocobalamin parenterally, and 10 μg cyanocobalamin parenterally. His initial vitamin B_{12} levels in the 4 trials was 228 ± 64 pg/ml. The results were as follows:

Route	Maximum increase from baseline	24-hour urinary excretion
Oral	43%	0.009%
Sublingual	34%	0.004%
Parenteral (hydroxycobalamin)	106%	2.7%
Parenteral (cyanocobalamin)	78%	4.2%

"These observations indicated that the amount of vitamin B_{12} recovered from an oral or sublingual dose is negligible as compared to an injected dose, and is not an effective alternative to a parenteral injection. The area under the curve is highest with the parenteral hydroxycobalamin, followed by the parenteral cyanocobalamin. The sublingual and oral curves were considerably less in area with the area of the oral curve being least" *(Sohler A, Pfeiffer CC, Kowalski T. Effectiveness and route of administration of vitamin B_{12}. Int Clin Nutr Rev 9(2):64-5, 1989).*

Oral cobalamin, given without intrinsic factor, at daily doses of at least 100-250 μg daily (2000 μg twice daily for the first month to be assured of replenishing body stores) provides adequate treatment of vitamin B_{12} deficiency, probably because there is an inefficient mechanism of cobalamin absorption that is independent of intrinsic factor. Previous concerns about unpredictable absorption are no longer relevant due to more recent absorption data *(Lederle FA. Commentary. Oral cobalamin for pernicious anemia. Medicine's best kept secret? JAMA 265(1):94-5, 1991).*

Note: Tablets may be more bioavailable if they are chewed before swallowing.

Experimental Study: 16 pts. with below normal serum B_{12} levels related to following a total vegetarian (vegan) diet received a 100 μg tablet once weekly of cyanocobalamin (Bronson, St. Louis, MO). After 6 wks., in the 7 pts. who chewed the tablets, the serum B_{12} level increased significantly (p<0.01). However, in the 9 pts. who gulped the pills down with water, the ave. B_{12} level failed to increase significantly, although there was a slight increase. When 7 of these 9 pts. chewed 5 of the tablets before swallowing for 10 days, the serum B_{12} rose to the normal range

(Crane MG, Sample C, Patchett S, Register UD. Vitamin B$_{12}$ studies in total vegetarians (vegans). J Nutr Med 4:419-30, 1994).

Note: In the elderly, a good diet and a daily 'multivitamin' may fail to maintain adequate vitamin B$_{12}$ nutriture, and intramuscular injections, or a higher dosage of oral B$_{12}$ than that found in most multivitamins, may be necessary.

Experimental Study: 228 ambulatory residents of a nursing home, mean age 87, who had not undergone major surgical procedures, ate a 'good' diet, and received at least one multivitamin pill daily for 3-5 of the preceding months, were compared to 204 healthy volunteers aged 20-50. 88/228 (39%) showed deficits of up to 5 of the B complex vitamins, one of which was vitamin B$_{12}$. Oral vitamin supplementation was stopped and a single IM injection of multivitamins was given. After 3 mo., these deficits were no longer detectable in the blood of 89-100% of the previously vitamin-deficient pts. *(Baker H, Frank O, Jaslow SP. Oral versus intramuscular vitamin supplementation for hypovitaminosis in the elderly. J Am Geriatr Soc 28(1):42-5, 1980).*

Note: Oral preparations containing intrinsic factor have been tried, but antibody production caused some patients to become refractory and relapse (Lowenstein L, Cooper BA, Brunton L, et al. An immunological basis for acquired resistance to oral administration of hog intrinsic factor and vitamin B$_{12}$ in pernicious anemia. J Clin Invest 40:1656-62, 1961).

Experimental Study: 64 pts. with pernicious anemia and other cobalamin deficiency states were treated with 1000 µg oral cyanocobalamin daily, with 61/64 treated for >3 years. Clinical and hematological remission, normalization of serum levels, and full replenishment of hepatic stores were observed in all pts. *(Berlin R, Berlin H, Brante G, Pilbrant A. Vitamin B$_{12}$ body sotres during oral and parenteral treatment of pernicious anemia. Acta Med Scand 204:81-4, 1978).*

See Also:

Berlin H, Berlin R, Brante G. *Oral treatment of pernicious anemia with high doses of vitamin B$_{12}$ without intrinsic factor. Acta Med Scand 184:247-58, 1968*

Waife SO, Jansen CJ, Crabtree RE, et al. *Oral vitamin B$_{12}$ without intrinsic factor in the treatment of pernicious anemia. Ann Intern Med 58:810-17, 1963*

McIntyre PA, Hahn R, Masters JM, Krevans JR. *Treatment of pernicious anemia with orally administered cyanocobalamin (vitamin B$_{12}$). Arch Intern Med 106:280-92, 1960*

Intranasal cobalamin may be more effective than oral cobalamin.

Experimental Study: Pharmacokinetic studies were performed by Nastech Pharmaceutical Company, the manufacturer of an intranasal cyanocobalamin gel hoping to receive US Food and Drug Administration approval as a new drug. For healthy volunteers, intranasal application of a 500 mg of the gel was significantly more effective than an oral tablet based by peak plasma increment over baseline (1177 pg/mL vs. 130 pg/mL, respectively) (*results summarized in: Romeo VD, Sileno A, Wenig DN. Intranasal cyanocobalamin. Letter. JAMA 268(10):1268-9, 1992*).

Experimental Study: The summary report by Nature's Bounty (NY, USA), the manufacturer of a brand of intranasal cyanocobalamin, of its clinical studies suggests that the rise in serum cobalamin levels after a single 400 µg intranasal dose approximates that from a 100 µg intramuscular dose, suggesting that, when used monthly, a single dose would be sufficient to maintain adequate levels of the vitamin in most pts. with pernicious anemia (*unpublished study summarized in Heimburger DC. Intranasal cobalamin: a warning. Letter. JAMA 265(17):2190, 1991*).

> *Note: There are no known adequate and well-controlled studies proving the safety and efficacy of this product which the US Food and Drug Administration considers to be an unapproved new drug and therefore illegally marketed* (*Hathcock JN, Troendle GJ. Intranasal cobalamin: a warning. Letter. JAMA 265(17):2190, 1991*).

Sublingual cobalamin does not appear to be more bioavailable than oral cobalamin for people without vitamin B_{12} malabsorption.

Case Report: A healthy, 23 year-old, fasting male received two 1000 µg tablets of B_{12} resin as cyanocobalamin orally, the same preparation sublingually, 10 µg hydroxocobalamin parenterally, and 10 µg cyanocobalamin parenterally. For the oral dose, there was a 43% increase from baseline and a 24-hr. urinary excretion of 0.009% of the dose. For the sublingual dose, there was a 34% increase from baseline and a 24-hr. excretion of 0.004%. The parenteral hydroxocobalamin preparation gave a maximum of a 106% increase in blood level and urine recovery was 2.7%, while the parenteral cyanocobalamin preparation gave a maximum blood level of 78% and urine recovery was 4.2% of the dose (*Sohler A, Pfeiffer CC, Kowalski T. Effectiveness and route of administration of vitamin B$_{12}$. Int Clin Nutr Rev 9(2):64-5, 1989*).

- Formulations

Cyanocobalamin may be better absorbed in liquid form than in a gelatin capsule.

Experimental Study: 42 subjects received simultaneous doses of cyanocobalamin in capsule and liquid form labeled with cobalt-57 and cobalt-60, respectively. Excretion was 2-66% greater with the liquid form. *In vitro* dissolution studies showed that the capsules had a tendency to collapse into a stringy mass and to dissolve slowly (*Baun DC, Bowen BM, Wood DE. Comparison of the* *bioavailability of cyanocobalamin from capsule and liquid dosage forms. Am J Hosp Pharm 32(10):1047-9, 1975).*

Absorption of oral vitamin B$_{12}$ is improved by the use of a resin adsorbate *(Davis BP, Gerstein LM, Rozeboom DL, Cranwell RW. Enhanced absorption of oral vitamin B$_{12}$ from a resin adsorbate administered to normal subjects. J Manipulative Physiol Ther 5(3):123-7, 1982).*

Vitamin C

Ascorbic acid absorption, under normal physiological conditions, shows saturation characteristics. Doses of up to 180 mg are 80-90% absorbed, but 1.5 g loads are only half absorbed while 12 g loads are only 16% absorbed *(Brown LAS, Jones DF. The biology of ascorbic acid, in E Cadenas, L Packer, Eds. Handbook of Antioxidants. New York, Marcel Dekker, 1996:118).*

- When to Provide Oral Supplementation

A water-soluble vitamin, ascorbic acid is absorbed with or without food although food, by slowing the rate of absorption, may increase the length of time that blood levels are increased and thereby reduce its eventual excretion. A similar improvement in absorption can be achieved by dividing the total dosage into several portions and taking them throughout the day.

Experimental Study: 3 healthy volunteers ingested 1 g vitamin C daily. The control subject took it in a single dose, the second took it in 8 small doses, and the third took it in a single dose after eating a high-fat meal. "The divided doses and after-meal treatments produced a significant increase in AA absorption compared to the corresponding control experiment, 72 percent and 69 percent, respectively. . . . Efficiency of AA absorption may be improved by either dividing up a daily dose into several smaller doses taken during the day or by ingesting the vitamin after a meal." *(Yung S, Mayersohn M, Robinson JB. Ascorbic acid absorption in man: influence of divided dose and food. Life Sci 28(22):2505-11, 1981).*

- Natural vs. Synthetic

Natural food sources of vitamin C and synthetic vitamin C are equally bioavailable *(Brown LAS, Jones DF. The biology of ascorbic acid, in E Cadenas, L Packer, Eds. Handbook of Antioxidants. New York, Marcel Dekker, 1996; Mangels AR, Block G, Frey CM, et al. The bioavailability to humans of ascorbic acid from oranges, orange juice and cooked broccoli is similar to that of synthetic ascorbic acid. J Nutr 123:1054-61, 1993; Pelletier O, Keith MO. Bioavailability of synthetic and natural ascorbic acid. J Am Diet Assoc 64:271-5, 1993).*

- Disintegration Time

Although US Pharmacopeia guidelines specify 30 minutes as the maximum disintegration time for vitamin C tablets, and the European compendia a maximum of 15 minutes, tablets that disintegrate in 60 minutes have the greatest bioavailability as compared to tablets with shorter and longer disintegration times and a vitamin C solution *(Bhagvan HN, Wolkoff BI. Correlation between the disintegration time and the bioavailability of vitamin C tablets. Pharm Res 10(2):239-42, 1993).*

- Sustained Release

Experimental Study: 4 healthy young adults received 1 g vitamin C orally daily for 2 weeks in several forms. 85% of a 1-gm IV dose was recovered as ascorbic acid and its metabolites in a 24-hr. urine collection while, when given as a single dose on an empty stomach, about 30% was recovered when solution and tablet (both chewable and non-chewable) forms were given, and only 14% was recovered after a timed-release capsule. There was considerable intersubject variability in absorption (*Yung S, Mayersohn M, Robinson JB. Ascorbic acid absorption in humans: A comparison among several dosage forms. J Pharm Sci 71(3):282-5, 1982*).

Experimental Study: When 1 gm of ascorbic acid was given orally, essentially complete absorption from a sustained-release capsule of vitamin C was found compared to 70% from a regular capsule (*Zetler G, Seidel G, Siegers CP, Iven H. Pharmacokinetics of ascorbic acid in man. Eur J Clin Pharmacol 10:273-82, 1976*).

- Formulations

Ascorbyl palmitate

A fat-soluble form of vitamin C, ascorbyl palmitate may be more bioavailable than ascorbic acid; however, questions about its efficacy remain.

Experimental Study: After a single dose of 2 g of ascorbic acid or ascorbyl palmitate, ascorbyl palmitate did not appear in the plasma vitamin C pool as rapidly as ascorbic acid. By 24 hrs., plasma vitamin C values were similar. However, following 2 wks. of supplementation, plasma vitamin C levels were slightly higher for ascorbyl palmitate than for ascorbic acid, while mean 24-hr. urinary excretion was 33% lower, suggesting that ascorbyl palmitate was better utilized (*Johnston CS, Monte WC, Bolton RS, et al. Nutr Res 14:1465-71, 1994*).

Animal Experimental Study: Ascorbic acid or ascorbyl palmitate was given for the treatment of scurvy in guinea pigs. Tissue levels of ascorbic acid and ascorbyl palmitate were not significantly different, while plasma vitamin C levels were higher in the ascorbyl palmitate group. Changes in bone structure were equally reversed by both forms of vitamin C; however, ascorbyl palmitate was 50% as potent as ascorbic acid in preventing weight loss (*Johnston CS, Monte WC, Bolton RS, et al. Nutr Res 14:1465-71, 1994*).

Ester-C®

Ester-C® is a proprietary product composed of a mixture of calcium ascorbate and dehydroascorbate along with 3 metabolites: calcium threonate and small amounts of xylonate and lyxonate. There is some evidence that Ester-C® may produce higher tissue levels of vitamin C than ordinary ascorbic acid.

Note: There may be as yet identified dangers (such as adverse effects due to the presence of dehydroascorbic acid) in taking Ester-C®. Moreover, Ester-C®, which is pH neutral, is being compared to ascorbic acid, which is acidic and does not contain calcium; a more appropriate comparison would be to calcium ascorbate. Ingesting a higher dosage of ascorbic acid is probably more cost-effective, and possibly safer, than purchasing this proprietary mixture (Gaby AR. Ester-C. Townsend Letter for Doctors 8-9/95, p. 115).

Note: Dehydroascorbic acid, the oxidized product of ascorbic acid, is not normally found in the plasma and serum (Dhariwal KR, Hartzell WO, Levine M. Ascorbic acid and dehydroascorbic acid measurements in human plasma and serum. Am J Clin Nutr 54:712-16, 1991), and it appears unknown whether the dehydroascorbic acid in Ester-C® causes this substance to appear.

Experimental Controlled Study: 17-18 healthy men received a low-ascorbic acid diet for 12 days. They then received a single oral dose of pure ascorbic acid, Ester-C® calcium ascorbate with standardized 3% calcium threonate, or Ester-c® calcium ascorbate without standardized 3% calcium threonate. White cell ascorbate in the ascorbic acid gp. declined by 24 h but remained high in the other 2 groups. At 24 h, both Ester-C® gps. showed white cell levels about twice as great as those in the ascorbic acid group; this difference was statistically highly significant. The Ester-C® product with standardized threonate produced higher white cell ascorbate levels than the non-standardized product (Hunt H, Rice T. Comparative efficacy of Ester-C® ascorbate. Unpublished Study. The Life Management Group, La Jolla, CA, January, 1995).

Negative Experimental Double-blind Study: Ester-C® was compared under randomized double-blind conditions to ascorbic acid and ascorbic acid plus hesperidin-rutin-buckwheat citrus bioflavonoids. Following ingestion by 9 healthy subjects, measurements of plasma and urinary vitamin C were comparable with all 3 items, as were 24-hr. vitamin C urinary excretions. Compared to the other 2 items, plasma vitamin C levels decreased more rapidly following ingestion of Ester-C® and, at 6 and 8 hrs. post-dose, plasma vitamin C levels were lower. "These results indicate that vitamin C from Ester-C . . . was not more bioavailable than simple ascorbic acid" (Johnston CS, Luo B. Comparison of the absorption and excretion of three commercially available sources of vitamin C. J Am Diet Assoc 94(7):779-81, 1994).

Experimental Placebo-controlled Study: 12 men aged 27-45 were placed on a low ascorbic acid diet for one week. They were then divided into 3 gps. of 4 and, after an overnight fast, gp. 1 received ascorbic acid 3000 mg, gp. 23 received Ester-C® calcium ascorbate (3000 mg of ascorbic acid equivalents), and gp. 3 received 3000 mg of citric acid placebo. After 24 hrs., Ester-C® produced higher serum ascorbate levels (56.2% increase vs. 24.6% increase with ascorbic acid and 5.9% increase with citrate) and higher intracellular ascorbate levels (measured in white blood cells) (18.2% increase vs. 5.3% decrease with ascorbic acid and 6.3% decrease with citrate). Also, 24-hr. urinary ascorbate output was lower in the Ester-C® gp., suggesting that more Ester-C® was retained (Wright JV, Suen RM. A human bioavailability study of Ester-C® ascorbate. Int Clin Nutr Rev 10(1), Jan. 1990).

- Mixed with <u>Bioflavonoids</u>

Vitamin C supplements are sometimes formulated with bioflavonoids, supposedly to enhance the bioavailabiity of the vitamin. While bioflavonoids can enhance the bioavailability of vitamin C, the dosages of bioflavonoids available in commercial preparations are generally too low to be effective.

Negative Experimental Double-blind Study: Ascorbic acid alone was compared under randomized double-blind conditions to a commercial preparation of ascorbic acid plus hesperidin-rutin-buckwheat citrus bioflavonoids having a ratio (weight per weight) of bioflavonoids to vitamin C of 0.05 to 1 (which is typical of commercial sources). Following ingestion by 9 healthy subjects, measurements of plasma and urinary vitamin C were comparable, as were 24-hr. vitamin C urinary excretions *(Johnston CS, Luo B. Comparison of the absorption and excretion of three commercially available sources of vitamin C. <u>J Am Diet Assoc</u> 94(7):779-81, 1994).*

Experimental Study: Healthy subjects received solutions of either vitamin C alone or vitamin C plus bioflavonoids with a 4 to 1 weight per weight ratio of bioflavonoids to vitamin C. The addition of bioflavonoids was found to enhance the bioavailability of vitamin C as it was more readily absorbed and remained longer in the body *(Vinson JA, Bose P. Comparative bioavailability of synthetic and natural vitamin C in guinea pigs. <u>Nutr Rep Int</u> 27:875-80, 1983).*

Experimental Study: Compared to the ingestion of vitamin C alone, the addition of 25 mg bioflavonoids to 500 mg vitamin C (ratio of 1 to 20) increased urinary vitamin C excretion in 5 young male volunteers, suggesting that oral absorption of vitamin C was enhanced *(Jones E, Hughes RE. <u>IRCS Med Sci</u> 12:320, 1984).*

Animal Experimental Study: Guinea pigs received solutions of either vitamin C alone or vitamin C plus bioflavonoids with a 0.7 to 1 weight per weight ratio of bioflavonoids to vitamin C. The addition of bioflavonoids was found to enhance the bioavailability of vitamin C as it was more readily absorbed and remained longer in the body *(Vinson JA, Bose P. Comparative bioavailability of synthetic and natural vitamin C in guinea pigs. <u>Nutr Rep Int</u> 27:875-80, 1983).*

See Also:

> *Vinson JA, Bose P. Bioavailability of synthetic ascorbic acid and a citrus extract. <u>Ann N Y Acad Sci</u> 498:525-6, 1987*

<u>Vitamin D</u>

<u>Vitamin D$_3$</u> (cholecalciferol; natural vitamin D) is naturally formed in skin by photochemical conversion of a precursor via the energy of ultraviolet light. It is commonly available as a supplement derived from fish liver oils.

<u>Vitamin D$_2$</u> (ergocalciferol; synthetic vitamin D) is produced by ultraviolet irradiation of the fungal steroid ergosterol and differs from vitamin D$_3$ by the presence of a double bond.

Note: The original antirachitic substance known as <u>vitamin D₁</u> was found to be merely a mixture of ergocalciferol and other steroids, so the term is no longer used.

Note: Vitamin D$_2$ is believed to behave metabolically like vitamin D$_3$ (Reichel H, Koeffler HP, Norman AW. The role of the vitamin D endocrine system in health and disease. <u>N Engl J Med</u> 320(15):980-91, 1989).

Vitamin D, regardless of its source, must be activated in a two-step process. It is first hydroxylated in the liver to 25 hydroxyvitamin D (calcidiol); then it is hydroxylated once again in the kidney to 1,25 dihydroxyvitamin D (calcitriol). For patients with liver and kidney disorders, calcitriol is available as an oral supplement.

Efficient absorption of fat-soluble vitamins depends upon the presence of adequate bile, pancreatic enzymes and bicarbonate as well as a normal small intestine (Gallo-Torres HE. *Obligatory role of bile for the intestinal absorption of vitamin E.* <u>Lipids</u> 5:379, 1970).

Topical application of vitamin D$_3$ is as effective as oral supplementation in increasing serum levels (Vieth R, Milojevic S. *Application of vitamin D to the skin is a viable alternative to its oral nutrition. Abstract.* <u>J Bone Miner Res</u> 8:S224, 1993).

- When to Provide Oral Supplementation

Since dietary fats generally promote absorption of oil-soluble substances, vitamin D supplements should be taken with a meal. Taking the supplement in portions several times a day will usually increase its utilization (<u>Vitamin E Fact Book</u>. VERIS (Vitamin E Research & Information Service, 5325 S. 9th Ave., LaGrange, IL 60525, 1994).

<u>Vitamin E</u>

Efficient absorption of fat-soluble vitamins depends upon the presence of adequate bile, pancreatic enzymes and bicarbonate as well as a normal small intestine (Gallo-Torres HE. *Obligatory role of bile for the intestinal absorption of vitamin E.* <u>Lipids</u> 5:379, 1970).

- When to Provide Oral Supplementation

Since dietary fats generally promote absorption of oil-soluble substances, vitamin E supplements should be taken with a meal. Taking the supplement in portions several times a day will usually increase its utilization (<u>Vitamin E Fact Book</u>. VERIS (Vitamin E Research & Information Service, 5325 S. 9th Ave., LaGrange, IL 60525, 1994).

- Gelation Capsules, Soft

<u>Alpha-tocopherol</u>, an oil, loses potency when exposed to air, heat and light. When enclosed in a soft gelatin capsule that excludes air, and the capsules are stored in a cool, dark place, it will retain potency for at least 3 years (<u>Vitamin E Fact Book</u>. VERIS [Vitamin E Research & Information Service], 5325 S. 9th Ave., LaGrange, IL 60525, 1994).

- Natural Versus Synthetic

"Natural source vitamin E [d-alpha-tocopherol] is officially recognized as having 36% greater potency than its synthetic counterpart [dl-alpha-tocopherol] as determined by studies in animals. However, recent studies of animals and human subjects indicate that natural-source vitamin E is almost twice as effective as synthetic vitamin E" *(Vitamin E Fact Book*. *VERIS (Vitamin E Research & Information Service, 5325 S. 9th Ave., LaGrange, IL 60525, 1994).*

Experimental Double-blind Crossover Study: 12 men received two 400 mg soft-gelatin capsules of either RRR alpha-tocopherol (natural source) or all racemic stereoisomers of alpha-tocopherol (synthetic) in random order. Mean plasma alpha-tocopherol concentrations were greater for RRR than all rac from 10-96 hrs. post-administration with Cmax for RRR (4.8 µg/mL) significantly greater than for all rac (4.0 µg/mL; p<0.05). The RRR ACC0-96 for both plasma and RBC were significantly greater than the all rac AUC0-96 (p<0.05), indicating a greater bioavailability of RRR vs. all rac alpha-tocopherol *(Ferslew KE, Acuff RV, Daigneault EA, et al. Pharmacokinetics and bioavailability of the RRR and all racemic stereoisomers of alpha-tocopherol in humans after single oral administration. J Clin Pharmacol 33(1):84-8, 1993).*

See Also:

> *Acuff RV, Thedford SS, Hidiroglou NN, et al. Relative bioavailability of RRR- and all-rac-a-tocopheryl acetate in humans: studies using deuterated compounds. Am J Clin Nutr 60:397-402, 1994*

Natural vitamin E may be more effective than the synthetic because there are specific protein receptors for d-alpha-tocopherol that make its transport and retention more efficient *(Kitabchi AE et al. Specific receptor sites for alpha-tocopherol in purified isolated adrenocortical cell membrane. Biochem Biophys Res Commun 96:1739-46, 1980).*

Animal Experimental Studies: Labeled alpha-tocopherol from natural sources remained in the tissues much longer than the similarly labeled synthetic product. For example, after 32 days, the ratio of the two compounds in the lung, liver and brain of rats was 1.9, 1.2 and 3.2, respectively, in favor of the alpha-tocopherol from natural sources. These ratios tended to increase in time and, after 154 days, were 2.6, 1.2 and 5.4, respectively *(Burton GW, Ingold KU. Vitamin E: Application of the principles of physical organic chemistry to the exploration of its structure and function. Acc Chem Res 19:194-201, 1986; Ingold KU et al. Biokinetics of and discrimination between dietary RRR- and SRR-alpha-tocopherols in the male rat. Lipids 22:163-72, 1987).*

Natural and synthetic vitamin E appear to be equally effective as antioxidants.

Experimental Study: 16 men and women received 1,600 mg of either natural or synthetic vitamin E. After 8 wks., alpha-tocopherol levels rose two-fold from baseline in both gps. and the susceptibility of LDL to oxidation was decreased by equivalent amts. *(Reaven P, Witztum J. Comparison of supplementation of RRR-alpha-tocopherol and racemic alpha-tocopherol in humans. Arter Throm 13:601-8, 1993).*

- Esters Versus Free Tocopherol

As vitamin E esters are resistant to oxidative destruction, they are considerably more stable than free alpha tocopherol *(Flodin NW. Pharmacology of Micronutrients. New York, Alan R. Liss, Inc., 1988)*, yet their bioavailability is adequate. They are therefore generally used in preference to the easily oxidizable alcohol in liquid and tablet preparations of vitamin E *(Flodin NW. Pharmacology of Micronutrients. New York, Alan R. Liss, Inc., 1988)*.

> **Experimental Study:** In 5 adults, competitive uptake studies of RRR-alpha-tocopherol and RRR-alpha-tocopheryl acetate after a single dose taken with a meal showed that the amt. of alpha-tocopherol from the free phenol form was equal to that from the acetate in plasma and blood cells *(Burton GW, Ingold KU, Foster DO, et al. Comparison of free alpha-tocopherol and alpha-tocopheryl acetate as sources of vitamin E in rats and humans. Lipids 23(9):834-40, 1988).*

> **Experimental Study:** Serum concentrations of alpha-tocopherol after ingestion of 800 IU of various vitamin E preparations were studied in 20 adult subjects. The mean increase in concentration of alpha-tocopherols (mg/g lipid) in 24 hrs. was 71% after RRR-alpha tocopherol, 63% after RRR-alpha-tocopherol acetate, and 41% after RRR-alpha-tocopherol succinate *(Horwitt MK, Elliott WH, Kanjananggulpan P, Fitch CD. Serum concentrations of alpha-tocopherol after ingestion of various vitamin E preparations. Am J Clin Nutr 40(2):240-5, 1984).*

Although, *in vitro*, vitamin E esters lack the antioxidant properties of the alcohol form *(Flodin NW. Pharmacology of Micronutrients. New York, Alan R. Liss, Inc., 1988)*, *in vivo* pancreatic enzymes assist in the removal of the acetate or succinate moiety prior to absorption, so that the free tocopherol is absorbed *(Bjorneboe A et al. Absorption, transport of vitamin E. J Nutr 120:233-42, 1990; Burton GW, Ingold KU, Foster DO, et al. Comparison of free alpha-tocopherol and alpha-tocopheryl acetate as sources of vitamin E in rats and humans. Lipids 23(9):834-40, 1988; Burton GW, Traber MG. Vitamin E: Antioxidant activity, biokinetics, and bioavailability. Annu Rev Nutr 10:357-82, 1990).*

> *Note: Results of an in vitro study suggest that, if the succinate were absorbed intact, it would actually be superior to free alpha tocopherol as an antioxidant:*

> > **In vitro Experimental Study:** Isolated liver cells were exposed to a free radical-rich environment. While added vitamin E failed to protect liver cells from free radical damage, incubation of the liver cells with vitamin E succinate completely protected them from the toxic effects of free radicals. These cells were found to contain both vitamin E and vitamin E succinate *(Fariss M. Oxygen toxicity: Unique cytoprotective properties of vitamin E succinate in hepatocytes. Free Rad Biol Med 9:333-43, 1990).*

Commonly available alpha tocopherol esters are the acetate and the succinate. Because of its greater stability, vitamin E acetate, an oil, can be used in liquid vitamin drops and in cosmetics, as well as in soft gelatin capsules. Vitamin E succinate is a solid at room temperature, and thus can be used in multivitamin tablets and hard gelatin capsules *(Vitamin E Fact Book. VERIS (Vitamin E Research & Information Service, 5325 S. 9th Ave., LaGrange, IL 60525, 1994).*

- Oil Versus Aqueous Solution

Aqueous solutions or dispersions of both alpha-tocopherol and its esters are available for oral administration and provide better absorption than oily vehicles, particularly when there is a deficiency of biliary or pancreatic secretions (*Machlin LJ. Vitamin E, in LJ Macklin, Ed. Handbook of Vitamins. New York, Marcel Dekker, 1984:99-145*).

Experimental Study: 500 IU vitamin E was administered as an oil, emulsion and as Emusol® (Bioglan, CA) ('micellized E'). After 5 days, the increase from baseline to steady state plasma vitamin E levels was set at 1.0 for d-alpha tocopherol (the oil). Compared to oil E, the increase was 0.5 for emulsified d,l-alpha-tocopheryl acetate, 1.5 for emulsified d-alpha tocopherol, 2.6 for micellized d-alpha-tocopheryl acetate, and 3.7 for micellized d-alpha tocopherol, suggesting not only that micellized E produces higher steady state plasma vitamin E levels than the oil and emulsified forms but that, when micellized, the free alcohol produces higher steady state plasma vitamin E levels than the ester. Also, micellized E had an absorption rate 370% faster than the oil and 200% faster than emulsified E (*Regtop HL, Beaumont PE - summarized in Rutolo DA Jr. Nutrition delivery systems II: micellization and fat soluble nutrients. Int Clin Nutr Rev 9(4):206-12, 1989*).

Experimental Crossover Study: 7 subjects (ave. age 27±3 yrs.), after an overnight fast, received 500 mg vitamin E equivalent in the morning in conjunction with a standard breakfast. All capsules were punctured and squeezed into the mouth to prevent differences in dissolution time. All subjects randomly consumed each of 4 substances: vitamin E oil, emulsified vitamin E, and two forms of water-soluble vitamin E, Emusol® (Bioglan, CA) ('micellized E') and polyethylene glycol succinate) with a 1 wk. lag between each trial. Micellized E was the first to appear in the serum, followed by polyethylene glycol succinate, then emulsified vitamin E, and finally the vitamin E oil. There was a nearly linear uptake of mycellized E into the serum and red cell after ingestion. If absorption were two or more phases (such as emulsification followed by lymphatic uptake and serum distribution), the kinetics would not have been linear. This suggests that mycellized E is being transported directly into the hepatoportal blood to the liver by way of small intestine absorption, attachment to lipoproteins and release to the blood, rather than through the lymphatic pathway and emulsification, a route that is inhibited in many fat malabsorbers (*Bland J, Prestbo E. Vitamin E: Comparative absorption studies. Int Clin Nutr Rev 4(2):82-6, 1984*).

See Also:

Regtop H. Perspective on vitamin E. Int Clin Nutr Rev 3:2:7-21, 1983

For intramuscular injection, an aqueous alcohol solution of synthetic alpha-tocopherol or of alpha-tocopheryl acetate (Ephynal®, Roche), but not of alpha-tocopheryl acetate in oil, is effective in rapidly elevating the plasma vitamin E level without undesirable overshoot (*Flodin NW. Pharmacology of Micronutrients. New York, Alan R. Liss, Inc., 1988*).

Vitamin K

Decomposed by sunlight.

Efficient absorption of fat-soluble vitamins depends upon the presence of adequate bile, pancreatic enzymes and bicarbonate as well as a normal small intestine (*Gallo-Torres HE. Obligatory role of bile for the intestinal absorption of vitamin E. Lipids 5:379, 1970*).

- When to Provide Oral Supplementation

Since dietary fats generally promote absorption of oil-soluble substances, vitamin K supplements should be taken with a meal. Taking the supplement in portions several times a day will usually increase its utilization (*Vitamin E Fact Book. VERIS (Vitamin E Research & Information Service, 5325 S. 9th Ave., LaGrange, IL 60525, 1994*).

Zinc

- When to Provide Oral Supplementation

Supplementation is best taken away from meals, as eggs, milk, and cereal (as well as possibly other foods) will greatly decrease its bioavailability (*Moser PB, Gunderson CJ. Changes in plasma zinc following the ingestion of a zinc multivitamin-mineral supplement with and without breakfast. Nutr Res 3:279-84, 1983; Oelshlegel FS Jr, Brewer GJ. Absorption of pharmacological doses of zinc, in GJ Brewer, AS Prasad, Eds. Zinc Metabolism: Current Aspects in Health and Disease. New York, Alan R. Liss, Inc., 1977:299-311*).

- Formulations

Zinc sulfate in a gelatin capsule without excipients is about as bioavailable as an aqueous solution of zinc when the entire daily dose is given at one time (*Neve J, Hanocq M, Peretz A, et al. [Some factors influencing the bioavailability of zinc in oral pharmaceutical dosage forms.] J Pharm Belg 48(1):5-11, 1993*).

> *Note: Zinc sulfate may produce gastric irritation and is less well tolerated than zinc acetate or gluconate* (*Prasad AS. Clinical, biochemical and pharmacological role of zinc. Ann Rev Pharmacol Toxicol 19:393-426, 1979*).

A form of *microencapsulated* zinc sulfate, by prolonging the period of zinc release, has improved bioavailability (*Oner L, Arcasoy A, Kas HS, Hincal AA. Studies on zinc sulphate microcapsules: III. In vivo evaluation. Eur J Drug Metab Pharmacokinet 14(2):107-10, 1989*).

The formulation of one brand of *enteric-coated* zinc aspartate (Taurizine) seemed to obstruct zinc absorption as it failed to increase plasma zinc levels (*Duisterwinkel FJ, Wolthers BG, Koopman BJ, et al. Bioavailability of orally administered zinc, using Taurizine. Pharm Weekbl [Sci] 8(1):85-8, 1986*).

Zinc-histidine complexes may be more bioavailable than zinc sulfate.

> **Experimental Study:** 10 healthy volunteers received zinc sulfate or zinc complexed with histidine. Zinc complexed with histidine at a ratio of 1:2 or 1:12 increased serum zinc concentration 25% more than zinc sulfate and its calculated

uptake was 30-40% higher, while urinary zinc excretion was similar. 15 mg of zinc as zinc histidine 1:2 gave an identical serum zinc response as 45 mg zinc as zinc sulfate (*Scholmerich J, Freudemann A, Kottgen E, et al. Bioavailability of zinc from zinc-histidine complexes. I. Comparison with zinc sulfate in healthy men. Am J Clin Nutr 45(6):1480-6, 1987*).

The importance of the physiological roles of picolinic and citric acids in zinc absorption is controversial.

Review Article: "Even at supplemental levels, citrate is apparently not a major regulator of zinc absorption, and normal intakes of citrate-containing foods do not influence zinc status significantly" (*Zinc bioavailability of human and cow's milk. Nutr Rev 44:181-3, 1986*).

Observational Study: Findings that the concentration of picolinic acid in human milk is extremely low and apparently absent in pancreatic juice and intestines suggest that it is not the zinc binding ligand of human milk and does not have an important physiological role in intestinal zinc absorption (*Rebello T, Lonnerdal B, Hurley LS. Picolinic acid in milk, pancreatic juice, and intestine: inadequate for role in zinc absorption. Am J Clin Nutr 35(1):1-5, 1982*).

Review Article: In humans and animals consuming a diet that contains physiological levels of zinc, the quantity of zinc transported across the absorptive cell is directly related to the availability of picolinic acid, a tryptophan metabolite. In the intestinal lumen, picolinic acid secreted by the exocrine cells of the pancreas coordinates with zinc to form a complex that facilitates the passage of zinc through the luminal membrane, across the absorptive cell and through the basolateral membrane of the cell (*Evans GW. Normal and abnormal zinc absorption in man and animals: the tryptophan connection. Nutr Rev 38(4):137-41, 1980*).

See Also:

> **Review Article:** *Hurley LS, Lonnerdal B. Zinc binding in human milk: citrate versus picolinate. Nutr Rev 40(3):65-71, 1982*

> *Hurley LS, Lonnerdal B. Picolinic acid as a zinc-binding ligand in human milk: an unconvincing case. Pediatr Res 15(2):166-7, 1981*

> *Evans GW, Johnson PE. Characterization and quantitation of a zinc-binding ligand in human milk. Pediatr Res 14(7):876-80, 1980*

Zinc picolinate may be more bioavailable than certain other zinc supplements, especially in patients with pancreatic insufficiency.

> **WARNING:**   Doses above 5 mg/d of zinc picolinate are not recommended as picolinic acid may interfere with iron utilization, resulting in anemia (*Evans GW. The Picolinates. New Canaan, CT, Keats Publishing, 1989:22-3; Fernandez-Pol JA. Iron: possible cause of the G1 arrest induced in HRK cells by picolinic acid. Biochem Biophys Res Commun 78(1):136, 1977*).

Experimental Double-blind Crossover Study: 15 healthy subjects received 50 mg elemental zinc in 3 different complexed forms and placebo for 4 wks. each in random order. Zinc picolinate supplementation showed significant increases in zinc levels of the hair, urine and erythrocytes, but no significant increase in the serum. Zinc citrate, zinc gluconate and placebo showed no significant changes (*Barrie SA, Wright JV, Pizzorno JE, et al. Comparative absorption of zinc picolinate, zinc citrate and zinc gluconate in humans. Agents Actions 21(1-2):223-8, 1987*).

Experimental Study: 5 pts. with pancreatic insufficiency and controls received zinc tolerance tests (ZTT) with zinc sulfate and zinc picolinate. Healthy controls had normal ZTT curves, with no significant difference between the 2 forms of zinc, while pts. with chronic illnesses had significantly depressed ZTT curves with both forms of zinc compared to the healthy controls. In contrast, pancreatic insufficiency pts. had significantly depressed ZTT curves with zinc sulfate but not with zinc dipicolinate, suggesting that normal pancreatic functioning may play a role in zinc metabolism (*Boosalis MG, Evans GW, McClain CJ. Impaired handling of orally administered zinc in pancreatic insufficiency. Am J Clin Nutr 37(2):268-71, 1983*).

Zinc gluconate may be more bioavailable than zinc sulfate.

Experimental Study: 10 subjects ingested 45 mg elemental zinc in various forms. For gelatin capsules without excipients taken in a non-divided dose, zinc gluconate was more bioavailable than zinc sulfate (*Neve J, Hanocq M, Peretz A, et al. [Some factors influencing the bioavailability of zinc in oral pharmaceutical dosage forms.] J Pharm Belg 48(1):5-11, 1993*).

Experimental Study: In comparing the rate of increase of zinc levels in serum, plasma and urine for a group of patients with anorexia nervosa and low zinc levels, citrate >gluconate >orotate >sulfate (results not significant) (*Ward NI. Assessment of zinc status and oral supplementation in anorexia nervosa. J Nutr Med 1:171-7, 1990*).

Zinc oxide is poorly absorbed in both hypochlorhydric and hyperchlorhydric patients, while zinc acetate is more consistently absorbed (*Brewer GJ. Effect of intragastric pH on the absorption of oral zinc acetate and zinc oxide in young volunteers. J Parenter Enter Nutr 19(5):393-7, 1995*).

Note: Perhaps 20-50% of patients aged 60 and over are hypochlorhydric.

Zinc monomethionine (OptiZinc, Inter Health) has proven efficacy in animals. In a human study, when taken away from a meal, it raised plasma zinc levels above those achieved by zinc sulfate and zinc polyascorbate (*Rosado JL et al. Zinc absorption from different forms of zinc supplements in the presence and absence of a rural Mexican diet. Abstract. 9th Latin American Congress of Nutrition, ?1992*).

Chapter Four

ADVERSE EFFECTS OF NUTRITIONAL SUPPLEMENTS

GENERAL

When micronutrients are taken at high doses, the <u>excipients and additives</u> included in the preparations may cause adverse effects.

> **Observational Study:** 34 mostly healthy subjects, ave. age 43 yrs., 17 of whom were smokers and 6 of whom were moderate drinkers, were studied for 4-5 years. Most consumed a balanced diet. Their range of micronutrient doses was generally 500%-10,000% greater than the level usually found in a balanced American diet; a small number used doses of some micronutrients as high as 20,000-40,000% greater. Daily ranges were as follows: ascorbic acid 2-8 g, alpha-tocopherol 600-2400 IU, niacin 80-160 mg, pantothenic acid 480-960 mg, pyridoxine 160-320 mg, riboflavin 16-32 mg, thiamine 160-320 mg, vitamin B_{12} 800-1600 µg, beta-carotene 15-60 mg, glutathione 200-400 mg, and the RDA for calcium and vitamin D. While excipients and additives do not normally cause adverse reactions if only 1 or 2 tablets are taken, the majority of subjects who consumed large quantities of micronutrients eventually reacted adversely to the excipients, binders, fillers, lubricants, oils, and some form of residues from natural sources. Most subjects, in order to continue to take large doses of micronutrients, eventually were forced to switch to relatively pure preparations due to progressive symptoms of <u>gastrointestinal pain</u>, <u>nausea</u>, <u>rhinitis</u>, <u>malaise</u>, <u>diarrhea</u>, <u>headaches</u> and <u>skin rashes</u>. After substituting relatively pure forms of micronutrients, these symptoms, which were not specific to a nutrient, no longer appeared (*Demopoulos HB, Santomier JP, Seligman ML, et al. Free radical pathology: rationale and toxicology of antioxidants and other supplements in sports medicine and exercise science, in <u>Free Radical Pathology</u>, Ca. 1985; Demopoulos HB, Santomier JP. Safety of large-dose antioxidant regimes in man. Abstract. <u>Med Sci Sports Exer</u>c 17(2):201-2, 1985).*

<u>Lactose</u> is one of the most commonly used fillers in nutritional supplements. Lactase deficiency occurs in about 75% of adults in all ethnic groups except those of Northwestern European origin, where the incidence is less than 20% (*Spiro HM. <u>Clinical Gastroenterology</u>. 3rd Edition*) and results in the inability to split lactose into glucose and galactose. Symptoms of lactose intolerance include digestive disturbances, abdominal distension and pain, diarrhea and gaseous stools.

> **Case Report:** A 24 year-old lactase-deficient woman using cromolyn sodium (Intal) through a turbo-inhaler for exercise-induced asthma had 2 episodes of bloating, nausea, abdominal cramps and flatulence. She read the label and discovered that each capsule contained 20 mg of lactose. Her physician then conducted a double-blind trial testing her nebulized Intal against 2 lactose-free solutions, lactose-free Intal and isotonic saline. Only the inhaled lactose-containing Intal induced her previously-experienced gastrointestinal

symptoms *(Brandstetter RD, Conetta R, Glazer B. Lactose intolerance associated with Intal capsules. N Engl J Med 315(25):1613-14, 1986).*

In multivitamin/multimineral preparations, vitamin B12 (cyanocobalamin), through an interaction with the combination of thiamine, vitamin C and copper, may be converted into inactive analogs which may fail to stimulate or even inhibit cobalamin-dependent enzymes, suggesting that vitamins and minerals should be provided separately *(Kondo H, Mitchell JB, Kolhouse FJ, et al. Presence and formation of cobalamin analogs in multivitamin-mineral pills. J Clin Invest 70(4):889-98, 1982).*

"Slow dissolving [nutrient] preparations may sit on the sensitive gastric mucosa and liberate their contents, actually producing gastric irritation. This has certainly been the case with iron preparations and may be also the case with other acidic vitamin supplements such as pantothenic acid, nicotinic acid, and folic acid" *(Bland J. Nutrient bioavailability and fast acting formulas. Int Clin Nutr Rev 5(1):25-9, 1985).*

Beta-Carotene

Recent clinical trials have raised concern about possible long-term adverse effects of beta-carotene supplements in regard to degenerative diseases. Beta-carotene has pro-oxidant activity at higher oxygen tensions such as those found in the lung. Only one of several carotenoids found in the human diet and plasma, ingestion of large amounts of beta-carotene may decrease uptake of other carotenoids that have a greater potential to prevent oxidative stress. Epidemiological evidence for a protective role of beta-carotene in cancer prevention may simply reflect the association of beta-carotene with a generally more healthy diet *(Woodall AA, Jack CI, Jackson MJ. Caution with β-carotene supplements. Letter. Lancet 347:967-8, 1996).*

Beta-carotene is very susceptible to oxidative damage (such as occurs during smoking and excess alcohol consumption) which results in its conversion to retinoic acid and retinaldehyde derivatives that can adversely influence the expression of various cell regulatory factors *(Krinsky NI. Antioxidant functions of carotenoids. Pure Appl Chem 66(5):1003-10, 1994).* The presence of adequate amounts of numerous antioxidant factors protects beta-carotene from such oxidative damage *(Krinsky NI. Antioxidant functions of carotenoids. Free Rad Biol Med 7:617-35, 1989).*

Alcohol-fed baboons given beta-carotene develop histological changes in the liver *(Leo MA, Kim C, Lowe N, Lieber CS. Interaction of ethanol with b-carotene: delayed blood clearance and enhanced hepatotoxicity. Hepatology 15:883-91, 1992),* suggesting that supplementation, while it may be justified in alcoholics with liver damage, should be coupled with control of drinking *(Ahmed S, Leo MA, Lieber CS. Interactions between alcohol and b-carotene in patients with alcoholic liver disease. Am J Clin Nutr 60:430-6, 1994).*

Largely anecdotal reports have related large intakes of beta-carotene to cause reversible leukopenia, enlarged liver, weakness, low blood pressure and weight loss *(Vakil DV et al. Hypercarotenaemia: A case report and review of the literature. Nutr Res 5:911-17, 1985),* as well as reproductive disorders, increased risk of prostate cancer, retinopathy and allergic reactions. None of these reports has been substantiated in clinical trials; thus no such reported side effects need be of concern *(Diplock AT. Safety of antioxidant vitamins and b-carotene. Am J Clin Nutr 62(suppl):1510S-16S, 1995).*

Note: Reports of carotenoid-associated toxicity were the result of the consumption of foods containing carotenoids rather than a pure product; thus other components of these foods are likely to be the major cause of the reported adverse effects. This pro-vitamin has been taken by many individuals at doses between 30 and 180 mg daily over a 15 year period without any adverse effects being noted (Bendich A. The safety of beta-carotene. Nutr Cancer 11:207-14, 1988).

Hypercarotenemia is associated with <u>orange discoloration of the skin</u> (especially palms, soles and naso-labial folds) (Vakil DV et al. Hypercarotenaemia: A case report and review of the literature. Nutr Res 5:911-17, 1985).

Experimental Placebo-controlled Study: 5 men randomly received carotenoid supplementation either as 30 mg purified beta-carotene, 12 mg beta-carotene, 272 g cooked carrots, 300 g cooked broccoli, 180 g tomato juice or placebo. Definite carotenodermia was first noted between 25-42 days and persisted 14 to >42 days post-treatment. It was only observed after plasma total carotenoid levels exceeded 4.0 mg/L (Micozzi MS et al. Carotenodermia in men with elevated carotenoid intake from foods and beta-carotene supplements. Am J Clin Nutr 48:1061-4, 1988).

Among smokers, former smokers and workers exposed to asbestos, long-term supplementation may <u>increase the risk of death</u>, especially from lung cancer and cardiovascular disease (Albanes D, Heinonen OP, Huttunen JK, et al. Effects of α-tocopherol and β-carotene supplements on cancer incidence in the Alpha-Tocopherol Beta-Carotene Cancer Prevention Study. Am J Clin Nutr 62(suppl):1427S-30S, 1995; Alpha-tocopherol, Beta-carotene Cancer Prevention Study Group. The effect of vitamin E and beta-carotene on the incidence of lung cancer and other cancers in male smokers. N Engl J Med 330:1029-35, 1994; Omenn GS, Goodman GE, Thornquist MD, et al. Effects of a combination of beta carotene and vitamin A on lung cancer and cardiovascular disease. N Engl J Med 334:1150-5, 1996).

Bismuth

Adverse side-effects appear limited to mild <u>dizziness</u>, <u>headache</u> and <u>diarrhea</u>. Anacids or milk should not be taken within 30 minutes before or after ingestion. Bismuth compounds should not be given to patients with renal or hepatic impairment. Due to lack of safety data, they should not be given during pregnancy (Wagstaff AJ et al. Colloidal bismuth subcitrate: A review of its pharmacodynamic and pharmacokinetic properties, and its therapeutic use in peptic ulcer disease. Drugs 36:132-57, 1988).

Calcium

A dietary calcium to phosphorus ratio above 2:1 due to excess calcium results in <u>reduced bone strength</u> and interferes with vitamin K synthesis and/or absorption, which could theoretically cause <u>internal bleeding</u> (Calcium: How much is too much? Nutr Rev 43(11):345, 1985).

Animal Experimental Study: Pigs who received a 3:1 ratio of calcium to phosphorus (in the form of calcium carbonate and dicalcium phosphate) all died with internal bleeding. However, when vitamin K was administered, clotting time was increased and there were no deaths (Hall et al. J Animal Sci 61(Suppl 1):319-20, 1985).

Primary <u>hyperparathyroidism</u> may be caused by a daily calcium intake of over 2 grams.

Case Report: A pt. with a daily calcium intake of >2 g presented with very high concentrations of intact parathyroid hormone, severe hypercalcemia and low circulating concentrations of 1,25-dihydroxyvitamin D. Following calcium restriction, serum calcium returned to normal concomitant with a pronounced rise in serum 1,25-dihydroxyvitamin D and a dramatic fall in circulating parathyroid hormone (*Shaker JL, Krawczyc KW, Finding JW. Primary hyperparathyroidism and severe hypercalcaemia with low circulating 1,25-dihydroxyvitamin D levels. J Clin Endocrinol Metab 62:1305-8, 1986*).

Supplementation for women receiving estrogens, in the face of commonly low magnesium intake, increases the risk of thrombosis (*Seelig MS. Interrelationship of magnesium and estrogen in cardiovascular and bone disorders, eclampsia, migraine and premenstrual syndrome. J Am Coll Nutr 12(4):442-58, 1993*).

Supplementation may increase the risk of urinary tract infections by increasing bacterial adherence to uroepithelial cells (*Apicella LL, Sobota AE. Increased risk of urinary tract infection associated with the use of calcium supplements. Urol Res 18:213-17, 1990; Peleg I, McGowan J, McNagny S. Dietary calcium supplementation increases the risk of urinary tract infection. Clin Res 40:A562, 1992*).

Calcium citrate markedly enhances dietary aluminum absorption (*Coburn JW et al. Am J Kidney Dis 17(6):708-11, 1991; Nestel AW et al. Effect of calcium supplement preparation containing small amounts of citrate on the absorption of aluminum in normal subjects and in renal failure patients. Nephron 68:197-201, 1994*).

> **Experimental Study:** 30 healthy women received calcium citrate (800 mg elemental calcium) daily. Compared to baseline, urinary aluminum excretion and plasma aluminum levels increased significantly, suggesting that calcium citrate increases absorption of aluminum from dietary sources (*Nolan CR et al. Aluminum and lead absorption from dietary sources in women ingesting calcium citrate. South Med J 87(9):894-8, 1994*).

Calcium carbonate, including the less-purified calcium carbonate in ground oyster shells, tends to increase fecal transit time and thus may cause constipation (*Kohls KJ, Kies C. Calcium bioavailability: a comparison of several different commercially available calcium supplements. J Appl Nutr 44(3&4):50-61, 1992*).

> *Note: Dolomite, which contains both calcium carbonate and magnesium carbonate, has less of an effect on fecal transit time, probably because of the irritant effect of magnesium carbonate (Kohls KJ, Kies C. Calcium bioavailability: a comparison of several different commercially available calcium supplements. J Appl Nutr 44(3&4):50-61, 1992).*

Calcium supplements, especially those from natural sources, may be a source of toxic metals.

> **Laboratory Study:** The lead content of 70 brands of calcium supplements was measured and ranged from 0.03-8.83 µg/g. Based on daily lead ingestion rates, about one-quarter of the products exceeded 6 µg lead daily, the US FDA's provisional total tolerable daily intake of lead for children aged 6 and under. 41/45 (91%) of products in the categories of refined calcium carbonate, chelated calcium, dolomite and bonemeal contained acceptable amts. of lead; however, only 11/25 (44%) of products in the category of natural source calcium carbonate (limestone rock derived from fossilized oyster shell) met this criterion. Since calcium supplements are sometimes used as a calcium source in children when cow's milk is avoided, it was notable that less than one-fifth of the supplements had normalized lead levels comparable to or lower than that reported for cow's milk (*Bourgoin BP, Evans DR, Cornett JR, et al. Lead content in 70 brands of dietary calcium supplements. Am J Public Health 83(8):1155-60, 1993*).

Laboratory Study: 10 randomly selected tablets of one brand of dolomite were analyzed. They were found to contain (mean weights/gm): 900 μg aluminum, 1.3 μg arsenic, 0.16 μg cadmium, and 1.9 μg lead (*Boulos FM, von Smolinski A. Alert to users of calcium supplements as antihypertensive agents due to trace mineral contaminants. Am J Hypertens 1(3 Pt 3):127S-142S, 1988*).

See Also:

> Roberts HJ. *Potential toxicity due to dolomite and bonemeal.* South Med J 76:556, 1983

Carnitine

In clinical studies of L-carnitine, 41% of patients developed gastrointestinal side-effects and 11% developed a body odor. In no patient was it discontinued due to these side-effects, and a decrease in dosage reduced or eliminated them (*FDA Drug Bull, June, 1986*).

Supplementation with D,L-carnitine 900-1200 mg daily (but not with L-carnitine) has been associated with a myasthenia-like syndrome in patients with renal impairment (*McCarty MF. A note on 'orthomolecular' aids for dieting - myasthenic syndrome due to DL-carnitine. Med Hypotheses December, 1982, pp. 661-2; Bazzato G et al. Myasthenia-like syndrome after DL - but not L - carnitine. Lancet i:1209, 1981*).

High dosages of carnitine in nutritional supplements may stimulate lipid peroxidation (*Hu M, Chen Y, Lin Y. the antioxidant and prooxidant activity of some B-vitamins and vitamin-like compounds. Chem Biol Interact 97:63-73, 1995*).

Choline

Choline chloride has a bitter taste and causes a "dead fish" body odor due to the action of intestinal bacteria that convert unabsorbed free choline into amines; phosphatidyl choline does not have these problems (*Lecithin and its uses. Advanced Nutritional Technology, Inc., P. O. Box 3225, Elizabeth, NJ 07207, 1986*).

Choline chloride, soy lecithin and phosphatidyl choline may all cause occasional gastrointestinal irritation (reduced appetite, vomiting, abdominal bloating, belching, and diarrhea with fatty stools). However, phosphatidyl choline almost never produces this side effect unless the daily doses are well above 40 gm (*Effects of consumption of choline chloride and lecithin on neurological and cardiovascular systems. Life Sciences Research Office, Bethesda, MD, USA. FASEB report prepared for the FDA Bureau of Foods, 1981*).

Chromium

Usual supplemental doses (50-200 μg) may cause irritability and insomnia (*Schrauzer G, Shrestra KP, Arce MF. Somatopsychological effects of chromium supplementation. J Nutr Med 3:43-8, 1992*).

Chromium picolinate is suspected of causing chromosomal damage.

Review Article: Cr^{3+} may accumulate and be retained in human tissue for extended periods, and its long-term biological effects are poorly understood. Moreover, the possibility that it may be involved in chromium-induced human cancers has not been ruled out; thus the long-term use of chromium dietary supplements in excessive doses should be viewed with caution (*Stearns DM et al. A prediction of chromium (III) accumulation in humans from chromium dietary supplements. FASEB J 9:1650-7, 1995*).

In vitro Experimental Study: Chinese hampster ovary cells were treated with chromium picolinate or chromium nicotinate for 24 hrs. and the results were compared to those of obtained in cells treated with ligands alone or with chromium chloride. Chromium picolinate was found to cause significant chromosomal damage at a non-toxic dose, and damage was dose-dependent. This damage was inferred to arise from the ligand since picolinate alone caused damage at a non-toxic dose, raising questions about the safety of chromium picolinate as a human dietary supplement (*Stearns DM, Wise JP Sr., Patierno SR, Wetterhahn KE. The dietary supplement chromium picolinate induces chromosome damage in Chinese hampster ovary cells. Abstract #2616. FASEB J 9(3):A451, 1995*).

> *Note: This study used an in vitro concentration of 100 micromoles, while 200 micrograms daily of chromium picolinate, the usual supplemental dosage, produces a serum chromium concentration of only 16 nanomoles, a concentration that is lower by a factor of 6,000* (*C. Leigh Broadhurst, Visiting Scientist, Beltsville Human Nutrition Research Center, USDA. Chromium picolinate. Letter. Townsend Letter October, 1995*).

Copper

Elevated levels (often due to contaminated drinking water) can be toxic, causing profound mental and physical fatigue, poor memory, severe depression and insomnia (*Nolan KB. Nutr Rev 41:318-20, 1983*).

Excess copper may increase susceptibility to infection (*Beisel WR. Single nutrients and immunity. Am J Clin Nutr 35:417-68 (suppl), 1982*).

L-Cysteine

May readily oxidize to insoluble cystine, a cause of kidney stones and tissue damage (*Higashi T et al. Sulfur Amino Acids: Biochemical and Clinical Aspects. New York, Alan R. Liss, 1983:419-34*).

L-Cystine

May cause kidney stones and tissue damage (*Higashi T et al. Sulfur Amino Acids: Biochemical and Clinical Aspects. New York, Alan R. Liss, 1983:419-34*).

Evening Primrose Oil   *See 'Omega-6 Fatty Acids' below.*

Fiber (dietary)

May increase the risk of osteoporotic hip fracture due to impairment of calcium absorption.

Observational Study: From an initial cohort of 65,000 Swedish women aged 40-75, 272 subsequent cases of hip fractures and 1024 matched controls were studied. There was only a weak association between high dietary fiber and hip fracture risk which only existed when calcium intake was high (*Michaelsson K, Holmberg L, Mallmin H, et al. Diet and hip fracture risk: case-control study. Int J Epidemiol 24(4):771-81, 1995*).

Fish Oils   *See 'Omega-3 Fatty Acids' below.*

Flavonoids

Cianidanol may induce intravascular or extravascular <u>immune hemolysis</u> and <u>fever</u> *(Jaeger A et al. Side effects of flavonoids in medical practice. <u>Prog Clin Biol Res</u> 280:379-94, 1988).*

Fluoride

In experimental animals, administration inhibits the enzyme phosphatase which is critically important for the assimilation of calcium and other minerals *(Yanick P. Solving problematic tinnitus. A clinical scientific approach. <u>Townsend Letter for Doctors</u>. February - March, 1985, p. 31).*

Damages the surface of the gastric mucosa at therapeutic dosages *(Spak C-J et al. Tissue response of gastric mucosa after ingestion of fluoride. <u>BMJ</u> 298:1686-7, 1989).*

May increase the risk of osteosarcoma.

> **Animal Experimental Study:** When 130 male rats drank water containing high levels of fluoride (>100 parts per million) over a lifetime, 4 developed osteosarcoma *(National Center for Toxicological Research, US Food and Drug Administration - noted in <u>FDA Consumer</u> May, 1991).*

Folic Acid

Daily oral supplements of 5-10 mg appear to be well-tolerated and without toxicity in normal non-pregnant subjects; some studies suggest ensuring adequate zinc intake if folate supplements are used during pregnancy *(Butterworth CE Jr, Tamura T. Folic acid safety and toxicity: A brief review. <u>Am J Clin Nutr</u> 50:353-8, 1989).*

> *Note: There have been several documented reports of hypersensitivity to folic acid, with oral doses of 1-10 mg producing <u>fever</u>, <u>urticaria</u>, <u>erythema</u>, <u>pruritis</u>, and <u>respiratory distress</u> (Zimmermann MB, Shane B. Supplemental folic acid. <u>Am J Clin Nutr</u> 58:127-8, 1993).*

Adverse effects may occasionally be seen at higher dosages.

> *Note: Such effects may reflect a tendency to overarousal as may occur with any antidepressant including its closely-related metabolite, S-adenosylmethionine (Crellin R, Bottiglierei T, Reynolds EH. Folates and psychiatric disorders. Clinical potential. <u>Drugs</u> 45(5):623-36, 1993).*

> **Case Reports:** 2 pts. are described who showed <u>exacerbation of psychotic behavior</u> during treatment with folic acid for folate deficiency which was associated with elevated RBC folate levels *(Prakash R, Petrie WM. Psychiatric changes associated with an excess of folic acid. <u>Am J Psychiatry</u>. 139(9):1192-3, 1982).*

> **Experimental Study:** 14 normal subjects received folic acid 15 mg daily. By 1 mo., 60% had developed <u>GI side-effects</u> (abdominal distension, flatulence, nausea, anorexia), <u>sleep</u>

disturbances with vivid dreams, malaise and irritability (*Hunter R, Barnes J, Oakeley HF, Matthews DM. Toxicity of folic acid given in pharmacological doses to healthy volunteers. Lancet i:61-3, 1970*).

High dose therapy may decrease vitamin B_{12} levels; thus B_{12} supplementation or regular monitoring is indicated (*Hunter R et al. Effect of folic-acid supplement on serum-vitamin-B_{12} levels in patients on anticonvulsants. Lancet ii:50, 1969*).

In patients with untreated cobalamin deficiency, dosages of folate >1 mg daily may ameliorate the anemia of pernicious anemia, but in about half the patients the neuropathy develops or progresses (*Chanarin I. Adverse effects of increased dietary folate. Relation to measures to reduce the incidence of neural tube defects. Clin Invest Med 17(3):131-7, 1994*).

Supplementation should be used with caution in drug-controlled epileptics as occasionally seizure activity may be induced (*Butterworth CE Jr, Tamura T. Folic acid safety and toxicity: A brief review. Am J Clin Nutr 50:353-8, 1989*).

Gamma-hydroxybutyrate

At doses ranging from 1/4 tsp to 4 tbsp, adverse effects have included coma and tonic-clonic seizure-like activity, abrupt drowsiness, dizziness, a 'high', headache, and nausea and vomiting. Following discontinuation of the supplement, there is full recovery. No clear dose-response effect has been observed (*Chin MY, Kreutzer RA, Dyer JE. Acute poisoning from gamma-hydroxybutyrate in California. West J Med 156(4):380-4, 1992*). Acute effects resolve within 7 hours (*Dyer JE. gamma-Hydroxybutyrate: a health-food product producing coma and seizurelike activity. Am J Emerg Med 9(4):321-4, 1991*).

Physical dependence may develop with chronic use (*Galloway GP, Frederick SL, Staggers J Jr. Physical dependence on sodium oxybate. Letter. Lancet 343:57, 1994*).

Germanium

Long-term ingestion of germanium dioxide may be nephrotoxic.

> **Review Article:** Acute renal failure or renal dysfunction associated with germanium-induced nephrotoxicity has been reported in 18 pts. since 1982. In 17/18 cases, biopsies showed vacuolar degeneration in renal tubular epithelial cells in the absence of glomerular changes, without proteinuria or hematuria. Although the mechanism for germanium-induced nephrotoxicity is unknown, the inorganic germanium salts, such as germanium dioxide, are the suspected cause. While sufficient evidence for a role of organogermanium compounds, such as carboxyethyl germanium sesquioxide ('Ge 132') or citrate-lactate germanate, is lacking, the introduction of germanium 'nutritional' supplements increases the risk of additional cases of germanium-induced nephrotoxicity, especially if appreciable levels of inorganic germanium salts are present and consumed for longer than 3 mo. at levels above the ave. daily estimated intake for germanium (*Schauss AG. Nephrotoxicity in humans by the ultratrace element germanium. Ren Fail 13(1):1-4, 1991*).

> **Case Reports:** Ingestion of germanium dioxide 50-250 mg daily for at least several mo. was associated with the development of renal failure in 2 patients. Renal function gradually improved after discontinuation of the germanium, but never recovered

completely. 8 other cases of germanium dioxide-induced nephropathy have been reported in the Japanese medical literature *(Matsusaka T et al. Germanium-induced nephropathy: Report of 2 cases and review of the literature. Clin Nephrol 30:341-5, 1988).*

L-Glutamine

Megadoses may cause <u>mania</u>.

Case Reports:
1. A pt. with no prior psychiatric history was hospitalized with a 1 wk. history of increasing motor and verbal activity culminating in grandiose delusions, hypersexuality, and insomnia. Two wks. earlier, he had begun to ingest up to 4 gm L-glutamine daily. Symptoms ceased within 1 wk. of stopping the supplement.
2. A pt. in psychotherapy with dysthymic disorder began to experience increasing sleep loss, unusually high energy and increased mental acuity and became unusually outgoing and talkative following 1 wk. of ingesting up to 2 gm daily of L-glutamine.
(Mebane AH. L-Glutamine and Mania. Letter. Am J Psychiatry 141(10), October, 1984).

Guar Gum

May adversely affect food absorption *(Meyer JH, Doty JE. Transit and absorption of solid food: Multiple effects of guar. Am J Clin Nutr 267-73, 1988).*

May cause <u>obstruction of the esophagus and small bowel</u> *(Lewis J. Esophageal and small bowel obstruction from guar gum-containing "diet pills" : Analysis of 26 cases reported to the Food and Drug Administration. Am J Gastroenterol 87:1424-8, 1992).*

L-5-Hydroxytryptophan

Gastrointestinal side effects (<u>nausea</u>, <u>vomiting</u>, <u>diarrhea</u>) are the only side effects of practical importance and are dose-dependent. They can be minimized by raising the dosage gradually and taking the supplement at mealtimes *(van Praag HM, Westenberg HGM. The treatment of depressions with l-5-hydroxytryptophan. Adv Biol Psychiatry 10:94-128, 1983).*

Too high a dosage may cause <u>hypomania</u> *(van Hiele LJ. L-5-Hydroxytryptophan in depression: the first substitution therapy in psychiatry? Neuropsychobiology 6(4):230-40, 1980).*

Iodine

Up to 1 mg daily may be consumed safely. The dosage that produces chronic iodine poisoning (iodism) varies greatly between individuals. Six mg or more daily may inhibit thyroid activity. Iodism includes the <u>unpleasant, brassy taste of iodine</u>, <u>burning in the mouth</u>, <u>sore mouth and throat</u>, <u>hypersalivation</u>, <u>painful sialadenitis</u>, <u>acne and other rashes</u>, <u>diarrhea</u>, <u>productive cough</u>, and <u>gynecomastia</u>. In patients with nontoxic nodular goiter, iodide administration may be followed by symptoms of <u>thyrotoxicosis</u> and an <u>increase in serum thyroid hormone concentrations</u> while, in patients with underlying autoimmune thyroiditis, <u>hypothyroidism</u> may occur. Acute poisoning is relatively rare but can occur in very sensitive individuals immediately or several hours after administration and may be marked by <u>angioedema</u> with <u>swelling of the larynx</u> and manifestations of serum sickness. The use of iodine during pregnancy is not recommended *(Drug Evaluations Subscription. Chicago, American Medical Association, Spring, 1990 & Summer, 1991)*.

Iron

Only supplement if deficient - otherwise supplementation can cause subclinical iron excess which may contribute to a wide variety of diseases by promoting oxidative damage *(Gordeuk V et al. Iron overload: causes and consequences. Annu Rev Nutr 7:485-508, 1987; Halliday J, Powell L. Iron overload. Sem Hematol 19:42-53, 1982)*, including cancer, infection *(Bergeron RJ et al. Influence of iron on in vivo proliferation and lethality of L1210 cells. J Nutr 115:369-74, 1985; Weinberg ED. Iron withholding: A defense against infection and neoplasia. Physiol Rev 64:65-102, 1984)* and growth retardation in children *(Idzradinata P, Watkins WE, Pollitt E. Adverse effect of iron supplementation on weight gain of iron-replete young children. Lancet 343:1252-4, 1994)*.

> *Note: Adequate tissue vitamin E levels may protect against oxidative damage due to iron (Linseman K, Larson P, Braughler J, et al. Iron-initiated tissue oxidation: Lipid peroxidation, vitamin E destruction and protein thiol oxidation. Biochem Pharmacol 45:1477-82, 1993; Omara FO, Blakley BR. Vitamin E is protective against iron toxicity and iron-induced hepatic vitamin E depletion in mice. J Nutr 123:1649-55, 1993).*

Gastrointestinal side effects (nausea, vomiting, epigastric discomfort, etc.) are commonly reported after iron supplementation *(Passmore R, Eastwood MA. Davidson and Passmore: Human Nutrition and Dietetics. Edinburgh, Churchill Livingstone, 1986:463)* which may turn the stools black.

A high iron intake may increase the risk of hip fractures.

> **Observational Study:** From an initial cohort of 65,000 Swedish women aged 40-75, 272 subsequent cases of hip fractures and 1024 matched controls were studied. There was an increased risk of fracture with high dietary intakes of iron which was greater when calcium intake was high *(Michaelsson K, Holmberg L, Mallmin H, et al. Diet and hip fracture risk: case-control study. Int J Epidemiol 24(4):771-81, 1995)*.

Lecithin

A study in rats suggests that soy lecithin supplementation in pregnant women could cause central nervous system damage in their children *(Bell JM, Lundberg PK. Effects of a commercial soy lecithin preparation on development of sensorimotor behavior and brain biochemistry in the rat. Dev Psychobiol 18(1):59-66, 1985)*.

Lithium

At doses of 900-1500 mg/d, may cause weight gain, tremor, thirst, diarrhea, frequent urination and hypothyroidism *(Jefferson JW. Lithium: a therapeutic magic wand. J Clin Psychiatry 50:81-6, 1989)*.

L-Lysine

May increase cholesterol and triglyceride levels.

> **Animal Experimental Study:** Chicks fed diets with 4% L-lysine developed elevated total cholesterol and triglycerides. No other amino acid had this effect. Addition of arginine failed to reverse these changes; thus they are not mediated by the antagonism between

lysine and arginine *(Schmeisser DD et al. Effect of excess dietary lysine on plasma lipids of the chick. J Nutr 113(9):1777-83, 1983).*

Magnesium

Supplementation with many magnesium salts may cause gastrointestinal side effects, especially diarrhea *(Fine KD, Santa Ana CA, Fordtran JS. Diagnosis of magnesium-induced diarrhea. N Engl J Med 324:1012-7, 1991; Lowenthal DT. Clinical pharmacology of magnesium chloride, in TD Giles, MS Seelig, Eds. The Role of Magnesium Chloride Therapy in Clinical Practice. Clifton NJ, Oxford Health Care, 1988; Steinberg W. Magnesium-induced diarrhea: more firm data on loose stools. Am J Gastroenterol 87(5):675-6, 1992).* This risk can be minimized by enteric coating *(Lowenthal DT. Clinical pharmacology of magnesium chloride, in TD Giles, MS Seelig, Eds. The Role of Magnesium Chloride Therapy in Clinical Practice. Clifton NJ, Oxford Health Care, 1988),* although enteric coating may reduce magnesium bioavailabilty *(Fine KD, Santa Ana CA, Porter JL, Fordtran JS. Intestinal absorption of magnesium from food and supplements. J Clin Invest 88:(2)396-402, 1991).*

> *Note: Most likely to cause digestive disturbances are the inorganic salts (ex. magnesium sulfate; magnesium carbonate) and some organic acid salts (ex. magnesium citrate) while magnesium aspartate-ascorbate complex and magnesium diglycinate (Albion's chelated magnesium) are two of the formulations that are generally very well tolerated (Amni® newsline. Summer, 1995. Advanced Medical Nutrition, Inc., 2247 National Ave., Hayward, CA 94545).*

Supplementation may cause dizziness or faintness due to hypotension. In excess, supplementation may cause sluggishness, cognitive impairment and depression *(Edwards N. Mental disturbances related to metals, in RCW Hall, Ed. Psychiatric Presentations of Medical Illness. Jamaica, NY, Spectrum Publications, 1980:283-308).*

A high magnesium intake may increase the risk of hip fractures.

> **Observational Study:** From an initial cohort of 65,000 Swedish women aged 40-75, 272 subsequent cases of hip fractures and 1024 matched controls were studied. There was an increased risk of fracture with high dietary intakes of magnesium which was more pronounced when calcium intake was low *(Michaelsson K, Holmberg L, Mallmin H, et al. Diet and hip fracture risk: case-control study. Int J Epidemiol 24(4):771-81, 1995).*

Age, abnormal renal function, gastrointestinal tract disease and the administration of concomitant medications (especially those with anticholinergic and narcotic effects) are risk factors for hypermagnesemia due to the widespread use of magnesium-containing over-the-counter products. These include magnesium supplements, antacids, laxatives and analgesics *(Fung MC, Weintraub M, Bowen DL. Hypermagnesemia. Elderly over-the-counter drug users at risk. Arch Fam Med 4(8):718-23, 1995).*

Manganese

Supplementation may occasionally elevate blood pressure in people over 40 or cause hypertensive headaches *(Pfeiffer CC, LaMola S. Zinc and manganese in the schizophrenias. J Orthomol Psychiatry 12:215-34, 1983).*

Chronic manganese intoxication may cause potentially irreversible movement and other neurologic disorders *(Donaldson J, Barbeau A. Manganese neurotoxicity: Possible clues to the etiology of human brain disorders, in S Gabay et al, Eds. Metal Ions in Neurology and Psychiatry. New York, Alan R. Liss, 1985:259-85; Weiner WJ et al. Regional brain manganese levels in an animal model of tardive dyskinesia, in WE Fann et al, Eds. Tardive Dyskinesia: Research and Treatment. New York, SP Medical and Scientific Books, 1980:159-63).*

N-Acetylcysteine

May act as a pro-oxidant in healthy subjects.

Experimental Study: 6 healthy volunteers received 1.2 g NAC daily for 4 wks. followed by 2.4 g daily for 2 weeks. Compared to controls, glutathione concentration in treated subjects was reduced by 48% and oxidized glutathione was 80% higher. The percent of glutathione to reduced glutathione, a marker of oxidative stress, was 83% lower in treated subjects. Also, there was no effect on oxidized LDL, suggesting that NAC was not acting as an antioxidant *(Kleinveld HA, Demacker PNM, Stalenhoef AFH. Failure of N-acetylcysteine to reduce low-density lipoprotein oxidizability in healthy subjects. Eur J Clin Pharmacol 43:639-42, 1992).*

Niacin

Note: *"The principal side effects of nicotinic acid . . . must be attributable to the high doses necessary to achieve a therapeutic effect, and can as a rule be prevented or alleviated by the use of nicotinic acid derivatives"* *(Hotz W. Nicotinic acid and its derivatives: A short survey. Adv Lipid Res 20:195-217, 1983).*

Experimental Study: 43% of 110 hypercholesterolemic pts. receiving regular niacin and 42% of those receiving sustained-release niacin were forced to discontinue the medication due to side effects *(Gibbons LW et al. The prevalence of side effects with regular and sustained-released nicotinic acid. Am J Med 99:378-85, 1995).*

Adverse effect of niacin:

1. <u>Histamine flush</u>: Common side effect due to histamine release from mast cells. Starts in 20 minutes and can last 1-1 1/2 hours. Usually lessened after 3 days and may disappear at higher doses. Can be minimized by taking niacin with meals, avoiding hot liquids and alcohol immediately after ingestion, and raising the dosage gradually. ASA 325 mg or ibuprofen 200 mg 30 minutes before ingestion may prevent or ameliorate it

2. <u>Hyperuricemia</u> due to its competition with uric acid for renal excretion is common, although exacerbation of gout or uric acid stone formation is rare *(Buist RA. Editorial: Vitamin toxicities, side effects and contraindications. Int Clin Nutr Rev 4(4):159-71, 1984; Pfeiffer CC. Mental and Elemental Nutrients. New Canaan, Conn. Keats Publishing, 1975:121).*

3. <u>Hyperglycemia</u> *(Schwartz M. Severe reversible hyperglycemia as a consequence of niacin therapy. Arch Intern Med 153:2050-2, 1993)* and <u>deterioration of oral glucose tolerance</u> *(Balasse EO, Neef A. Metabolism 22:1193, 1973; Gaut QN et al, in KF Gey, LA Carlson, Eds. Metabolic Effects Of Nicotinic Acid and Its Derivatives. Bern, Huber, 1971:923; Mosher LR. Am J Psychiatry 126:1290, 1970).*

4. Ocular side effects: <u>macular edema</u>, <u>sicca syndrome</u> and <u>proptosis</u>, all of which are usually reversible with a decrease in dosage *(Fraunfelder FW, Fraunfelder FT, Illingworth DR. Adverse ocular effects associated with niacin therapy. Br J Ophthalmol 79:54-6, 1995).*

5. Other side effects: Pruritis, hyperpigmentation, rash, acanthosis nigricans, nausea, diarrhea, aggravation of peptic ulcers, hypotension, and atrial fibrillation (*Coronary Drug Project Research Group: Clofibrate and niacin in coronary heart disease. JAMA 231:360-81, 1975*).

See Also:

> Goldstein MR. *Potential problems with the widespread use of niacin. Am J Med 85:881, 1988*

> *The Medical Letter Vol. 27, No. 695, August 30, 1985*

Sustained release niacin is associated with the risk of additional side effects following long-term ingestion:

1. Hepatic toxicity is a rare complication which usually occurs with ingestion of over 3 gm daily of sustained release niacin (perform baseline liver function studies and repeat every 6-8 mo.) (*Mullin GE et al. Fulminant hepatic failure after ingestion of sustained-release nicotinic acid. Ann Intern Med 111(3):253-5, 1989; Patterson DJ et al. Niacin hepatitis. South Med J 76(2):239-41, 1983; Rader JI, Calvert RJ, Hathcock JN. Hepatic toxicity of unmodified and time-release preparation of niacin. Am J Med 92:77-81, 1992*).

See Also:

> Rader JI, Calvert RJ, Hathcock JN. *Hepatic toxicity of unmodified and time-release preparation of niacin. Am J Med 92:77-81, 1992*

> Coppola A, Brady P, Nord J. *Niacin-induced hepatotoxicity: unusual presentations. South Med J 87:30-2, 1994; Henkin Y et al. Rechallenge with crystalline niacin after drug-induced hepatitis from sustained-release niacin. JAMA 264(2):241-3, 1990*

> Mullin GE et al. *Fulminant hepatic failure after ingestion of sustained-release nicotinic acid. Ann Intern Med 111(3):253-5, 1989*

> Christensen NA et al. *Nicotinic acid treatment of hypercholesterolemia, comparison of plain and sustained action preparations, and report of two cases of jaundice. JAMA 177:546-50, 1961*

2. Prolonged bleeding may occur along with a prolonged thrombin time (*Dearing BD, Lavie CJ, Lohmann TP, Genton E. Niacin-induced clotting factor synthesis deficiency with coagulopathy. Arch Intern Med 152:861-3, 1992*).

3. Lactic acidosis may occur with nausea and vomiting (*Earthman T, Odom L, Mullins C. Lactic acidosis associated with high-dose niacin therapy. South Med J 84:496-7, 1991*).

Niacinamide (nicotinamide)

Sedation is a common side effect.

Large doses may cause <u>hepatic toxicity</u> *(Winter SL, Boyer JL. Hepatic toxicity from large doses of vitamin B$_3$ (nicotinamide). <u>N Engl J Med</u> 289(22):1180-2, 1973).*

Omega-3 Fatty Acids

Due to water pollution, some fatty fish and thus commercial fish oil supplements may contain concentrated quantities of mercury or polychlorinated dibenzodioxins and dibenzofurans if they are not removed during processing. Similarly, some fish oils contain large quantities of cholesterol that should be removed during processing *(Anastasios Salachas, M.D. - interviewed in <u>Clinical Pearls News</u> 5(5), May, 1995).*

Supplementation may require additional vitamin E intake to prevent increased membrane peroxidation and immune suppression.

Experimental Study: 9 healthy volunteers received a daily fish oil supplement providing 2.1 g DHA and 0.8 g EPA. Fish oil supplementation markedly decreased plasma vitamin E levels to below the normal range, even though the supplement contained additional vitamin E and synthetic antioxidants. Plasma vitamin E levels did not return to baseline values for 20 wks. after the supplement was discontinued *(Sanders TAB, Hinds A. The influence of a fish oil high in docosahexaenoic acid on plasma lipoprotein and vitamin E concentrations and hemostatic function in healthy male volunteers. <u>Br J Nutr</u> 68:163-73, 1992).*

Review Article: The major safety concern regarding omega-3 fatty acid supplements is their potential to undergo oxidation in the body. Susceptibility of fatty acids to oxidative damage increases proportionally to the degree of unsaturation, and these fatty acids are among the most unsaturated in the diet. However, this problem is easily overcome by increasing the coingestion of more vitamin E, beta-carotene, or other lipid-soluble antioxidants *(Leaf A. Health claims: omega-3 fatty acids and cardiovascular disease. <u>Nutr Rev</u> 50(5):150-2, 1992).*

Experimental Placebo-controlled Crossover Study: Healthy males ate a controlled basal diet providing a total of 40% of energy from fat when fed in conjunction with 15 g/d of either placebo oil (PO) or fish-oil concentrate (FOC) fortified with 15 mg all-*rac*-α-tocopherol/d for 3 periods. Subjects were supplemented with PO for 10 wks., with FOC for 10 wks., and with FOC plus an additional 200 mg α-tocopherol/d for 8 weeks. During FOC supplementation mitogenic responsiveness of peripheral blood mononuclear cells to concanavalin A stimulation was suppressed, but this effect was reversed by concurrent supplementation with α-tocopherol. There was a significant positive relationship ($p < 0.001$) between plasma α-tocopherol concentrations and responsiveness of T lymphocytes to concanavalin A *(Kramer TR et al. Increased vitamin E intake restores fish oil-induced suppressed blastogenesis of mitogen-stimulated T lymphocytes. <u>Am J Clin Nutr</u> 54:896-902, 1991).*

Experimental Study: 15 young women (aged 33-35) and 10 older women (aged 51-71) were supplemented with commercially available fish oil capsules. Plasma lipid peroxide levels significantly increased in both gps. through 2 mo. of supplementation and then declined but remained at higher levels than before supplementation. Older women had significantly higher lipid peroxide concentrations than younger women after 2 months. While plasma vitamin E concentrations did not change significantly after fish oil supplementation, plasma vitamin E levels were significantly lower in young women after 3 mo. of supplementation than after 1 month. There was also a significant decrease in the ratio of plasma vitamin E to EPA + DHA (which are present in the fish oils). These data suggest that long-term fish oil supplementation may potentiate susceptibility of plasma lipids to free radical attack, and that the vitamin E content of fish oil capsules may not be sufficient to provide adequate antioxidant protection (*Meydani M et al. Effect of long-term fish oil supplementation on vitamin E status and lipid peroxidation in women. J Nutr 121:484-91, 1991*).

Animal Experimental Study: Gps. of lupus-prone mice were fed diets similar in kcal., containing either 20% corn oil or 20% mehaden (fish) oil (which is high in omega-3 fatty acids). Both diets were supplemented with 75 IU of dl-alpha tocopherol acetate. When the fish diet was consumed, serum vitamin E levels dropped to 20% of the level on the corn oil diet. *In vitro* experiments equated this decline with increased free radical-induced peroxidation of cellular membranes. Both the drop in serum vitamin E and the increase in cellular damage were reversed within 1 mo. after vitamin E supplementation (*Laganiere S, Fernandes G. High peroxidizability of subcellular membrane induced by high fish oil diet is reversed by vitamin E. Clin Res 35:A565, 1987*).

See Also:

> *Meydani SN et al. Effect of age and dietary fat (fish, corn and coconut oils) on tocopherol status of C57BL/6Nia mice. Lipids 22:345-50, 1987*

Gastrointestinal side effects from fish oil ingestion are common (mild dyspepsia, belching, increased flatulence, diarrhea or a fishy aftertaste) which will cause about 10% of patients to discontinue the preparation. These side effects can be minimized by taking the supplement with food (*Anastasios Salachas, M.D. - interviewed in Clinical Pearls News 5(5), May, 1995*). An enteric-coated preparation (Purepa, Tillotts Pharma, Ziefen, Switzerland) reduces most gastrointestinal side-effects; however, 10% of patients still drop out due to specifically to diarrhea (*Belluzzi A, Brignola C, Campieri M, et al. Effect of an enteric-coated fish-oil preparation on relapses in Crohn's disease. N Engl J Med 334(24):1557-60, 1996*).

Supplementation may cause a temporary thrombocytopenia (*Goodnight S. The antithrombotic effects of fish oil, in AP Simopoulos et al, Eds. Health Effects of Polyunsaturated Fatty Acids in Seafoods. New York, Academic Press, 1986:135-48*).

> *Note: There have been no reports of clinically significant bleeding from the ingestion of omega-3 fatty acids, even when ingested with aspirin (Gerster H. n-3 fish oil polyunsaturated fatty acids and bleeding. J Nutr Environ Med 5:281-96, 1995; Leaf A. Health claims: omega-3 fatty acids and cardiovascular disease. Nutr Rev 50(5):150-2, 1992).*

In type I (insulin-dependent) diabetics, supplementation may increase total cholesterol with increases in both HDL2 and LDL fractions (*Vandongen R et al. Hypercholesterolaemic effect of fish oil in insulin-dependent diabetic patients. Med J Aust 148:141-3, 1988*).

While there is evidence that supplementation may increase fasting plasma glucose and triacylglycerol levels and decrease insulin activity in normals (*Bhathena SJ, Berlin E, Judd JT, et al. Effects of w-3 fatty acids and vitamin E on hormones involved in carbohydrate and lipid metabolism in men. Am J Clin Nutr 54(4):684-8, 1991*). there is also evidence that glucose metabolism may be unaffected by supplementation (*Toft I, Bonaa*

KH, Ingebretsen OC, et al.   Effects of N-3 polyunsaturated fatty acids on glucose homeostasis and blood pressure in essential hypertension: a randomized, controlled trial. Ann Intern Med 123(12):911-18, 1995).

In type II (non-insulin-dependent) diabetics, supplementation may increase <u>fasting plasma glucose concentrations</u>.

> *Note: The addition of extra vitamin E to fish oil may prevent adverse effects on the pancreatic insulin response.*

> **Experimental Double-blind Crossover Study:** 12 healthy males were given 30 ml per day of fish oil stabilized with vitamin E 1.5 IU/g (FO) or the same fish oil supplemented with an additional 4.5 IU vitamin E/g (FO+E), each for 4 wks., in random order. Fasting blood glucose levels increased significantly by 9.1% during the FO period, but did not change significantly after FO+E. Moreover, while the fasting insulin/glucose ratio did not change after FO, it increased significantly after FO+E, suggesting a more adequate pancreatic insulin response to glucose *(Luostarinen R et al. Vitamin E supplementation counteracts the fish oil-induced increase of blood glucose in humans. Nutr Res 15:953-68, 1995).*

Review Article: 13 studies examining the effects of fish oils in pts. with type II diabetes were reviewed. An increase in fasting plasma glucose was observed in 2/6 controlled studies and in 4/7 uncontrolled studies *(Puhakainen I, Ahola I, Yki-Järvinen H. Dietary supplementation with n-3 fatty acids increases gluconeogenesis from glycerol but not hepatic glucose production in patients with non-insulin-dependent diabetes mellitus. Am J Clin Nutr 61:121-6, 1995).*

Supplementation may decrease several indices of <u>cell-mediated immunity</u>.

> *Note: There have been no reports of undue reductions in immune or inflammatory responses to omega-3 fatty acid supplementation (Leaf A. Health claims: omega-3 fatty acids and cardiovascular disease. Nutr Rev 50(5):150-2, 1992).*

Experimental Study: Subjects consumed a typical American diet (15% saturated, 15% monounsaturated, 5% omega-6 fatty acids, 1% omega-3 fatty acids, and 180 mg cholesterol/1000 calories) for 6 wks. and were then switched to a low-fat, low-cholesterol diet containing 5% saturated, 12% monounsaturated, 7.5% omega-6 fatty acids, 2.5% omega-3 fatty acids from fish oils, and 60 mg cholesterol/1000 calories. On the latter diet, omega-3 fatty acid plasma levels rose and prostaglandin E_2 levels decreased. Helper and suppressor T cell activity and numerous other indices of immune function also decreased, suggesting that an omega-3-enriched, low-fat diet may increase susceptibility to infection and disease *(Meydani S et al. Effect of low-fat, low cholesterol (LF-FCHL) diet enriched in N-3 fatty acids (FA) on the immune response of humans. FASEB J 5:1449A, 1991).*

Omega-6 Fatty Acids

Supplementation may require additional vitamin E to minimize the potential damage of excessive <u>lipid peroxidation</u> *(Reddy ACP, Lokesh BR. Dietary unsaturated fatty acids, vitamin E, curcumin and eugenol alter serum and liver lipid peroxidation in rats. Nutr Res 14:1423-37, 1994).*

Prolonged supplementation with high doses (ex. 2 g/d) of gamma-linolenic acid may increase the serum phospholipid content of <u>arachidonic acid</u>, the primary precursor for several pro-inflammatory prostaglandins and leukotrienes (*Phinney S. Potential risk of prolonged gamma-linolenic acid use. Letter. <u>Ann Intern Med</u> 120(8):692, 1994*).

Gamma-linolenic acid may exacerbate <u>temporal lobe epilepsy</u> (*Holman CP, Bell AFJ. A trial of evening primrose oil in the treatment of chronic schizophrenia. <u>J Orthomol Psychiatry</u> 12:302-4, 1983; Vaddadi KS. The use of gamma-linolenic acid and linoleic acid to differentiate between temporal lobe epilepsy and schizophrenia. <u>Prostaglandins Med</u> 6:375-9, 1981*).

Gamma-linolenic acid may exacerbate <u>mania</u> (*Horrobin DF. The regulation of prostaglandin biosynthesis by the manipulation of essential fatty acid metabolism. <u>Rev Pure Appl Pharmacol</u> 4:339-83, 1983*).

Para-amino Benzoic Acid

Potential side-effects include <u>skin rash</u>, <u>anorexia</u>, <u>nausea</u> and <u>fever</u> (*<u>Physicians' Desk Reference</u>. Oradell, NJ, Med. Economics Co., Inc., 1986*) as well as <u>vitiligo</u> (*Hughes CG. Oral PABA and vitiligo. <u>J Am Acad Dermatol</u> 9:770, 1983*) and <u>liver toxicity</u> (*Kantor GR, Ratz JL. Liver toxicity from potassium para-aminobenzoate. Letter. <u>J Am Acad Dermatol</u> 13(4):671-2, 1985*).

Phenylalanine

Supplementation may cause <u>anxiety</u>, <u>headache</u> and <u>hypertension</u> and should be avoided by <u>phenylketourics</u> and women who are pregnant or lactating.

Potassium

Supplementation may be dangerous for the elderly and for patients suffering from <u>renal impairment</u> and those taking certain drugs such as potassium-sparing diuretics, angiotensin converting enzyme inhibitors and non-steroidal anti-inflammatory drugs (*Swales JD. Salt substitutes and potassium intake. Too much potassium intake may be disastrous for some. <u>Br J Med</u> 303:1084-5, 1991*).

Quercetin

Review Article: Although found to be mutagenic *in vitro*, quercetin has been shown to be anticarcinogenic *in vivo* (*Stavric B. Quercetin in our diet: from potent mutagen to probably anticarcinogen. <u>Clin Biochem</u> 27(4):245-8, 1994*).

Review Article: Has been shown to be mutagenic to mammalian cells *in vitro*; however all but one *in vivo* study of carcinogenicity have been negative, and numerous researchers have been unable to confirm the results of that study despite using markedly greater dosages. In addition, the one positive study found an increase in bladder cancer in a strain of rat known to have an extremely high rate of spontaneous bladder cancer. More recent research seems to support quercetin as a <u>suppressor</u> of tumor formation (*Murray MT. "Disinformation" concerning quercetin. Letter. <u>Townsend Letter for Doctors</u> 53:377-78, 1987*).

See Also:

> *Nishino H et al. Interaction between quercetin and Ca^{++}-calmodulin complex: Possible mechanism for anti-tumor-promoting action of the flavonoid.* <u>Gann</u> *74:311-16, 1984*

S-Adenosylmethionine

Side effects, usually mild and transient, include <u>dry mouth</u>, <u>thirst</u>, <u>nausea</u>, <u>gas</u>, <u>urinary delay</u>, <u>blurred vision</u>, <u>headache</u>, <u>sweating</u>, <u>anxiety</u>, and <u>restlessness</u>. In perhaps 10-15% of patients, <u>hypomania</u> or <u>mania</u> may develop, especially if they have a history of mania (*Rosenbaum JF et al. An open-label pilot study of oral S-adenosyl-L-methionine in major depression: interim results.* <u>Psychopharmacol Bull</u> *24(1):189-94, 1988*).

Selenium

Toxicity may be associated with <u>hair loss</u>, <u>thickened, fragile fingernails</u>, <u>muscle discomfort</u>, <u>dermatitis</u>, <u>nausea</u>, <u>garlic breath odor</u>, <u>fatigue</u> and <u>suppression of phagocytic and natural killer cell function</u>.

> **Case Reports:** About a dozen cases of selenium toxicity were reported to the Centers for Disease Control (U.S.) after a manufacturing error led to the distribution of a selenium supplement containing 25,000 µg instead of the intended 150 µg. One of these was published. Symptoms included loss of hair and nails, nausea and fatigue (*MMWR Mortal Wkly Rep 33(12):157-8, 1984*).

<u>Selenite</u> has been shown in a Japanese study to interact with glutathione in the presence of oxygen to generate free radicals. Since glutathione is found in all cells, this form of selenium may be unsuitable for human use (*Schrauzer GN. Benefits of nutritional selenium. Report of presentation from the Fourth International Symposium on Selenium in Biology and Medicine, Tubingen U., W. Germany, July, 1988.* <u>Anabolism</u> *7(4):5, 1988*).

Sodium <u>selenate</u> in high dosage is less likely to be toxic as it is more rapidly excreted in the urine than selenite (*Thompson CD, Robinson MF. Urinary and fecal excretions and absorption of a large supplement of selenium: Superiority of selenate over selenite.* <u>Am J Clin Nutr</u> *44:659-63, 1986*).

Thiamine

Toxic side-effects have mostly occurred after intramuscular or parenteral injections which occasionally cause an acute allergic reaction including <u>generalized urticaria</u>, <u>facial edema</u>, <u>dyspnea</u>, <u>cyanosis</u>, <u>wheezing</u> and <u>anaphylactic shock</u>.

Oral supplementation has very rarely produced side-effects, although <u>nervousness</u>, <u>itching</u>, <u>flushing</u>, <u>shortness of breath</u>, <u>tachycardia</u>, a <u>sensation of heat</u> and <u>perfuse perspiration</u> have been reported. (*Buist RA. Editorial: Vitamin toxicities, side effects and contraindications.* <u>Int Clin Nutr Rev</u> *4(4):159-71, 1984*). Other symptoms include <u>headache</u>, <u>insomnia</u>, <u>irritability</u>, <u>muscle tremors</u> and <u>weakness</u> (*Clarence Mills, professor, U. of Cincinnati College of Medicine, 1940 - reported in Hausman P.* <u>The Right Dose: How to Take Vitamins and Minerals Safely</u>. *New York, Ballantine Books, 1987*).

High dosages of thiamine in nutritional supplements may stimulate lipid peroxidation (*Hu M, Chen Y, Lin Y. the antioxidant and prooxidant activity of some B-vitamins and vitamin-like compounds. Chem Biol Interact 97:63-73, 1995*).

L-Tryptophan

In recent years, the ingestion of tryptophan supplements has been associated with the eosinophilia-myalgia syndrome (*Martin RW et al. The clinical spectrum of the eosinophilia-myalgia syndrome associated with L-tryptophan ingestion. Ann Intern Med 113:124-34, 1990*). While most cases are now known to be due to a contaminant introduced during the manufacturing process by one manufacturer (*Mayeno AN et al. Characterization of 'peak E' a novel amino acid associated with exposure of tryptophan from a single manufacturer. JAMA 264:213-17, 1990*), tryptophan has been removed from the market in many countries until its safety is better proven.

It has been suggested (*Soukes TL. Toxicology of serotonin precursors. Adv Biol Psychiatry 10:160-75, 1983*) that the following groups not receive large, chronic doses of tryptophan:

1. Patients with cancer or a history of it
2. Patients with any source of irritation of the urinary bladder
3. Children and pregnant women
4. Diabetics and patients with a family history of diabetes
5. Patients with a history of any scleroderma-like condition
6. Patients with large flora high in the intestinal tract (e.g. those with achlorhydria)

High doses are frequently associated with nausea (*Greenwood MW et al. The acute effects of oral tryptophan in human subjects. Br J Clin Pharmacol 2:165-72, 1975*).

Supplementation may aggravate bronchial asthma.

> **Experimental Double-blind Study:** Pts. with bronchial asthma on a low-tryptophan diet improved (*Urge G et al. Effect of dietary tryptophan restrictions on clinical symptoms in patients with endogenous asthma. Allergy 38:211-2, 1983*).

Lupus patients are said to have decreased serotonin levels, perhaps due to deficient conversion of tryptophan to serotonin. The tryptophan breakdown products may lead to auto-antibody production (*McCormick JP et al. Characterization of a cell-lethal product from the photooxidation of tryptophan: Hydrogen peroxide. Science 191:468-9, 1976*).

> **Review Article:** Lupus pts. demonstrated an abnormal tryptophan metabolism with high excretion particularly of kynurenines and xanthurenic acid (*Cardin de' Stefani E, Costa C. [Changes in the metabolism of tryptophan in erythematosus.] Boll Soc Ital Biol Sper 60(8):1535-40, 1984*).

Supplementation may be harmful during pregnancy (*Meier AH, Wilson JM. Tryptophan feeding adversely influences pregnancy. Life Sci 32:1193, 1983*).

Supplementation may promote bladder cancer in patients who are vitamin B_6-deficient (*Birt DF et al. Effect of L-tryptophan excess and vitamin B_6 deficiency on rat urinary bladder cancer promotion. Cancer Res 47:1244-50, 1987*).

Supplementation may be toxic to patients with adrenal insufficiency (*Trulson ME et al. Low doses of L-tryptophan are lethal in rats with adrenal insufficiency. Life Sci 41:349-53, 1987*).

Supplementation may reduce the efficacy of <u>morphine analgesia</u> (*Franklin KB et al. Tryptophan-morphine interactions and postoperative pain. Pharmacol Biochem Behav 35(1):157-63, 1990*).

Tyrosine

May have a mild <u>stimulant</u> effect (*Elwes RDC et al. Treatment of narcolepsy with L-tyrosine: double-blind placebo-controlled trial. Lancet ii:1067-9, 1989*).

Vanadium

Studies of diabetic rats treated with vanadyl or vanadate to improve glucose homeostatis found tissue accumulation and evidence of serious toxicity at the dosages utilized (*Domingo JL, Gomez M, Llobet JM, et al. Toxicology 66:279-87, 1991; Domingo JL, Gomez M, Llobet JM, et al. Toxicology 68:249-53, 1991*), while human studies have yet to be published proving the safety of pharmacological dosages.

Vitamin A

> *Note:* *Vitamin E ameliorates the adverse side effects of hypervitaminosis A* (*Graf N et al. Retinoids in the treatment of acute promyelocytic leukemia: review of the literature. Klin Pediatr 207:43-7, 1995; Tappel AL. Nutrition Today July-August 1973; Weiser H, Probst HP, Bachmann H. Vitamin E prevents side effects of high doses of vitamin A in chicks. Ann N Y Acad Sci 669:396-8, 1992*).

> *Note:* *"The synthetic retinoids are comparable to vitamin A in their spectrum of toxicity"* (*Lippman SM, Hong WK. Chemoprevention of aerodigestive epithelial cancers. Adv Exp Med Biol 320:151-61, 1992*).

Hypervitaminosis A is by far the most common cause of vitamin toxicity. The dosage required to produce toxicity is highly variable. While it is possible to receive as much as 1 million IU daily for 5 years without developing toxicity (*Hruban Z et al. Am J Pathol 76:451-61, 1974*), doses of ≥100,000 IU/d for days to weeks, or doses as low as 25,000-50,000 IU/d for several months or longer can produce toxic effects, especially in persons with liver function compromised by drugs, viral hepatitis, or protein-energy malnutrition. Reports of toxicity in adults with supplemental intakes <50,000 IU/d mainly involve persons with unusually high dietary intakes or with confounding medical conditions (*Hathcock JN et al. Evaluation of vitamin A toxicity. Am J Clin Nutr 52:183-202, 1990*).

Worldwide, the incidence of vitamin A excess, or hypervitaminosis A, is estimated to be only 200 cases annually (*Bauernfeind JC. The Safe Use Of Vitamin A: A Report of the International Vitamin A Consultative Group. Washington, DC, The Nutrition Foundation, 1980*). Over the last 50 years, the number of reported cases has remained relatively constant despite the significant growth in production and use of vitamin A supplements (*Bendich A, Langseth L. Safety of vitamin A. Am J Clin Nutr 49:358-71, 1989*).

When vitamin A toxicity has developed following administration under medical supervision, so that the level of reported intake is likely to be more accurate, manifestations of hypervitaminosis A were abstract or slight (*Bauernfeind JC. The Safe Use Of Vitamin A: A Report of the International Vitamin A Consultative Group. Washington, DC, The Nutrition Foundation, 1980*).

Reported manifestations of chronic toxicity include <u>fatigue, malaise and lethargy</u>, <u>headaches</u>, <u>abdominal discomfort</u>, <u>constipation</u>, <u>insomnia</u> and <u>restlessness</u>. Later, <u>night sweats</u>, <u>alopecia</u>, brittle nails, irregular menses, emotional lability, mouth fissures, dry, scaly, rough, yellowish skin, superficial retinal hemorrhages, exophthalmos, peripheral edema and increased intracranial pressure with headaches, nausea and vomiting may develop *(Buist RA. Editorial: Vitamin toxicities, side effects and contraindications. Int Clin Nutr Rev 4(4):159-71, 1984).*

Daily doses higher than 10,000 IU of preformed vitamin A are contraindicated during pregnancy as they appear to be teratogenic *(Rothman KJ, Moore LL, Singer MR, et al. Teratogenicity of high vitamin A intake. N Engl J Med 333(21):1369-73, 1995).*

May cause abnormal bone growth in young children due to premature epiphyseal closing and thickening of the cortical regions *(Buist RA. Editorial: Vitamin toxicities, side effects and contraindications. Int Clin Nutr Rev 4(4):159-71, 1984).*

Very high doses of vitamin A have been shown to produce more than 70 types of congenital abnormalities in experimental animals, and 5 cases of human birth defects have been reported where unusually high doses of vitamin A had been taken during pregnancy; however, no clear cause-and-effect relationship was demonstrated in any of these cases *(Bauernfeind JC. The Safe Use Of Vitamin A: A Report of the International Vitamin A Consultative Group. Washington, DC, The Nutrition Foundation, 1980).*

Hypervitaminosis A is often associated with hypercalcemia and hypercalciuria and calcium deposition in soft tissues may occur *(Buist RA. Editorial: Vitamin toxicities, side effects and contraindications. Int Clin Nutr Rev 4(4):159-71, 1984).*

Hyperplasia of both liver and spleen may occur with chronic consumption as low and 25,000 IU/d with elevation of AST. Liver biopsies reveal hepatic fibrosis, fat deposition, obstruction of portal blood flow with portal hypertension and sclerosis of vessels *(Iatrogenic liver disease from vitamin A. Nutr Rev 49(10):309-12, 1991; Buist RA. Editorial: Vitamin toxicities, side effects and contraindications. Int Clin Nutr Rev 4(4):159-71, 1984; Krasinski SD et al. Relationship of vitamin A and vitamin E intake to fasting plasma retinol, retinol-binding protein, retinyl esters, carotene, α-tocopherol, and cholesterol among elderly people and young adults: increased plasma retinyl esters among vitamin A-supplement users. Am J Clin Nutr 49:112-20, 1989).*

Elevated retinol levels may play an important role in the development of some attacks of gouty arthritis *(Marson AR. Letter. Lancet i:1181, 1984).*

In most cases, when vitamin A intake is discontinued, many symptoms are relieved within a few days or a week, and full recovery usually follows within weeks or months. Irreversible effects include bone changes and cirrhosis *(Bauernfeind JC. The Safe Use Of Vitamin A: A Report of the International Vitamin A Consultative Group. Washington, DC, The Nutrition Foundation, 1980).*

Vitamin B₆

Supplementation may cause a sensory neuropathy in doses as low as 200 mg daily over 3 years (usually 2-5 gm daily). The neurotoxicity is believed to be due to exceeding the liver's ability to phosphorylate pyridoxine to the active coenzyme, pyridoxal phosphate. The resulting high pyridoxine blood level could be directly neurotoxic or may compete for binding sites with pyridoxal phosphate resulting in a relative deficiency of the active metabolite *(Parry GJ, Bredesen DE. Sensory neuropathy with low-dose pyridoxine. Neurology 35:1466-8, 1985; Waterston JA, Gilligan BS. Pyridoxine neuropathy. Med J*

Aust 146:640-2, 1987). Supplementation in the form of pyridoxal phosphate should thus avoid this danger.

> **Experimental and Observational Study:** 103/172 (60%) women with premenstrual syndrome who had elevated blood pyridoxine levels complained of neurological symptoms (paresthesias, hyperesthesia, bone pain, muscle weakness, numbness, fasciculations). On average, their daily dose had been 117 mg for 2.9 years. 3 mo. after stopping B_6 supplements (and following a program of PMS treatment), 55% reported partial or complete symptom relief. After 6 mo., all women were asymptomatic. 7 pts. who failed to stop B_6 continued to have symptoms *(Dalton K, Dalton MJT. Characteristics of pyridoxine overdose neuropathy syndrome. Acta Neurol Scand 76:8, 1987).*

> *Note: Vague neurological complaints are common among PMS sufferers and may be due to numerous causes. This uncontrolled study on patients who were simultaneously in active multi-faceted treatment program fails to demonstrate that symptom relief was due to stopping pyridoxine supplements. The patients who failed to improve and also failed to stop pyridoxine may well have been treatment failures because of their failure to comply with other aspects of the treatment program (Gaby AR. Editorial: Vitamin B_6 toxicity: How much is too much? Townsend Letter for Doctors, May, 1988, p. 184).*

Supplementation with 100 mg or more daily may impair <u>memorization</u>.

> **Experimental Placebo-controlled Study:** 58 students took 100 or 500 mg of pyridoxine or a placebo. After 10 days, the 500 mg/d gp. scored significantly worse on a standard memorization test than the placebo group. While the 100 mg/d gp. also scored worse than the placebo gp., the difference failed to reach significance *(Molimard R et al. Impairment of memorization by high doses of pyridoxine in man. Biomedicine 32:88-92, 1980).*

Supplementation may cause an <u>acneiform eruption</u> or worsening of <u>acne vulgaris</u>.

> **Observational Study:** Deterioration of acne vulgaris or eruption of an acneiform exanthema could be established during treatment with vitamin B_6 and/or vitamin B_{12} in 14 patients. Females were by far the more frequently affected. Characteristic is the appearance of lesions outside the typical age group affected by acne vulgaris. Lesions consisted of loosely disseminated small papules or papulopustules on the face (especially on the forehead and chin), on the upper parts of the back and chest and spreading to the upper arm and usually faded shortly after B_6 or B_{12} was stopped *(Braun-Falco O, Lincke H. [The problem of vitamin B_6/B_{12} acne. A contribution on acne medicamentosa. MMW 118(6):155-60, 1976).*

See Also:

> *Sheretz EF. Acneform eruption due to megadose vitamins B_6 and B_{12}. Cutis 48:19-20, 1991*

Supplementation at doses of at least 100 times the recommended daily allowance of 1.6-2 mg may be toxic to the central nervous system.

Animal Experimental Study: 12 female rats received 1, 10, 100, 200 or 300 times the requirement of vitamin B_6 for 7 weeks. Their startle reflex was significantly weakened at the 3 highest levels of intake. When a prepulse (a nonstartling stimulus) proceeded the startle stimulus, the gps. fed the 2 highest doses demonstrated weakened reflexes as compared to the gps. fed the lower doses (*Schaeffer M. Excess dietary vitamin B_6 alters startle behavior of rats. J Nutr 123:1444-52, 1993*).

High dosages of pyridoxine, but not of pyridoxal, in nutritional supplements may stimulate lipid peroxidation (*Hu M, Chen Y, Lin Y. the antioxidant and prooxidant activity of some B-vitamins and vitamin-like compounds. Chem Biol Interact 97:63-73, 1995*).

Vitamin B_{12}

In multivitamin/multimineral preparations, vitamin B_{12} (cyanocobalamin), through an interaction with the combination of thiamine, vitamin C and copper, may be converted into inactive analogs which may fail to stimulate or even inhibit cobalamin-dependent enzymes, suggesting that vitamins and minerals should be provided separately (*Kondo H, Mitchell JB, Kolhouse FJ, et al. Presence and formation of cobalamin analogs in multivitamin-mineral pills. J Clin Invest 70(4):889-98, 1982*).

In vitro and Animal Experimental Studies: 3 popular multivitamin-mineral pills were homogenized in water, incubated at 37^0 C for 2 hrs., and the cobalamin isolated. 20-90% of the cobalamin was in the form of cobalamin analogs formed by the concerted action of thiamine, vitamin C and copper on cyanocobalamin. In mice, these analogs are absorbed from the GI tract and either fail to stimulate or actually inhibit cobalamin-dependent enzymes when injected parenterally. Results suggest that the existence of these interactions in multivitamin-mineral pills may be responsible for the presence of cobalamin analogs in human blood and tissues, and the presence of them in animal chow may be responsible for the analogs in animal blood and tissues (*Kondo H, Mitchell JB, Kolhouse FJ, et al. Presence and formation of cobalamin analogs in multivitamin-mineral pills. J Clin Invest 70(4):889-98, 1982*).

Supplementation may cause an acneiform eruption or worsening of acne vulgaris.

Observational Study: Deterioration of acne vulgaris or eruption of an acneiform exanthema could be established during treatment with vitamin B_6 and/or vitamin B_{12} in 14 patients. Females were by far the more frequently affected. Characteristic is the appearance of lesions outside the typical age group affected by acne vulgaris. Lesions consisted of loosely disseminated small papules or papulopustules on the face (especially on the forehead and chin), on the upper parts of the back and chest and spreading to the upper arm and usually faded shortly after B_6 or B_{12} was stopped (*Braun-Falco O, Lincke H. [The problem of vitamin B_6/B_{12} acne. A contribution on acne medicamentosa. MMW 118(6):155-60, 1976*).

See Also:

Sheretz EF. Acneform eruption due to megadose vitamins B_6 and B_{12}. Cutis 48:19-20, 1991

Vitamin C

High supplemental doses appear to be safe for healthy people (*Diplock AT. Safety of antioxidant vitamins and β-carotene. Am J Clin Nutr 62(suppl):1510S-16S, 1995; Rivers JM. Safety of high-level vitamin C ingestion. Ann N Y Acad Sci 498:445-54, 1987*).

Diarrhea, or abdominal cramping, is the major side-effect of large doses (*Korner WF, Weber F. Tolerance of high ascorbic acid doses. Int J Vitam Res 42:528, 1972*).

The risk of hip fractures in older women may be increased by a high vitamin C intake if calcium intake is high.

> **Observational Study:** From an initial cohort of 65,000 Swedish women aged 40-75, 272 subsequent cases of hip fractures and 1024 matched controls were studied. There was an increased risk of fracture with high dietary intakes of vitamin C which was non-significant when calcium intake was low and more pronounced when calcium intake was high (*Michaelsson K, Holmberg L, Mallmin H, et al. Diet and hip fracture risk: case-control study. Int J Epidemiol 24(4):771-81, 1995*).

Enhances aluminum absorption; therefore should not be taken with aluminum-containing substances, especially when the patient has renal insufficiency (*Domingo JL et al. Effect of ascorbic acid on gastrointestinal aluminum absorption. Letter. Lancet 338:1467, 1991*).

In vitro, mixtures of ascorbic acid with iron or copper can accelerate oxidative damage. This is often dismissed as irrelevant *in vivo* because such ions are usually safely protein-bound, and any danger can be futher mitigated by ingesting ascorbic acid with food (whose buffering action increases gastric pH which increases protein binding). However, free iron or copper ions may be released at sites of tissue injury, in which case, theoretically at least, high ascorbate levels may promote oxidative damage (*Halliwell B, Cross CE, Gutteridge JM. Free radicals, antioxidants and human disease: where are we now? J Lab Clin Med 119:598-620, 1992; Halliwell B, Gutteridge JM. The antioxidants of human extracellular fluids. Arch Biochem Biophys 280:1-8, 1990; Halliwell B, Gutteridge JM. Free Radicals in Biology and Medicine, second edition. Oxford, Clarendon Press, 1989; Maskos Z, Koppenol WH. Oxyradicals and multivitamin tablets. Free Rad Biol Med 11:609-10, 1991*).

High dose supplementation may interfere with certain laboratory tests for glucose, uric acid, creatinine, and inorganic phosphate, and can interfere with the detection of occult blood in feces (*Bendich A, Langseth L. The health effects of vitamin C supplementation: a review. J Am Coll Nutr 14(2):124-36, 1995*).

Megadoses do not appear to increase the risk of urinary oxalate stones in most instances.

> *Note:* "The apparent increase [found in some studies] in the urine samples during ascorbate supplementation could be more than accounted for by nonenzymatic conversion during analysis of ascorbate present in the urine sample into oxalate. Furthermore, making the assumption that the oxalate increase measured reflects the actual urine oxalate content and not that generated from nonenzymatic conversion of ascorbate into oxalate during the analysis of oxalate, the increase in the level of urinary oxalate due to ascorbate ingestion . . . is small and of equivocal physiological importance" (*Wandzilak TR et al. Effect of high dose vitamin C on urinary oxalate levels. J Urol 151(4):834-7, 1994*).

Note: It has been argued that any increase in urinary oxalate can be prevented by taking supplemental vitamin B_6 (The Linus Pauling Newsletter 1(4), Fall, 1978).

Case Report: When a pt. began taking 8 g/d of vitamin C, his urinary oxalate level increased from 40 to 383 mg/24 hr., thus demonstrating that he had an unusual tendency towards hyperoxaluria. However, 2 wks. after adding vitamin B_6 50 mg twice daily, his 24 hr. urinary oxalate had dropped to 57 mg *(Wright JV. High-dose vitamin C and kidney stones, in Dr. Wright's Book of Nutritional Therapy. Emmaus, PA, Rodale Press, 1979:272-7).*

Review Article: "The formation of urinary oxalate stones in subjects ingesting large amounts of vitamin C over a long period proved to be without foundation. . . . Excretion of oxalate derived from ascorbate accounts for ≈35-40% of the daily excretion of oxalate, but ingestion of large amounts of vitamin C does not result in any more than a small increase in the excretion of oxalate. . . . No dose-response relation exists between administered vitamin C and excreted oxalate. . . . The conversion of ascorbate to oxalate in vivo is thus considered to be minimal and cannot be detected when fresh samples of urine are analyzed" *(Diplock AT. Safety of antioxidant vitamins and β-carotene. Am J Clin Nutr 62(suppl):1510S-16S, 1995).*

Review Article: Several studies have found no evidence that vitamin C increases the risk of kidney stone formation *(Bendich A, Langseth L. The health effects of vitamin C supplementation: a review. J Am Coll Nutr 14(2):124-36, 1995).*

Review Article: Urinary oxalate excretion generally does not increase significantly for both normal subjects and stone-formers with ascorbic acid supplementation unless doses exceed 6 gm daily; however, oxalate excretion even at those high doses is still usually in the range achievable by dietary influences alone. The exceptions derive from anecdotal reports of a small number of cases and from one poorly-controlled trial with unstated methodology and questionable assay techniques *(Piesse JW. Nutritional factors in calcium containing kidney stones with particular emphasis on vitamin C. Int Clin Nutr Rev 5(3):110-29, 1985).*

The regulation of body iron stores appear to be unaffected by any increased availability of iron from the diet that might be caused by excess ascorbate; even in patients with hemochromatosis there is almost no effect of vitamin C *(Diplock AT. Safety of antioxidant vitamins and β-carotene. Am J Clin Nutr 62(suppl):1510S-16S, 1995).*

The evidence does <u>not</u> support claims that ascorbic acid promotes uricosuria. Even in patients with gout or hyperuricosuria, it is doubtful that large doses of ascorbic acid would lead to increased uric acid excretion *(Rivers JM. Safety of high-level vitamin C ingestion. Ann N Y Acad Sci 498:445-54, 1987).*

There is <u>no</u> support for earlier concerns that large daily intakes of ascorbic acid will induce vitamin B_{12} deficiency, as vitamin B_{12} in food and the body is not destroyed by ascorbic acid *(Rivers JM. Safety of high-level vitamin C ingestion. Ann N Y Acad Sci 498:445-54, 1987).*

Early reports of rebound scurvy after withdrawal of high doses of vitamin C supplements were uncontrolled and have not been substantiated. Moreover, studies in guinea pigs have failed to find evidence of increased catabolism of ascorbate following withdrawal from high doses *(Diplock AT.*

Safety of antioxidant vitamins and β-carotene. Am J Clin Nutr 62(suppl):1510S-16S, 1995; (Rivers JM. Safety of high-level vitamin C ingestion. Ann N Y Acad Sci 498:445-54, 1987).

Vitamin D

Excessive intake may cause hypercalcemia due to increased intestinal absorption of calcium which can quickly lead to reduction of kidney function (due to nephrocalcinosis from deposition of calcium phosphate) and soft tissue calcifications, especially in the joints, blood vessels, stomach, lungs and heart *(Buist RA. Editorial: Vitamin toxicities, side effects and contraindications. Int Clin Nutr Rev 4(4):159-71, 1984).*

Vitamin E

In reviewing over 10,000 cases of subjects consuming 200-3000 IU/d for up to 11 years, the incidence of nonspecific side effects was 0.8%, a level expected in untreated populations *(Salkald RM. Safety and tolerance of high-dose vitamin E administration in man: A review of the literature. Fed Register (US) 44:16172, 1979).*

Reports of adverse symptoms from large supplemental doses are largely subjective and based on limited observations; they include diarrhea, fatigue, weakness, intestinal cramps, breast soreness, thrombophlebitis and acne. In fact, doses as high as 3200 mg/d have not been found to induce adverse side effects. However, vitamin E supplementation has been shown to exacerbate the effects of vitamin K deficiency *(Bendich A, Machlin LJ. Safety of oral intake of vitamin E. Am J Clin Nutr 48:612-19, 1988).*

The most common complaint following large supplemental doses is transient gastrointestinal disturbances (nausea, flatulence, or diarrhea) *(Bieri JG. Medical uses of vitamin E. N Engl J Med 308(18):1063-71, 1983).*

Supplementation may exacerbate hypertension. When the oily form is used, this effect is accompanied by an increase in the serum triglycerides:vitamin E ratio; thus the water miscible form is preferred for patients with cardiovascular disorders and diabetes mellitus *(Buist RA. Editorial: Vitamin toxicities, side effects and contraindications. Int Clin Nutr Rev 4(4):159-71, 1984).*

As Vitamin E may reduce the insulin requirement, diabetics on insulin should be started on 100 IU or less daily and the dosage raised slowly with adjustment of the insulin dose *(Vogelsang A. Vitamin E in the treatment of diabetes mellitus. Ann N Y Acad Sci 52:406, 1949).*

Vitamin E at high intakes only affects blood clotting if a vitamin K deficiency is present; otherwise it does not cause coagulation abnormalities *(Kappus H, Diplock AT. Tolerance and safety of vitamin E: a toxicological position report. Free Radic Biol Med 13:55-74, 1992).*

During pregnancy, daily doses of 40,000 IU or more may be teratogenic *(Martinez-Frias ML, Salvador J. Megadose vitamin A and teratogenicity. Letter. Lancet i:236, 1988),* while doses lower than 10,000 IU appear to be safe *(Smithell RW. Spina bifida and vitamins. Br Med J 286:388-9, 1983).*

A double-blind study *(Kitagawa M, Mino M. Effects of elevated d-alpha (RRR)-tocopherol dosage in man. J Nutr Sci Vitaminol (Tokyo):35(2):133-42, 1989)* has failed to confirm reports that megadoses of vitamin E may cause a decrease in thyroid hormone *(Roberts HJ. Thrombophlebitis associated with vitamin E therapy with commentary on other medical side effects. Angiology 30:169-76, 1979; Tsai AC et al. Study on the effect of megavitamin E supplementation in man. Am J Clin Nutr 31:831-7, 1978).*

Zinc

Pharmacological doses of zinc (≈100-300 mg daily) for several months can produce a severe copper deficiency causing <u>hypocupremia</u>, <u>anemia</u>, <u>leukopenia</u> and <u>neutropenia</u> *(Copper deficiency induced by megadoses of zinc. Nutr Rev 43(5):148-9, 1985; Broun RE et al. Excessive zinc ingestion: a reversible cause of sideroblastic anemia and bone marrow depression. JAMA 264:1441-3, 1990; Forman WB et al. Zinc abuse: an unsuspected cause of sideroblastic anemia. West J Med 152:190-2, 1990; Hoffman HN II et al. Zinc-induced copper deficiency. Gastroenterology 94:508-12, 1988; Prasad AS et al. Hypocupremia induced by zinc deficiency in adults. JAMA 240:2166-8, 1978).*

> *Note: Concurrent supplementation with 1.0 mg daily of copper will prevent copper deficiency due to zinc supplementation; also copper status can be easily monitored by following serum ceruloplasmin levels (Yuzbasiyan-Gurkan V, Brewer GJ. The therapeutic use of zinc in macular degeneration. Letter. Arch Ophthalmol 107:1723, 1989).*

Similarly, the lowering of copper levels in response to high doses of zinc (>150 mg daily) may be responsible for causing a marked <u>decrease in HDL cholesterol</u> *(Hooper PL et al. Zinc lowers high-density lipoprotein-cholesterol levels. JAMA 244:1960, 1980; Klevey LM. Interactions of copper and zinc in cardiovascular disease. Ann N Y Acad Sci 355:140-51, 1980; Fischer P et al. The effect of dietary copper and zinc on cholesterol metabolism. Am J Clin Nutr 33:1019-25, 1980).*

Abnormalities in cardiac function are common when zinc is supplemented without concurrent copper supplementation.

> **Review Article:** In published studies, nearly 16% of 51 subjects who appeared to have normal cardiac status at baseline displayed cardiac abnormalities that were associated with a dietary zinc to copper ratio of ≥ 16 as compared to a ratio of 5-14 in the diets consumed by many Americans (8-12 mg Zn; 0.8-1.5 mg Cu). However, prior copper status was unknown. Based on the limited research done, it is suggested that supplementation with more than 9 mg zinc daily may be unsafe *(Sandstead HH. Requirements and toxicity of essential trace elements, illustrated by zinc and copper. Am J Clin Nutr 61(suppl):621S-4S, 1995).*

See Also:

> **General Review Article:** *Fosmire GJ. Zinc toxicity. Am J Clin Nutr 51:225-7, 1990*

Pharmacological doses of zinc (≈100-300 mg daily) for several weeks can <u>impair immune responses</u>.

> **Experimental Study:** 11 healthy adult men ingested 150 mg of elemental zinc twice daily. After 6 wks., there was a reduction in lymphocyte stimulation response to phytohemagglutinin as well as a reduction in chemotaxis and phagocytosis of bacteria by polymorphonuclear leukocytes *(Chandra RK. Excessive intake of zinc impairs immune responses. JAMA 252(11):1443-6, 1984).*

Pharmacological levels of supplementation may increase susceptibility to <u>bacterial infections</u>.

> **Experimental Study:** 11 healthy adult men ingested 150 mg of elemental zinc twice daily. After 6 wks., there was a reduction in chemotaxis and phagocytosis of bacteria by polymorphonuclear leukocytes *(Chandra RK. Excessive intake of zinc impairs immune responses. <u>JAMA</u> 252(11):1443-6, 1984).*

Other possible side-effects of pharmacologic dosages are occasional <u>nausea</u>, <u>increased sweating</u>, <u>alcohol intolerance</u> and transient worsening of <u>depression</u> or <u>hallucinations</u>. In addition, zinc supplementation may increase <u>grand mal seizures</u> in epileptics, possibly due to a reduction in blood manganese levels; thus, for epileptics, manganese supplementation should be started prior to zinc supplementation *(Pfeiffer CC, LaMola S. Zinc and manganese in the schizophrenias. <u>J Orthomol Psychiatry</u> 12:215-34, 1983).*

Zinc picolinate is suspected of causing <u>chromosome damage</u>.

> **In vitro Experimental Study:** Chinese hamster ovary cells were treated with chromium picolinate or chromium nicotinate for 24 hrs. and the results were compared to those of obtained in cells treated with ligands alone or with chromium chloride. Chromium picolinate was found to cause significant chromosomal damage at a non-toxic dose, and damage was dose-dependent. This damage was inferred to arise from the ligand since picolinate alone caused damage at a non-toxic dose, raising questions about the safety of chromium picolinate as a human dietary supplement *(Stearns DM, Wise JP Sr., Patierno SR, Wetterhahn KE. The dietary supplement chromium picolinate induces chromosome damage in Chinese hamster ovary cells. Abstract #2616. <u>FASEB J</u> 9(3):A451, 1995).*

Chapter Five
NUTRIENT-NUTRIENT INTERACTIONS

Beta-carotene

MAY BE INFLUENCED BY

- Fat

Enhances absorption (*Dimitrov NV, Meyer C, Ullrey DE, et al. Bioavailability of beta-carotene in humans. Am J Clin Nutr 48(2):298-304, 1988*).

- Vitamin E

Interact synergistically to inhibit lipid peroxidation (*Palozza P, Krinsky NI. B-carotene and alpha-tocopherol are synergistic antioxidants. Arch Biochem Biophys 297(1):184-7, 1992*).

Biotin

MAY BE INFLUENCED BY

- Ethanol

Inhibits the intestinal transport of biotin and is associated with a significant decrease in plasma biotin concentrations (*Said HM et al. Chronic ethanol feeding and acute ethanol exposure in vitro: effect on intestinal transport of biotin. Am J Clin Nutr 52:1083-6, 1990*).

Calcium

MAY BE INFLUENCED BY

- Caffeine

Increases urinary calcium excretion (*Kynast-Gales SA, Massey LK. Effect of caffeine on circadian excretion of urinary calcium and magnesium. J Am Coll Nutr 13(5):467-72, 1994; Yeh JK et al. Influence of injected caffeine on the metabolism of calcium and the retention and excretion of sodium, potassium, phosphorus, magnesium, zinc and copper in rats. J Nutr 116(2):273-80, 1986*).

- Fatty Acids

Decrease calcium absorption due to the formation of calcium soaps in the GI tract (*Weiser NM, in NW Solomons, IH Rosenberg, Eds. Absorption and Malabsorption of Mineral Nutrients. New York, Alan R. Liss, 1984:15*).

Negative Experimental Study: 6 male volunteers were given rectal infusions of isotonic saline with and without the addition of calcium and short chain fatty acids (SCFA). When SCFA were added, serum calcium increased, most likely as the result of enhanced calcium absorption in the distal colon (*Trinidad TP, Wolever TMS, Thompson LU. Interactive effects of calcium and short chain fatty acids on absorption in the distal colon of man. Nutr Res 13:417-25, 1993*).

> *Note: Fermentation of dietary fiber by colonic bacteria produces short chain fatty acids.*

- Fiber

Decreases intestinal calcium absorption (*Heaney RP et al. Calcium nutrition and bone health in the elderly. Am J Clin Nutr 36(5 Suppl):986-1013, 1982*).

Negative Experimental Study: Under conditions that mimic those in the intestines, the binding of calcium to soluble fibers (pectin, alginate, carrageenan, guar gum) is extremely weak. If calcium is bound to fiber in the duodenum, it will be released again as it enters the jejunum and ileum, where it can still be effectively absorbed (*Schlemmer U. Studies of the binding of copper, zinc, and calcium to pectin, alginate, carrageenan, and guar gum in HCO_3-CO_2 buffer. Food Chem 32:223-34, 1989*).

- Iron

Enhances calcium absorption.

Animal Experimental Study: Utilizing a brush border membrane vesicle model, when iron and calcium were present in the US RDA ratio of 1:1, no decrease in calcium intake into rat brush border membrane vesicles was seen. At high concentrations, iron enhanced calcium uptake (*Roth-Bassell HA, Clydesdale FM. The influence of zinc, magnesium, and iron on calcium uptake in brush border membrane vesicles. J Am Coll Nutr 10(1):44-9, 1991*).

- Lactose

Appears to enhance calcium absorption, but the evidence is controversial (*Allen LH. Calcium and osteoporosis. Nutr Today 21(3):6-10, 1986*).

- Lysine

Concurrent administration of 4-800 mg lysine enhances calcium absorption without increasing urinary calcium excretion (*Civitelli R et al. Dietary L-lysine and calcium metabolism in humans. Nutrition 8(6):400-5, 1993*).

- Magnesium

> *Note: Supplementation does not appear to affect calcium balance.*

Experimental Study: Since conflicting results have been reported, calcium absorption studies were carried out under strictly controlled conditions. The magnesium intake in control studies ranged from 240-264 mg daily and was increased to about 800 mg daily due to the intake of magnesium oxide tablets. The studies were carried out during 3 calcium intakes of 240, 800, and 1400 mg daily. Intestinal calcium absorption did not change during the high magnesium intake regardless of the calcium intake. Also, although urinary calcium increased during the addition of magnesium supplementation, calcium balance did not change (*Spencer H, Fuller H, Norris C, Williams D. Effect of magnesium on the intestinal absorption of calcium in man. J Am Coll Nutr 13(5):485-92, 1994*).

Negative Experimental Study: Subjects given a diet of sustained calcium content received supplementation with 1 gm magnesium daily. The intestinal absorption and the net retention by the body of both metals was increased, the effect being quantitatively greater for calcium than for magnesium (*Anne M. Briscoe, Ragan C. Effect of magnesium on calcium metabolism in man. Am J Clin Nutr 19(5):296-3061966*).

Magnesium regulates the neuromuscular activity of the Ca^{++} ion. As a magnesium deficiency enhances the availability of ionic calcium, magnesium supplementation is a natural calcium-channel blocker (*Iseri LT, French JH. Magnesium: Nature's calcium blocker. Am Heart J 108:H366-H388, 1984*).

Magnesium depletion may cause hypocalcemia (*Leicht E, Biro G. Mechanisms of hypocalcaemia in the clinical form of severe magnesium deficit in the human. Magnes Res 5(1):41-4, 1992; The Merck Manual. Sixteenth Edition. Rahway, NJ, Merck & Co., 1992*).

Observational Study: 22% of pts. with below normal serum calcium levels were magnesium-deficient (*Whang R et al. Predictors of clinical hypomagnesemia: Hypokalemia, hypophosphatemia, hyponatremia, and hypocalcemia. Arch Intern Med 144:1794-6, 1984*).

- Oxalates

Note: High in certain leafy green vegetables which are also high in calcium such as spinach, but not in Brassica oleracea (broccoli, turnip greens, collard greens, mustard greens).

May inhibit the absorption of calcium contained in its food source, but not the absorption of calcium from other foods simultaneously ingested (*Allen LH. Calcium and osteoporosis. Nutr Today 21(3):6-10, 1986*).

See Also:

Heaney RP, Weaver CM. Calcium absorption from kale. Am J Clin Nutr 51:656-7, 1990

- Phosphorus

The ideal dietary calcium to phosphorus ratio is 1:1 *(Linkswiler HM, Zemel MB. Calcium to phosphorus ratios. Contemp Nutr 4(5), May, 1979).*

A dietary calcium to phosphorus ratio above 2:1 due to excess calcium results in <u>reduced bone strength</u> and interferes with vitamin K synthesis and/or absorption, which could theoretically cause <u>internal bleeding</u> *(Calcium: How much is too much? Nutr Rev 43(11):345, 1985).*

High phosphorus intakes (meat, grains, potatoes and soft drinks) promote calcium loss through the induction of 'nutritional hyperparathyroidism' in order to maintain normal serum calcium levels in the face of decreased Ca/P ratios *(Jowsey J. Osteoporosis. Postgrad Med 60:75-9, 1976).*

> *Note: A phosphorus intake of up to 2000 mg/d does not have adverse effects on calcium metabolism; however the type of phosphate contained in carbonated beverages may not behave in the same manner (Spencer H et al. Do protein and phosphorus cause calcium loss? J Nutr 118:657-60, 1988).*

Fecal phosphorus appears to bind calcium and reduce its intestinal absorption *(Franz KB. Influence of dietary phosphorus on absorption of dietary calcium and magnesium in humans. Abstract. J Am Coll Nutr 6(5):444, 1987).*

- Phytates

> *Note: Found in the bran layer of <u>cereal grains</u>.*

Decrease intestinal calcium absorption *(Goodhart RS, Shils ME. Modern Nutrition in Health and Disease. 6th Edition. Philadelphia, Lee & Febiger, 1980).*

> **Experimental Study:** Absorption of calcium from soybeans with low and high phytate contents was measured in 16 normal women and compared in 15 of these subjects with absorption of calcium from milk. Calcium absorption was reduced about 25% by the high phytate beans compared to the low phytate beans (p<0.001) *(Heaney RP et al. Soybean phytate content: effect on calcium absorption. Am J Clin Nutr 53:745-7, 1991).*

- Potassium

Increases calcium retention.

> **Review Article:** A fall in urinary calcium during potassium administration is accompanied by an increase in serum calcium and implies that potassium either directly or indirectly enhances renal tubular calcium absorption. Apart from its natriuretic effects, potassium inhibits renal calcitriol synthesis thereby causing renal phosphate retention. This inhibits intestinal calcium absorption and thus contributes to the decrease in urinary calcium excretion which over time would dampen continuously positive calcium balances. Because the ability of potassium to reduce urinary calcium is sustained, it has the potential of protecting bone

(Lemann J, Pleuss JA, Gray RW. Potassium causes calcium retention in healthy adults. J Nutr 123:1623-6, 1993).

- <u>Protein</u>

Increases urinary calcium excretion *(Allen LH. Calcium and osteoporosis. Nutr Today 21(3):6-10, 1986).*

Negative Review Article: Controlled human studies show that commonly used complex dietary proteins, which have a high phosphorus content, do not cause calcium loss in adult humans. In contrast, a diet low in protein and phosphorus may have adverse effects on calcium balance in the elderly *(Spencer H et al. Do protein and phosphorus cause calcium loss? J Nutr 118:657-60, 1988).*

- <u>Sodium</u>

Increases urinary calcium excretion *(Heaney RP. Calcium bioavailability. Contemp Nutr 11(8), 1986).*

Observational Study: In a study of healthy adults aged 60 and older consuming self-selected diets, there was a positive association between salt intake and urinary calcium excretion for both males and females. This association remained significant even when controlled for gender, age, body mass, alkaline phosphatase levels and protein intake. Urinary calcium excretion was found to increase about 1 mmol/d per 100 mmol increase in urinary sodium excretion *(Itoh R et al. The interrelation of urinary calcium and sodium intake in healthy elderly Japanese. Int J Vitam Nutr Res 61:159-65, 1991).*

- <u>Sodium Bicarbonate</u>

Improves urinary calcium retention in protein-induced hypercalciuria.

Experimental Study: 6 normal women received 44 gm protein in their diets for 16 days followed by 102 gm for 24 days. Calcium, phosphorus and magnesium intakes were held constant at 500, 900 and 300 mg. During the last 10 days, 5.85 gm of sodium bicarbonate was ingested concomitantly. The increase in protein intake significantly increased urinary calcium and net renal acid excretion and the mean calcium balance became negative. The ingestion of sodium bicarbonate alkalinized the urine, reversed the increase in urinary calcium, and the mean net calcium balance became positive *(Lutz J. Calcium balance and acid-base status of women as affected by increased protein intake and by sodium bicarbonate ingestion. Am J Clin Nutr 39:281-8, 1984).*

- <u>Sugar</u>

Glucose increases calcium absorption.

Experimental Study: In a study of 8 normal subjects, oral coadministration of glucose with calcium increased the efficiency of intestinal calcium absorption by 20% *(Wood RJ et al. Effects of glucose and glucose polymers on calcium absorption in healthy subjects. Am J Clin Nutr 46(4):699-701, 1987).*

Increases urinary calcium concentration.

Experimental Study: When subjects consumed a sugary beverage, urinary calcium excretion increased and the calcium loss continued for several hours (*Holl M, Allen L. Sucrose ingestion, insulin response and mineral metabolism. J Nutr 117:1229-33, 1987*).

Experimental Study: In a study of 24 hr. urines of 18 normal subjects, an increase in refined carbohydrates (sugar and sugar products) in a standardized diet caused a significant increase in the number of urines with a calcium concentration above 9 mmol/l (*Thom JA et al. The influence of refined carbohydrate on urinary calcium excretion. Br J Urology 50:459-64, 1978*).

- Uronic Acid

Note: found in the hemi-cellulose fiber component of fruit and vegetables.

Inhibits intestinal calcium absorption (*Allen LH. Calcium and osteoporosis. Nutr Today 21(3):6-10, 1986*).

- Vitamin A

Nutriture is important to calcium metabolism and the formation of healthy bones and teeth (*Navia JM, Harris SS. Vitamin A influence on calcium metabolism and calcification, Ann N Y Acad Sci 355, 1980*).

- Vitamin B$_6$

Deficiency is associated with a negative calcium balance suggesting impaired absorption and/or utilization or possibly increased mobilization of calcium (*Turnlund JR, Betschart AA, Liebman M, et al. Vitamin B-6 depletion followed by repletion with animal- or plant-source diets and calcium and magnesium metabolism in young women. Am J Clin Nutr 56:905-10, 1992*).

- Vitamin D

Promotes calcium absorption and mobilizes calcium from bone (*Passmore R, Eastwood MA. Davidson and Passmore: Human Nutrition and Dietetics. Eighth Edition. London, Churchill Livingstone, 1986:139*).

- Zinc

Decreases calcium absorption when a high level of daily zinc supplementation (140 mg) is given along with a very low daily dietary calcium intake (200 mg) but not with a normal calcium intake (800 mg) (*Spencer H et al. Effect of zinc supplements on the intestinal absorption of calcium. J Am Coll Nutr 6(1):47-51, 1987; Spencer H et al. Am J Clin Nutr 35:829, 1982*), an intermediate, but still low level of calcium intake (500 mg), or a lower level of zinc intake (100 mg) (*Spencer H, Norris C, Osis D. Further studies of the effect of zinc on intestinal absorption of calcium in man. J Am Coll Nutr 11(5):561-6, 1992*).

Animal Experimental Study: Utilizing a brush border membrane vesicle model, when zinc and calcium were present in the US RDA ratio of 1:1, no decrease in calcium intake into rat brush border membrane vesicles was seen. At high ratios, however, zinc significantly reduced calcium uptake. This result is biologically significant as calcium uptake was affected when zinc was present at only 1/10 the molar concentration of calcium (Zn/Ca RDA ratio of 10:1); thus these results confirm the findings of Spencer et al (*Roth-Bassell HA, Clydesdale FM. The influence of zinc, magnesium, and iron on calcium uptake in brush border membrane vesicles. J Am Coll Nutr 10(1):44-9, 1991*).

Carnitine

MAY BE INFLUENCED BY

- Choline

Supplementary choline reduces serum and urinary carnitine concentrations (which may simulate carnitine deficiency) while promoting carnitine conservation (*Dodson WL, Sachan DS. Choline supplementation reduces urinary carnitine excretion in humans. Am J Clin Nutr 63:904-10, 1996*).

- Coenzyme Q_{10}

Their interactions produce a synergistic effect (*Bertilli A, Gonca G. Carnitine and coenzyme Q_{10}: biochemical properties and functions, synergism and complementary action. Int J Tiss React 12(3):183-6, 1990*).

- Vitamin C

Increases urinary excretion of carnitine.

> **Experimental Study:** In healthy elderly men, supplementation with 200 mg/day of ascorbic acid increased urinary carnitine excretion while, in elderly female hospital pts., urinary carnitine was positively correlated with leukocyte ascorbic acid (*Davies HEF et al. Ascorbic acid and carnitine in man. Nutr Rep Int 36:941, 1987*).

Carotenoids (general)

MAY BE INFLUENCED BY

- Beta-carotene

Supplementation may lower the plasma concentration of other carotenoids (*Kostic D, White WS, Olson JA. Am J Clin Nutr 62:604-10, 1995; Micozzi MS, Brown ED, Edwards BK, et al. Am J Clin Nutr 55:1120-5, 1992*) but does not appear to affect the distribution of carotenoids in lipoproteins (*Ribaya-Mercado JD, Ordovas JM, Russell RM. J Am Coll Nutr 14(6):614-20, 1995*).

Chromium

MAY BE INFLUENCED BY

- Calcium Carbonate

Reduces chromium absorption.

Experimental Controlled Study: Subjects were fasted and then given either water, ascorbic acid or a calcium carbonate antacid followed by chromium chloride. The chromium supplement was poorly absorbed, and absorption was further reduced when it was taken with calcium carbonate. As compared to the water and ascorbic acid gps., tissue chromium concentrations were lower. Results suggest that calcium carbonate might form insoluble complexes with chromium to decrease its absorption or might decrease chromium absorption by altering the intestinal pH (*Seaborn C, Stoecker B. Effects of antacid or ascorbic acid on tissue accumulation and urinary excretion of chromium. Nutr Res 10:1401-7, 1990*).

- Sugar

Increases urinary chromium loss.

Experimental Study: 27/37 normal subjects had an increase in urinary chromium excretion during a high sucrose diet (35% of calories from sucrose; 15% from complex carbohydrates) compared to a diet with 15% of calories from sucrose and 35% from complex carbohydrates, with the increase ranging from 10-300% (*Kozlovsky AS et al. Effects of diets high in simple sugars on urinary chromium losses. Metabolism 35:515, 1986*).

- Vanadium

May prevent chromium's potentiation of insulin by occupying chromium's receptor sites (*Hill CH. Mineral interrelationships, in AS Prasad, D Oberleas, Eds. Trace Elements in Human Health and Disease. Volume 2. New York, Academic Press, 1976:281-300*).

Cobalt

MAY BE INFLUENCED BY

- Iron

Competes with iron for absorption (*Pollack S et al. The absorption of nonferrous metals in iron deficiency. J Clin Invest 44:1470, 1965*).

Coenzyme Q10

MAY BE INFLUENCED BY

- Carnitine

Their interactions may produce a synergistic effect (*Bertilli A, Gonca G. Carnitine and coenzyme Q10: biochemical properties and functions, synergism and complementary action. Int J Tiss React 12(3):183-6, 1990*).

Copper

MAY BE INFLUENCED BY

- Alcohol

Aggravates copper deficiency (*Fields M, Lewis C. Alcohol consumption aggravates copper deficiency. Metabolism 39:610-13, 1990*).

- Egg

Egg yolk forms an insoluble copper sulfide with free copper in the digestive tract (*Schultze MO et al. Further studies on the availability of copper from various sources as a supplement to iron in hemoglobin formation. J Biol Chem 115:453-7, 1936*).

- Fructose

The fructose moiety of sucrose may contribute to copper deficiency when used as a major source of dietary carbohydrate.

> **Experimental Crossover Study:** 20 healthy male volunteers were fed fructose or starch as 20% of their diet while on a low-copper diet. After 11 wks., subjects on fructose developed significantly lower RBC superoxide dismutase levels (a very sensitive indicator of copper status); neither serum copper nor ceruloplasmin activity was significantly affected by the type of dietary carbohydrate (*Reiser S, Smith JC, Mertz W, et al. Indices of copper status in humans consuming a typical American diet containing either fructose or starch. Am J Clin Nutr 42:242-51, 1985*).

- Iron

Decreases gastrointestinal absorption of copper.

> **Experimental Study:** An iron-fortified infant formula, when compared to the unfortified formula, decreased copper absorption by over 50% (*Haschke F, Ziegler EE, Edwards BB, Fomon SJ. Effect of iron fortification of infant formula on trace mineral absorption. J Pediatr Gastroenterol Nutr 5:768-73, 1986*).

- Molybdenum

Increases copper excretion.

> **Experimental Study:** Molybdenum intakes as low as 1.5 mg/day increased copper excretion (*Doesthale YG, Gopalan C. The effect of molybdenum levels in sorghum (Sorghum Vulgare Pers.) on uric acid and copper excretion in man. Br J Nutr 31:351-5, 1974*).

- Sulfur Amino Acids

Increase the severity of copper deficiency (*Kato N, Saari JT, Schelkoph GM. Cystine feeding enhances defects of dietary copper deficiency by a mechanism not involving oxidative stress. J Nutr Biochem 5:99-105, 1994*).

- Vitamin B$_6$

Deficiency decreases gastrointestinal absorption (*Turnlund JR et al. A stable-isotope study of zinc, copper, and iron absorption and retention by young women fed vitamin B-6-deficient diets. Am J Clin Nutr 54:1059-64, 1991*).

- Vitamin C

High levels of supplementation decrease gastrointestinal absorption of copper (*Milne DB et al. Effects of ascorbic acid supplements and a diet marginal in copper on indices of copper nutriture in women. Nutr Res 8:865-73, 1988; Van Campen DR, Gross E. Influences of ascorbic acid on the absorption of copper in rats. J Nutr 95:617-22, 1968*).

> **Experimental Study:** Healthy volunteers received the following total ascorbic acid intakes in sequence: 65 mg/day x 2 wks., 5 mg/day x 4 wks., 605 mg/day x 3 wks., and 5 mg/day x 4 wks. Copper absorption, copper retention, total serum copper and serum ceruloplasmin levels were not significantly affected; however, the oxidase activity of serum ceruloplasmin was decreased during the high (605 mg/day) ascorbic acid intake period (*Jacob RA et al. Effect of varying ascorbic acid intakes on copper absorption and ceruloplasmin levels of young men. J Nutr 117(12):2109-15, 1987*).

> **Experimental Study:** Healthy volunteers consuming self-selected diets took 500 mg of ascorbic acid with each meal for 64 days. Serum ceruloplasmin activity was significantly reduced at every data point during supplementation, and a similar but non-significant trend was observed for serum copper. In addition, 20 days after supplementation ceased, there was a significant increase in serum copper (*Finley EB, Cerklewski FL. Influence of ascorbic acid supplementation on copper status in young adult men. Am J Clin Nutr 37(4):553-6, 1983*).

Ascorbate also has a postabsorption role in the transfer of copper ions into cells. It reacts with ceruloplasmin, a serum copper protein, labilizing the bound copper atoms and facilitating their cross-membrane transport, thus stimulating tissue copper utilization. Also, at physiological levels and above, ascorbate impedes the intracellular binding of copper to Cu,Zn superoxide dismutase - which may or may not have physiological significance (*Harris ED, Percival SS. A role for ascorbic acid in copper transport. Am J Clin Nutr 54:1193S-7S, 1991*).

- Zinc

Decreases copper nutriture.

> **Review Article:** Excessive zinc inhibits intestinal absorption, hepatic accumulation and placental transfer of copper and induces a copper deficiency; thus zinc supplementation should be avoided in areas where copper intakes are

suboptimal (*Bremner I, Beattie JH. Copper and zinc metabolism in health and disease: speciation and interactions. Proc Nutr Soc 54:489-99, 1995*).

Experimental Study: 6 healthy women supplemented their diet with 50 mg of elemental zinc for 12 days. Erythrocyte superoxide dismutase, a marker of copper status, showed a significant 20% decrease (*Abdallah SM, Samman S. The effect of increasing dietary zinc on the activity of superoxide dismutase and zinc concentration in erythrocytes of healthy female subjects. Eur J Clin Nutr 47:327-32, 1993*).

Case Report: A 35-year-old Caucasian woman ingested 110-165 mg elemental zinc as zinc sulfate for 10 months. She developed a slowly worsening microcytic-hypochromic anemia found to be due to copper deficiency. Zinc supplementation was eliminated and she was supplemented with 2 mg copper daily. After 2 mo., her anemia was unchanged. She received 10 mg copper chloride IV over a period of 5 days, and responded (*Hoffman HN 2nd et al. Zinc-induced copper deficiency. Gastroenterology 94:508-12, 1988*).

Experimental Study: 9 men consumed diets containing 2.6 mg copper and 1.8, 4.0, 6.0, 8.0, 18.5 or 20.7 mg of zinc daily for 1-2 wk. periods. While the weekly plasma copper concentration remained within the normal range during the 63-day study, fecal copper and apparent copper retention were influenced by the level of dietary zinc and the duration it was consumed. After a 1-wk. lag, an increase of zinc to 18.5 mg zinc daily, only 3.5 mg above the RDA for men, elevated fecal copper and thus reduced apparent copper retention (*Festa MD, Anderson H, Dowdy RP, et al. Effect of zinc intake on copper excretion and retention in men. Am J Clin Nutr 41:285-92, 1985*).

Negative Experimental Study: Healthy men and women consumed either 50 mg zinc 3 times daily or placebo. After 3 mo., there were no adverse effects on plasma copper levels (*Samman S, Roberts D. The effect of zinc supplements on plasma zinc and copper levels and the reported symptoms in healthy volunteers. Med J Aust 146:246-7, 1987*).

Experimental Study: Adult males who received zinc 50 mg daily for 6 wks. had a significant decrease in erythrocyte Cu,Zn-superoxide dismutase, suggesting that copper status was decreased (*Fischer PW, Giroux A, L'Abbe MR. Effect of zinc supplementation on copper status in adult men. Am J Clin Nutr 40(4):743-6, 1984*).

Review Article: It appears that tissues must be loaded with zinc before an effect on copper absorption is observed (*Brewer GJ et al. Biological roles of ionic zinc. Prog Clin Biol Res 129:35-51, 1983*).

Experimental Study: Daily ingestion of 150 mg zinc daily for 2 yrs. for the treatment of sickle-cell anemia produced hypocupremia in some pts. (*Prasad AS et al. Hypocupremia induced by zinc therapy in adults. JAMA 240:2166-8, 1978*).

Animal Experimental Study: Zinc supplementation decreased copper absorption in rats when the zinc to copper ratio was >2.5/1 (*Fischer PWF et al. The effect of dietary zinc on intestinal copper absorption. Am J Clin Nutr 34:1670-5, 1981; Van Campen DR, Scaife PU. Zinc interference with copper absorption in rats. J Nutr 91:473-6, 1967*).

Flavonoids

MAY BE INFLUENCED BY

- Vitamin C

The vitamin enhances their antioxidant protective capabilities (*Jacob R. The integrated antioxidant system. Nutr Res 15:755-66, 1995*).

Fluoride

MAY BE INFLUENCED BY

- Magnesium

Magnesium seems to compete with fluoride for absorption from the gut. Rat studies suggest that magnesium deficiency may promote higher bone fluoride levels causing adverse effects on bone strength and elasticity. Magnesium may thus protect against some of the adverse effects of fluoride (*Machoy-Mokrzynska A. Fluoride-magnesium interaction. Fluoride 28:175-7, 1995*).

Folic Acid

MAY BE INFLUENCED BY

- Pancreatic Enzymes

Bind with folic acid to form insoluble complexes, thus decreasing folate absorption (*Russell RM et al. Impairment of folic acid absorption by oral pancreatic extracts. Dig Dis Sci 25(5):369, 1980*).

- Vitamin B$_{12}$

Regulates folic acid metabolism (*Chanarin I, Deacon R, Lumb M, Perry J. Cobalamin-folate interrelations. Blood Rev 3(4):211-15, 1989; Chanarin I et al. Vitamin B$_{12}$ regulates folate metabolism by the supply of formate. Lancet ii:505-7, 1980*).

Vitamin B$_{12}$ deficiency may induce a functional folate deficiency (*Shane B, Stokstad EL. Vitamin B$_{12}$-folate interrelationships. Annu Rev Nutr 5:115-41, 1985*).

Glutathione

MAY BE INFLUENCED BY

- alpha-Lipoic acid

Data from animal and *in vitro* studies suggest that alpha-lipoic acid may increase intracellular glutathione (*Busse E, Zimmer G, Schopohl B, Kornhuber B. Influence of alpha-lipoic acid on intracellular glutathione in vitro and in vivo. Arzeimittelforschung 42(6):829-31, 1992; Han D, Tritschler JH, Packer L. Alpha-lipoic acid increases cellular glutathione in a human T-lymphocyte Jurkat cell line. Biochem Biophys Res Commun 207(1):258-64, 1995).*

- N-acetylcysteine

Depleted intracellular levels may be boosted by oral supplementation with N-acetylcysteine, perhaps because cysteine availability can become limiting in situations that increase the demand for intracellular glutathione utilization *(Smith CV. Will glutathione become a hot new supplement? Nutr Report 11(11), November, 1993).*

- Vitamin C

Acts together with glutathione to alleviate various oxidant stresses *(Jacob R. The integrated antioxidant system. Nutr Res 15:755-66, 1995).*

- Vitamin E

Supplementation may boost plasma glutathione levels.

> **Experimental Study:** 23 females and 8 males aged 24-78 yrs. ingested either 15, 60 or 120 IU alpha tocopherol daily. After 1 mo., subjects ingesting 60 and 200 IU daily showed significantly increased plasma glutathione levels, although no dose of vitamin E significantly affected DNA repair activities *(Hu JJ et al. Effects of dietary supplementation of alpha-tocopherol on plasma glutathione and DNA repair activities. Cancer Epidemiol Biomark Preven 5(4):263-70, 1996).*

Iron

MAY BE INFLUENCED BY

- Calcium

Excessive supplementation decreases iron absorption in a dose-defined manner leading to iron-deficiency anemia. Perhaps 23% of those ingesting more than 2 gm daily are at risk *(Read MH et al. Mineral supplementation practices of adults in seven western states. Nutr Res 6:375-83, 1986).*

> **Experimental Study:** Iron absorption from 2 identical 10-day periods was compared for 21 healthy females when the same amt. of calcium (937 mg) was distributed in two different ways. About 30-50% more iron was absorbed when no milk or cheese (rich in calcium) was served with lunch or dinner, a statistically significant difference *(Gleerup A, Rossander-Hulthén L, Gramatkovski E, Hallberg L. Iron absorption from the whole diet: comparison of the effect of two different distributions of daily calcium intake. Am J Clin Nutr 61:97-104, 1995).*

> **Experimental Study:** Including calcium-rich foods in a meal was found to reduce iron absorption by 50-60%, suggesting that such foods should be reduced or eliminated at meals that provide a large percentage of the day's iron *(Hallberg L,*

Rossander-Hulten L, Brune M, et al. Calcium and iron absorption: Mechanisms of action and nutritional importance. Eur J Clin Nutr 46:317-27, 1992).

Negative Experimental Study: 57 premenopausal women took 500 mg of calcium as the carbonate with each of 2 meals daily while 52 women served as controls. After 12 wks., there were no significant differences in any of several measures of iron stores between the 2 gps. *(Sokoll LJ, Dawson-Hughes B. Calcium supplementation and plasma ferritin concentrations in premenopausal women. Am J Clin Nutr 45:1045-8, 1992).*

Experimental Study: In a study of 126 subjects, addition of calcium chloride to wheat rolls significantly reduced iron absorption. Calcium added to the dough when making the rolls reduced phytate degradation during fermentation and baking, thus increasing the phytate content of the rolls to levels interfering with iron absorption. Calcium also had a direct dose-related inhibiting effect on iron absorption both for heme- nonheme-iron. Since the absorption of these 2 forms of iron is by different mechanisms, this result implies that the inhibition does not occur at the GI wall *(Hallberg L et al. Calcium: effect of different amounts on nonheme- heme-iron absorption in humans. Am J Clin Nutr 53:112-19, 1991).*

Experimental Study: Using a double-radioisotope technique, the influence of calcium supplements on the absorption of dietary nonheme iron and of iron supplements was evaluated. Results suggest that taking regular calcium supplements with meals makes it more difficult for women to meet their daily iron requirement *(Cook JD et al. Calcium supplementation: effect on iron absorption. Am J Clin Nutr 53:106-11, 1991).*

Experimental Placebo-controlled Study: 24 healthy postmenopausal women received capsules containing 500 mg calcium as calcium carbonate or hydroxyapatite or placebo along with a test meal. Based on a whole-body radioisotope counting technique, iron retention was decreased to 45% of control values by both calcium compounds *(Dawson-Hughes B, Seligson FH, Hughes VA. Effects of calcium carbonate and hydroxyapatite on zinc and iron retention in postmenopausal women. Am J Clin Nutr 44:83-8, 1986).*

- Chromium

Supplementation may reduce iron nutriture.

Animal Experimental Study: Iron uptake was reduced significantly in the presence of chromium. *In vivo* study showed that the serum levels of iron and total iron binding capacity (TIBC) were reduced by 28 and 11%, respectively, following daily administration of chromium (1 mg/kg) for 45 days, while serum ferritin was reduced by 22%. Hematocrit and hemoglobin levels were both reduced by 17%. Spectrophotometric titration of each individual amino acid located in the iron binding site of transferrin revealed that tyrosine might be the most suitable ligand for the binding of chromium to transferrin, suggesting that chromium may compete with iron in binding to apo-transferrin to influence iron metabolism and its related biochemical parameters *(Ani M, Moshtaghie AA. The effect of chromium on parameters related to iron metabolism. Biol Trace Elem Res 32:57-64, 1992).*

- Cobalt

Competes with iron for absorption *(Pollack S et al. The absorption of nonferrous metals in iron deficiency. J Clin Invest 44:1470, 1965).*

- Coffee

Decreases iron absorption.

Experimental Study: In a study of 37 healthy subjects, coffee 1 hr. before eating did not affect iron absorption, while coffee taken with the meal or up to 1 hr. after eating reduced absorbed iron by 39%. This effect was concentration-dependent *(Morck TA et al. Inhibition of food iron absorption by coffee. Am J Clin Nutr 37(3):416-20, 1983).*

- Fiber

Reduces absorption of inorganic iron *(Ricketts CD. Influence of fiber on the absorption from various types of iron tablets. J Optimal Nutr 3(3):126-31, 1994).*

- Fructose

Forms stable complexes with iron and promotes its absorption *(O'Dell BL. Fructose and mineral metabolism. Am J Clin Nutr 58(suppl):771S-8S, 1993).*

- Hydrochloric Acid

If deficient, impairs iron absorption.

Experimental Study: 25 diabetic pts. with blood counts 4.2 million or less who were under good diabetic control were randomly selected to receive glutamic acid HCl 5 gr 3 times daily before meals which, at the end of 1 mo., was replaced by ferrous carbonate 6 3/4 gr 3 times daily. At the end of another mo., both supplements were prescribed concomitantly. Following the first mo., the RBC increased significantly from 4.06 to 4.56 million, while iron supplementation failed to be followed by a significant change. Following combined supplementation, RBC again increased significantly by 1/4 million. The experiment was replicated with similar results *(Rabinowich IM. Achlorhydria and its clinical significance in diabetes mellitus. Am J Dig Dis 16:322-32, 1949).*

See Also:

Conrad ME, Schade SG. Ascorbic acid chelates in iron absorption: A role for hydrochloric acid and bile. Gastroenterol 55:35, 1968

Jacobs P et al. Role of hydrochloric acid in iron absorption. J Appl Physiol 19(2):187-8, 1964

- Manganese

Inhibits iron absorption *(Hurley LS, Keen CL. Manganese, in E Underwood and W Mertz, Eds. Trace Elements in Human Health and Animal Nutrition. New York, Academic Press, 1987:185-223; Rossander-Hultén L et al. Competitive inhibition of iron absorption by manganese and zinc in humans. Am J Clin Nutr 54:152-6, 1991).*

- Milk

Inhibits iron absorption *(Deehr MS et al. Effects of different calcium sources on iron absorption in postmenopausal women. Am J Clin Nutr 51:95-9, 1990).*

- Phenolics

Note: Usually tannins or polyphenols, these compounds are present in tea, coffee, certain spices, fruits and vegetables.

Powerfully inhibit nonheme-iron absorption *(Tuntawiroon M et al. Dose-dependent inhibitory effect of phenolic compounds in foods on nonheme-iron absorption in men. Am J Clin Nutr 53:554-7, 1991).*

- Phytates

Note: Present in cereals, certain vegetables, roots, nuts, etc.

The main cause of the inhibitory effect of bran on iron absorption *(Hallberg L et al. Phytates and the inhibitory effect of bran on iron absorption in man. Am J Clin Nutr 45:988-96, 1987).*

- Protein

Beef, lamb, chicken, pork and fish enhance iron absorption, while soy decreases it *(Kane AP, Miller DD. In vitro estimation of the effects of selected proteins on iron bioavailability. Am J Clin Nutr 393-401, 1984)* as do the two major milk proteins *(Hurrell RF et al. Iron absorption in humans as influenced by bovine milk proteins. Am J Clin Nutr 49:546-52, 1989).*

- Riboflavin

Iron absorption, the mobilization of intracellular iron, and the retention of absorbed iron are all sensitive to changes in riboflavin status *(Bates CJ et al. Vitamins, iron, and physical work. Lancet ii:313-14, 1989; Powers HJ. Riboflavin-iron interactions with particular emphasis on the gastrointestinal tract. Proc Nutr Soc 54:509-17, 1995).*

- Tea

Decreases iron absorption.

Note: Tannins in tea are one of many types of phenolic compounds in foods. Phenolics usually polymerize to large complex molecules (polyphenols), some of which bind iron which inhibits its absorption (Hallberg L. Search for nutritional confounding factors in the relationship between iron deficiency and brain function. Am J Clin Nutr 50:598-606, 1989).

Experimental Study: In a study of 37 healthy subjects, tea taken with a hamburger meal reduced iron absorption by 64% compared to a 39% reduction when coffee was substituted for tea (Morck TA et al. Inhibition of food iron absorption by coffee. Am J Clin Nutr 37(3):416-20, 1983).

- Vitamin A

Deficiency impairs mobilization of iron stores and decreases iron utilization for hemoglobin formation (Bloem MW et al. Vitamin A intervention: short-term effects of a single, oral, massive dose on iron metabolism. Am J Clin Nutr 51:76-9, 1990; Mejia LA, Arroyave G. The effect of vitamin A fortification of sugar on the iron metabolism in preschool children in Guatemala. Am J Clin Nutr 36:87-93, 1982).

- Vitamin B_6

Deficiency decreases iron status without reducing gastrointestinal absorption (Turnlund JR et al. A stable-isotope study of zinc, copper, and iron absorption and retention by young women fed vitamin B-6-deficient diets. Am J Clin Nutr 54:1059-64, 1991).

- Vitamin C

WARNING: When given concurrently with iron, there is the danger of hydroxyl radical production in the acidic environment of the stomach. This danger is mitigated if the supplement is ingested with food as food's buffering action increases gastric pH and, at higher pH, iron becomes bound to proteins and forms inactive complexes (Maskos Z, Koppenol WH. Oxyradicals and multivitamin tablets. Free Rad Biol Med 11:609-10, 1991).

When given concurrently, ascorbic acid markedly enhances non-heme iron absorption by keeping iron in the reduced (ferrous) state to prevent or delay the formation of insoluble or undissociated ferric compounds, thus keeping it soluble and available for absorption at the alkaline pH of the duodenum (Brise H, Hallberg L. Effect of ascorbic acid on iron absorption. Acta Med Scand Suppl 376, 171:51, 1962; Conrad ME, Schade SG. Ascorbic acid chelates in iron absorption: A role for hydrochloric acid and bile. Gastroenterology 55:35, 1968; Lynch SR, Cook JD. Interaction of vitamin C and iron. Ann N Y Acad Sci 355:32-44, 1980; Monsen ER. Ascorbic acid: An enhancing factor in iron absorption, in Nutritional Bioavailability of Iron. American Chemical Society, 1982:85-95).

Note: The addition of ascorbic acid does not affect clinical indicators of iron status, suggesting that its effects on body iron retention from whole diets are considerably more modest and gradual than effects predicted from studies of single meals (Hunt JR, Gallagher SK, Johnson LAK. Effect of ascorbic acid on apparent iron absorption by women with low iron stores. Am J Clin Nutr 59:1381-5, 1994). *Even in patients with hemochromatosis, there is almost no effect of vitamin C* (Diplock AT. *Safety of antioxidant vitamins and β-carotene. Am J Clin Nutr 62(suppl):1510S-16S, 1995*).

Ferritin regulates the bioavailability of iron within cells. It keeps iron in a relatively accessible form while providing storage capacity to reduce the threat of iron-catalyzed oxidant damage. By contrast, iron stored in hemosiderin is inaccessible. Ascorbate increases the proportion of iron stored in ferritin, which increases iron availability in the cell (Hoffman KE, Yanellki K, Bridges KR. *Ascorbic acid and iron metabolism: alterations in lysomal function. Am J Clin Nutr 54:1188S-92S, 1991*).

Counteracts the inhibition of iron absorption by phenols and phytates, suggesting that, in diets with a high phenol or phytate content, the desired levels of ascorbic acid should also be high (Hallberg L et al. *Iron absorption in man: ascorbic acid and dose-dependent inhibition by phytate. Am J Clin Nutr 49:140-4, 1989; Siegenberg D et al. Ascorbic acid prevents the dose-dependent inhibitory effects of polyphenols and phytates on nonheme-iron absorption. Am J Clin Nutr 53:537-41, 1991*).

- Vitamin D

By enhancing the absorption of calcium (which competes with iron for absorption), may decrease iron absorption (Pollack S et al. *The absorption of nonferrous metals in iron deficiency. J Clin Invest 44, 1965*).

- Vitamin E

Adequate tissue levels may protect against oxidative damage due to iron (Linseman K, Larson P, Braughler J, et al. *Iron-initiated tissue oxidation: Lipid peroxidation, vitamin E destruction and protein thiol oxidation. Biochem Pharmacol 45:1477-82, 1993; Omara FO, Blakley BR. Vitamin E is protective against iron toxicity and iron-induced hepatic vitamin E depletion in mice. J Nutr 123:1649-55, 1993*).

- Zinc

Supplementation impairs the intestinal absorption of iron (Crofton RW et al. *Inorganic zinc and the intestinal absorption of ferrous iron. Am J Clin Nutr 50:141-4, 1989; Meadows NJ et al. Oral iron and the bioavailability of zinc. Br Med J 287:1013-4, 1983*).

Note: Instead of competitive inhibition, an intraluminal reaction may occur - as a fivefold excess of zinc to iron reduced iron absorption by 56% when given in a water solution but not when given with a hamburger meal (Rossander-Hultén L et al. *Competitive inhibition of iron absorption by manganese and zinc in humans. Am J Clin Nutr 54:152-6, 1991*).

Supplementation may impair iron status.

Experimental Study: 10 wks. after starting supplementation with zinc gluconate containing 50 mg elemental zinc daily, 18 female subjects demonstrated significantly lower serum ferritin and hematocrit compared to pretreatment levels ($p < 0.05$) (Yadrick MK et al. *Iron, copper, and zinc status: response to supplementation with zinc or zinc and iron in adult females. Am J Clin Nutr 49:145-50, 1989*).

Magnesium

MAY BE INFLUENCED BY

- Caffeine

Increases urinary magnesium excretion *(Kynast-Gales SA, Massey LK. Effect of caffeine on circadian excretion of urinary calcium and magnesium. J Am Coll Nutr 13(5):467-72, 1994; Yeh JK et al. Influence of injected caffeine on the metabolism of calcium and the retention and excretion of sodium, potassium, phosphorus, magnesium, zinc and copper in rats. J Nutr 116(2):273-80, 1986).*

- Calcium

May impair magnesium absorption, probably due to competition for a common transport system *(O'Donnell JM, Smith DW. Uptake of calcium and magnesium by rat duodenal mucosa analyzed by means of competing metals. J Physiol 229:733, 1973).*

Negative Experimental Double-blind Study: For 14 days, 26 adolescent girls ate a controlled basal diet containing 667 mg calcium and 176 mg magnesium. In addition, they randomly received 1000 mg elemental calcium/day as calcium citrate malate or a placebo. Results "indicate that alterations in magnesium utilization should not be anticipated in adolescent females consuming a high-calcium diet" *(Andon MB, Ilich JZ, Tzagournis MA, Matkovic V. Magnesium balance in adolescent females consuming a low- or high-calcium diet. Am J Clin Nutr 63:950-3, 1996).*

Experimental Study: When dietary magnesium was maintained at 250 mg/day, and calcium was increased from 200 mg/day to 1400 mg/day, the magnesium balance became negative, but was restored when magnesium intake was increased to 500 mg/day *(Spencer H et al. Magnesium in Health and Disease. Jamaica, NY, SP Medical and Scientific Books, 1980:911-19).*

- Ethanol

Increases urinary magnesium excretion *(Lindeman RD et al. Magnesium in Health and Disease. Jamaica, NY, SP Medical and Scientific Books, 1980:236-45).*

- Fat

High levels of fat in the intestinal lumen interfere with magnesium absorption because soaps that are formed from fat and divalent cations like magnesium are not absorbed *(Seelig MS. Magnesium requirements in human nutrition. Magnes Bull 3(Suppl 1a):26-47, 1981).*

- Fiber (dietary)

"The results of metabolic balance studies suggest that fiber causes loss of minerals, including magnesium" *(Seelig MS. Magnesium requirements in human nutrition. Magnes Bull 3(Suppl 1a):26-47, 1981).*

- Fluoride

Fluoride interferes with the biological activities of magnesium, especially when magnesium intake is low and the environmental fluoride dose is high. Magnesium seems to compete with fluoride for absorption from the gut. Rat studies suggest that magnesium deficiency may promote higher bone fluoride levels causing adverse effects on bone strength and elasticity. Magnesium may thus protect against some of the adverse effects of fluoride (*Machoy-Mokrzynska A. Fluoride-magnesium interaction. Fluoride 28:175-7, 1995*).

- Folic Acid

Increases the metabolic need for magnesium by increasing the activity of glycolytic enzymes that require it (*RE Hodges, Ed. Human Nutrition: A Comprehensive Treatise. New York, Plenum Press, 1979*).

- Fructose

As compared to glucose, may increase magnesium absorption; however, a study on rats suggests that it also enhances magnesium excretion, resulting in reduced magnesium retention (*van der Heijden A, van den Berg G, Lemmens AG, Beynen AC. Dietary fructose vs. glucose in rats raises urinary excretion, true absorption and ileal solubility of magnesium but decreases magnesium retention. Br J Nutr 72:567-77, 1994*).

- Iron

May decrease serum magnesium levels (*Newhouse I, Clement D, Lai C. Effects of iron supplementation and discontinuation on serum copper, zinc, calcium and magnesium levels in women. Med Sci Sports 25:562-71, 1993*).

- Lithium

In (therapeutic) megadoses, may increase serum magnesium concentrations through changes in phosphates (*Anath J, Yassa R. Magnesium in mental illness. Compr Psychiatry 20(5):475-82, 1979*).

- Manganese

May decrease magnesium absorption and take the place of magnesium in some enzyme systems that require magnesium (*Watts DL. The nutritional relationships of magnesium. J Orthomol Med 3(4):197-201, 1988*).

- Phosphorus

Fecal phosphorus appears to bind magnesium and reduce its intestinal absorption (*Franz KB. Influence of dietary phosphorus on absorption of dietary calcium and magnesium in humans. Abstract. J Am Coll Nutr 6(5):444, 1987*).

Experimental Study: A negative magnesium balance was produced when phosphate was increased from the near RDA level of 975 mg daily to 1500 mg daily *(Spencer H et al. Magnesium in Health and Disease. Jamaica, NY, SP Medical and Scientific Books, 1980:911-19).*

- Potassium

Supplementation may increase urinary magnesium excretion.

> **Experimental Study:** Normotensive women received either a high-salt diet with 20 gm salt and 50 mEq potassium or the same diet with 100 mEq potassium. The high-potassium gp. showed substantial urinary losses of magnesium which paralleled urinary potassium excretion *(Saito N, Kuchiba A. The changes of magnesium under high salt diets and by administration of antihypertensive diuretics. Magnes Bull 9:53, 1987).*

- Protein

"During protein-synthesis and formation of new tissue by growing and developing children, by athletes-in-training, by pregnant or lactating women, and by those recovering from starvation or wasting illness, high-protein diets increase magnesium needs" *(Seelig MS. Magnesium requirements in human nutrition. Magnes Bull 3(Suppl 1a):26-47, 1981).*

- Riboflavin

High-dosage riboflavin increases the risk of magnesium deficiency *(Seelig MS. Magnesium requirements in human nutrition. Magnes Bull 3(Suppl 1a):26-47, 1981).*

- Sodium

Greater sodium loads, such as are provided when saline is used to expand the extracellular volume, decrease serum magnesium levels and increase urinary magnesium excretion. Magnesium deficiency is associated with sodium and water retention, while repletion produces sodium and water loss *(Seelig MS. Magnesium requirements in human nutrition. Magnes Bull 3(Suppl 1a):26-47, 1981).*

- Sugar

High intake of sugar increases the need for magnesium *(Durlach J. Le Diabete 19:99-113, 1971)* and increases urinary magnesium excretion *(Lindeman RB et al, in Magnesium in Health and Disease. Jamaica, NY, SP Medical and Scientific Books, 1980:236-45; Lindeman RB. Influence of various nutrients and hormones on urinary divalent cation excretion. Ann N Y Acad Sci 162:802-9, 1969).*

- Vitamin B$_6$

Magnesium and vitamin B$_6$ deficiency produce comparable clinical disorders, and treatment with either or both has been found effective in several clinical conditions in which one or the other has been investigated *(Seelig MS. Magnesium requirements in human nutrition. Magnes Bull 3(Suppl 1a):26-47, 1981).*

Deficiency is associated with a negative magnesium balance due to increased urinary magnesium excretion (*Turnlund JR, Betschart AA, Liebman M, et al. Vitamin B-6 depletion followed by repletion with animal- or plant-source diets and calcium and magnesium metabolism in young women. Am J Clin Nutr 56:905-10, 1992*).

Increases cell membrane transfer and utilization of magnesium (*Aikawa JK. Proc Soc Exp Biol Med 104:461-3, 1960; Durlach J. Donnees Actuelles Sur les mecanismes de Synergie entre Vitamin B$_6$ et Magnesium. J Medicine de Besancon 5:349, 1969*), resulting in increased tissue magnesium levels (*Majumdar P, Boylan M. Alteration of tissue magnesium levels in rats by dietary vitamin B$_6$ supplementation. Int J Vitam Nutr Res 59:300-3, 1989*).

Supplementation may normalize deficient intracellular magnesium levels.

> **Experimental Study:** 9 females with low red blood cell magnesium levels received vitamin B$_6$ 100 mg twice daily. After 4 wks., red cell magnesium levels had normalized (*Abraham GE et al. Effect of vitamin B$_6$ on plasma red blood cell magnesium levels in premenopausal women. Ann Clin Lab Sci 11(4):333-6, 1981*).

- Vitamin D

Stimulates intestinal magnesium absorption (*Nordin BEC. Plasma calcium and plasma magnesium homeostasis, in BEC Nordin, Ed. Calcium, Phosphorus and Magnesium Metabolism. New York, Churchill Livingstone, 1976*). It may enhance magnesium deficiency, however, as it increases calcium absorption more than it increases magnesium absorption; thus tissue calcium accumulation may displace magnesium (*Magnesium in Human Nutrition. US Department of Agriculture Home Econ. Res. Report No. 19, 1962*).

- Vitamin E

Deficiency may lower tissue magnesium levels (*Goldsmith LA. Relative magnesium deficiency in the rat. J Nutr 93:87-102, 1967; Seelig MS. Magnesium requirements in human nutrition. Magnes Bull 3(Suppl 1a):26-47, 1981*).

- Zinc

Supplementation may interfere with magnesium absorption and metabolic balance.

> **Experimental Study:** Supplementation of 21 healthy males (ave. age 58) with 142 mg zinc as zinc sulfate significantly decreased magnesium absorption and balance (*Spencer H, Norris C, Williams D. Inhibitory effects of zinc on magnesium balance and magnesium absorption in man. J Am Coll Nutr 13(5):479-84, 1994*).

Manganese

MAY BE INFLUENCED BY

- Calcium

Impairs plasma uptake.

Experimental Study: In a study of 6 adult subjects, the addition of calcium to a 40 mg oral manganese load essentially blocked the plasma uptake of manganese (*Freeland-Graves JH, Lin P-H. Plasma uptake of manganese as affected by oral loads of manganese, calcium, milk, phosphorus, copper, and zinc. J Am Coll Nutr 10(1):38-43, 1991*).

Reduces absorption.

Experimental Study: The addition of calcium to human milk resulted in a significant decrease in manganese absorption (*Davidsson L et al. The effect of individual dietary components on manganese absorption in humans. Am J Clin Nutr 54:1065-70, 1991*).

- Copper

Impairs plasma uptake.

Experimental Study: In a study of 6 adult subjects, the addition of copper to a 40 mg oral manganese load decreased the area under the curve for plasma manganese by about half (*Freeland-Graves JH, Lin P-H. Plasma uptake of manganese as affected by oral loads of manganese, calcium, milk, phosphorus, copper, and zinc. J Am Coll Nutr 10(1):38-43, 1991*).

- Iron

Accelerates the development of manganese deficiency (*Hurley LS, Keen CL. Manganese, in E Underwood and W Mertz, Eds. Trace Elements in Human Health and Animal Nutrition. New York, Academic Press, 1987:185-223*) by reducing absorption (*Finley JW, Johnson PE, Johnson LAK. Sex affects manganese absorption and retention by humans from a diet adequate in manganese. Am J Clin Nutr 60:949-55, 1994; Thomson ABR et al. Interrelation of intestinal transport system for manganese and iron. J Lab Clin Med 73:6422, 1971*).

Note: Iron status only appears to affect manganese absorption when it is below a certain point; above that point, manganese status may be independent of iron status, perhaps due to a low efficiency of iron absorption (Finley JW, Johnson PE, Johnson LAK. Sex affects manganese absorption and retention by humans from a diet adequate in manganese. Am J Clin Nutr 60:949-55, 1994).

Note: The negative effects of iron on manganese status refer to non-heme iron; heme-iron has no consistent effect on manganese nutriture (Davis CD, Malecki EA, Greger JL. Interactions among dietary manganese, heme iron, and nonheme iron in women. Am J Clin Nutr 56:926-32, 1992).

- Zinc

May increase plasma manganese levels.

Experimental Study: In a study of 6 adult subjects, the addition of zinc to a 40 mg oral manganese load produced a significant increase in plasma manganese (*Freeland-Graves JH, Lin P-H. Plasma uptake of manganese as affected by oral loads of manganese, calcium, milk, phosphorus, copper, and zinc. J Am Coll Nutr 10(1):38-43, 1991*).

N-acetylcysteine

MAY BE INFLUENCED BY

- nutrient minerals

Despite the ability of NAC to chelate heavy metals at high IV doses, it does not appear to reduce plasma concentrations of trace metals or increase their excretion when administered orally in therapeutic doses; thus additional supplementation with trace metals during oral administration is unnecessary (*Hjortso E, Fomsgaard JS, Fogh-Andersen N. Does N-acetylcysteine increase the excretion of trace metals (calcium, magnesium, iron, zinc and copper) with given orally? Eur J Clin Pharmacol 39(1):29-31, 1990*).

Niacin

MAY BE INFLUENCED BY

- Vitamin B6

A vitamin B6 deficiency often produces a niacin deficiency with pellagra-like clinical manifestations. The absence of improvement after IV niacin establishes the diagnosis (*Bousquet B, Larregue M, Barthelemy JP, et al. Syndrome pellagroide avec carence en vitamine B6 (étude biologique et clinique à propos d'un cas). Ann Biol Clin (Paris) 30:585-92, 1972*).

Omega-3 Essential Fatty Acids

MAY BE INFLUENCED BY

- Vitamin E

Supplementation may require additional vitamin E intake to prevent increased membrane peroxidation and immune suppression.

> *Note: Fish oil supplementation (rich in omega-3 fatty acids) markedly decreases plasma vitamin E levels to below the normal range, even if the supplement contains additional vitamin E and synthetic antioxidants* (*Sanders TAB, Hinds A. The influence of a fish oil high in docosahexaenoic acid on plasma lipoprotein and vitamin E concentrations and hemostatic function in healthy male volunteers. Br J Nutr 68:163-73, 1992*).

Review Article: The major safety concern regarding omega-3 fatty acid supplements is their potential to undergo oxidation in the body. Susceptibility of fatty acids to oxidative damage increases proportionally to the degree of unsaturation, and these fatty acids are among the most unsaturated in the diet. However, this problem is easily overcome by increasing the coingestion of more vitamin E, beta-carotene, or other lipid-soluble antioxidants (*Leaf A. Health claims: omega-3 fatty acids and cardiovascular disease. Nutr Rev 50(5):150-2, 1992*).

Omega-6 Essential Fatty Acids

MAY BE INFLUENCED BY

- Omega-3 Essential Fatty Acids

Omega-6 fatty acids cannot accumulate normally in cell membranes if the supply of omega-3 fatty acids is too low (*Bjerve KS et al. a-linolenic acid and long-chain w-3 fatty acid deficiency: effect on lymphocyte function, plasma and red cell lipids, and prostanoid formation. Am J Clin Nutr 49:290-300, 1989*).

- Vitamin E

Vitamin E prevents the peroxidation of polyunsaturated fatty acids and thus is recommended whenever they are heavily supplemented (*Chow CK. Nutritional influences on cellular antioxidant defense systems. Am J Clin Nutr 32:1066-81, 1979*).

Pantothenic acid

MAY BE INFLUENCED BY

- Biotin

Reduces the severity of symptoms of a pantothenic acid deficiency (*Sauberlich HE. Interactions of thiamin, riboflavin and other B-vitamins. Ann N Y Acad Sci 355:80-97, 1980*).

Phosphorus

MAY BE INFLUENCED BY

- Caffeine

Increases urinary excretion of inorganic phosphate and may cause a negative balance (*Yeh JK et al. Influence of injected caffeine on the metabolism of calcium and the retention and excretion of sodium, potassium, phosphorus, magnesium, zinc and copper in rats. J Nutr 116(2):273-80, 1986*).

- Calcium

Increases fecal phosphorus excretion by binding primarily dietary but also endogenous phosphorus (*Schiller LR et al. Effect of the time of administration of calcium acetate on phosphorus binding. N Engl J Med 320:1110-13, 1989*).

A calcium to phosphorus ratio above 2:1 due to excess calcium results in reduced bone strength and interferes with vitamin K synthesis and/or absorption, causing internal bleeding (*Calcium: How much is too much? Nutr Rev 43(11):345, 1985*).

- Vitamin D

Facilitates phosphate absorption (*Passmore R, Eastwood MA. Davidson and Passmore: Human Nutrition and Dietetics. Eighth Edition. London, Churchill Livingstone, 1986:139*).

Potassium

MAY BE INFLUENCED BY

- Caffeine

Increases urinary potassium excretion and may cause a negative balance (*Yeh JK et al. Influence of injected caffeine on the metabolism of calcium and the retention and excretion of sodium, potassium, phosphorus, magnesium, zinc and copper in rats. J Nutr 116(2):273-80, 1986*).

- Magnesium

Potassium deficiency may be refractory in the presence of magnesium depletion (*Rude RK. Physiology of magnesium metabolism and the important role of magnesium in potassium deficiency. Am J Cardiol 63(14):31G-34G, 1989; Whang R et al. Refractory potassium repletion: a consequence of magnesium deficiency. Arch Intern Med 152:40-5, 1992; Whang R et al. Magnesium depletion as a cause of refractory potassium repletion. Arch Intern Med 145(9):1686-9, 1985*) which has been found in 42% of patients with hypokalemia (*Whang R et al. Predictors of clinical hypomagnesemia. Hypokalemia, hypophosphatemia, hyponatremia, and hypocalcemia. Arch Intern Med 144(9):1794-6, 1984*).

Magnesium may have a regulatory role in the maintenance of cellular potassium concentration and may be required in addition to potassium supplementation for patients treated with diuretics (*Dorup I, Skajaa K, Thybo HK. Oral magnesium supplementation restores the concentrations of magnesium, potassium and sodium-potassium pumps in skeletal muscle of patients receiving diuretic treatment. J Intern Med 233:177-23, 1993*).

Protein

MAY BE INFLUENCED BY

- Calcium

Increases nitrogen excretion and thus may adversely affect protein status (*Kandiah J, Kies C. Calcium carbonate supplements may adversely affect protein nutriture. Nutr Res 14:177-84, 1994*).

Selenium

MAY BE INFLUENCED BY

- Vitamin B$_6$

Affects the distribution, transportation, and metabolism of selenium (*Yin S, Sato I, Yamaguchi K. Comparison of selenium level and glutathione peroxidase activity in tissues of vitamin B$_6$-deficient rats fed sodium selenite or DL-selenomethionine. J Nutr Biochem 3:633-43, 1992*).

- Vitamin C

An adequate ascorbic acid status is important in the maintenance of body selenium metabolism.

> **Experimental Study:** While levels of natural selenium in urine, plasma, and feces do not vary with the intake of low and high amts. of ascorbic acid, the selenite-exchangeable metabolic pool is reduced following ascorbic acid restriction (*Martin RF et al. Ascorbic acid-selenite interactions in humans studied with a oral dose of $^{74}SeO_3^{2-}$. Am J Clin Nutr 49:862-9, 1989*).

> **Experimental Study:** 30 Finnish female students aged 21-30 received with meals either sodium selenite 50 mg 3 times daily, sodium selenite and vitamin C 600 mg, or vitamin C 600 mg. After 4 wks., the largest plasma selenium increase was in the gp. receiving both selenium and vitamin C. As all 3 gps. had significant increases in glutathione peroxidase levels, results suggest that vitamin C increased the bioavailability of all dietary selenium, not just the sodium selenite supplement, in subjects who had a low baseline selenium status (*Mutanen M, Mykkanen HM. Effect of ascorbic acid supplementation on selenium bioavailability in humans. Hum Nutr Clin Nutr 39C:221-6, 1985*).

Sodium selenite is reduced by vitamin C *in vitro* to the ineffective elemental selenium, a reaction which is the basis for the analytical measurement of selenium (*Newberry & Christian, JOAC 48:322, 1965*).

> **Experimental Study:** In healthy subjects, absorption of 1 mg selenium as sodium selenite 2 hrs. given with breakfast or juice was measured by fecal and urinary excretion. When ascorbic acid 1 g was added to the selenium supplement and both were consumed 2 hrs. before a meal, absorption was significantly reduced. Ascorbic acid reduces selenite to elemental selenium which is poorly absorbed (*Robinson MF, Thomas CD, Huemmer PK. Effect of a megadose of ascorbic acid, a meal and orange juice on the absorption of selenium as sodium selenite. N Z Med J 98:627-9, 1985*).

- Vitamin E

Deficiency syndromes of both vitamin E and selenium overlap and most can be treated successfully with either nutrient due to their closely-related mechanisms of action (*Combs GF. Assessment of vitamin E status in animals and man. Proc Nutr Soc 40:187-94, 1981*).

Sodium

MAY BE INFLUENCED BY

- Caffeine

Increases urinary sodium excretion and may cause a negative balance (*Yeh JK et al. Influence of injected caffeine on the metabolism of calcium and the retention and excretion of sodium, potassium, phosphorus, magnesium, zinc and copper in rats. J Nutr 116(2):273-80, 1986*).

- Calcium

Increases urinary sodium excretion (*Nordin BEC, Needd AG, Morris HA, Horowitz M. The nature and significant of the relationship between urinary sodium and urinary calcium in women. J Nutr 123:1615-22, 1993*).

Thiamine

MAY BE INFLUENCED BY

- Magnesium

Necessary for the conversion of thiamine into thiamine pyrophosphate, its biologically active form (*Seelig MS. Nutritional status and requirements of magnesium with consideration of individual differences and prevention of cardiovascular disease. Magnesium Bull 8:170-84, 1986*).

> **Case Report:** A 44 year-old pt. with Crohn's disease and chronic diarrhea resulting in thiamine and magnesium deficiency failed to respond to massive IV doses of thiamine until the magnesium deficiency was corrected (*Dyckner T, Ek B, Nyhlin H, Wester PO. Aggravation of thiamine deficiency by magnesium depletion. A case report. Acta Med Scand 218:129, 1985*).

See Also:

> *Zieve L. Role of cofactors in the treatment of malnutrition as exemplified by magnesium. Yale J Biol Med 48:229-37, 1975*

> *Stendig-Lindberg G. Hypomagnesemia in alcohol encephalopathies. Acta Psychiatr Scand 50:465-80, 1974*

L-Tryptophan

MAY BE INFLUENCED BY

- Carbohydrate

Effects of tryptophan are potentiated by concurrent carbohydrate ingestion in order to stimulate insulin release which takes up the other amino acids into the tissues, thus improving brain tryptophan intake (*Fernstrom JD. Effects of the diet on brain neurotransmitters. Metabolism 26:207-33, 1977*).

- Niacinamide

The rationale for the addition of niacinamide to tryptophan is that the high rate of catabolism of tryptophan by the liver suggested by animal work can be inhibited with niacinamide (*Young SN, Sourkes TL. The antidepressant effect of tryptophan. Lancet ii:897-8, 1974*). Recent data, however, indicate that niacinamide will not inhibit breakdown of tryptophan in humans at clinical doses following an acute loading (*Green AR et al. Metabolism of an oral tryptophan load: Effect of pretreatment with the putative tryptophan pyrollase inhibitors nicotinamide or allopurinol. Br J Clin Pharmacol 10:611-15, 1980*). In addition, in pts. receiving up to 6 gm tryptophan daily along with niacinamide, tryptophan metabolism was still highly variable; thus it is unlikely that niacinamide is a useful adjunct (*Chouinard G et al. Tryptophan in the treatment of depression and mania. Adv Biol Psychiatry 10:47-66, 1983*).

- Protein

Effects of tryptophan are potentiated by avoiding protein for 90 minutes before or afterwards (*Fernstrom JD et al. Diurnal variations in plasma concentrations of tryptophan, tyrosine, and other neutral amino acids: Effects of dietary protein intake. Am J Clin Nutr 32:1912-22, 1979*).

- Riboflavin

Required for the conversion of tryptophan to nicotinic acid (*Sauberlich HE. Interactions of thiamin, riboflavin and other B-vitamins. Ann N Y Acad Sci 355:80-97, 1980*).

- Vitamin B$_6$

Supplementation may increase serotonin synthesis, perhaps due to an increase of tryptophan transport into serotonergic neurons.

> **Experimental Crossover Study:** 6 healthy females and 4 healthy males, aged 22-45, received 80 mg pyridoxine hydrochloride and/or 0.5 g, 1.0 g or 2.0 g L-tryptophan following a 2 hr. fast at 2200 hrs. and continued for 7 days with 1-wk. wash-out periods in-between each trial. A significant increase in the nocturnal excretion of urinary 5-HIAA (a serotonin metabolite) was measured following 7 days of treatment with pyridoxine and also after both single and repeated administration of 2 gm tryptophan together with pyridoxine (p<0.05). A single dose of 2 gm tryptophan led to a small, insignificant increase in 5-HIAA. The urinary 5-HIAA excretion rate decreased significantly after 7 days of administration of 2 gm tryptophan, but not when tryptophan was administered with pyridoxine. Comparable increases in urinary 5-HIAA excretion were also measured following single or repeated administration of 1 gm and 0.5 gm tryptophan in conjunction with 80 mg pyridoxine. Analysis of variance for dependent gps. showed neither a significant effect of the tryptophan dose nor of the time course of application. Also, a dose-dependent increase in urinary kynurenine excretions at night was measured following a single or subchronic

administration of tryptophan or tryptophan plus pyridoxine, while pyridoxine and subchronic administration of tryptophan did not lead to significant changes in urinary kynurenine. In conclusion, 1 wk. administration of 80 mg pyridoxine alone or together with tryptophan increased serotonin synthesis, perhaps due to an increase of tryptophan transport into serotonergic neurons. It appears unlikely that the increase was caused by a reduction in kynurenine levels since no effect of pyridoxine on urinary kynurenine excretion was found, although it is possible that pyridoxine led to reduced plasma kynurenine levels which was not reflected in urinary excretion *(Bemisch L, Kaczmarczyk P. Tryptophan metabolism in healthy subjects: influence on pyridoxine after single or repeated administrations. Adv Exp Med Biol 294:519-21, 1991).*

Supplementation may increase brain serotonin (5-hydroxytryptamine) content by influencing the decarboxylation of 5-hydroxytryptophan by pyridoxal phosphate *(Dakshinamurti K, Sharma SK, Bonke D. Influence of B vitamins on binding properties of serotonin receptors in the CNS of rats. Klin Wochenschr 68(2):142-5, 1990).*

Supplementation may increase brain tryptophan levels by reducing levels of kynurenine which competes with tryptophan for transport.

> **Review Articles:** Kynurenine is derived from tryptophan by the action of tryptophan pyrrolase in the liver and is taken up in the brain and transferred by the same transport carrier as tryptophan where it has a competitively inhibitory effect upon tryptophan equal to that of the competing amino acids *(Möller SE et al. Tryptophan availability in endogenous depression - relation to efficacy of L-tryptophan treatment. Adv Biol Psychiatry 10:30-46, 1983).* Supplementation with tryptophan increases the plasma concentration of kynurenine in proportion to the dose given and, after longer-term administration, there is a marked increase in basal kynurenine with a further substantial increase following a further dose of tryptophan. This large increase in kynurenine concentration might reflect a relative saturation of the kynurenine pathway, possibly because of vitamin B_6 depletion since many of the degradative enzymes down the pathway are B_6-dependent. Consistent with this hypothesis are findings that, when tryptophan is given for 7 days with pyridoxine, the basal plasma kynurenine is half that seen in subjects given tryptophan alone, and the peak kynurenine concentration following a single load is the same after long-term pretreatment with tryptophan plus pyridoxine as after no pre-treatment and only half that seen in subjects who have taken longer-term tryptophan without pyridoxine *(Green AR, Aronson JK. The pharmacokinetics of oral L-tryptophan: Effects of dose and concomitant pyridoxine, allopurinol or nicotinamide administration. Adv Biol Psychiatry 10:67-81, 1983).*

Vanadium

MAY BE INFLUENCED BY

- Chromium

Chromium is vanadium's principal antagonist *(Hill CH. Mineral interrelationships, in AS Prasad, D Oberleas, Eds. Trace Elements in Human Health and Disease. Volume 2. New York, Academic Press, 1976:281-300).*

Vitamin A

MAY BE INFLUENCED BY

- Vitamin C

Increases the availability of vitamin A (*Wilson RL. Free radical protection: why vitamin E, not vitamin C, beta-carotene or glutathione, in R Porter, J Whelan, Eds. Biology of Vitamin E. London, Pitman, 1983:19-37*).

- Vitamin E

Vitamin A absorption may be markedly impaired in vitamin E deficiency.

> **Animal Experimental Study:** Vitamin A levels of vitamin-E-deficient mice remained low after vitamin A injections until they also received vitamin E injections (*Ames SR. Factors affecting absorption, transport and storage of vitamin A. Am J Clin Nutr 22:934, 1969*).

Vitamin E supplementation may improve the therapeutic efficacy of vitamin A.

> **Review Article:** Tissue levels of retinol and retinol esters are increased following increased dietary levels of alpha tocopherol. Experimental work with rats suggests that the increase in vitamin A levels is due to inhibition of vitamin E of the hydrolysis of vitamin A esters such as retinyl palmitate at physiological concentrations (*Alpha-tocopherol influences tissue levels of vitamin A and its esters. Nutr Rev 43:55-6, 1985*).

> **Case Report:** 200,000 units of vitamin A daily produced only slight improvement in a case of Darier's Disease. However, after the addition of 1600 units of vitamin E, 100,000 units of vitamin A produced dramatic improvement (*Ayres S. Darier's Disease: Update on an effective new therapy. Arch Dermatol 119:710, 1983*).

See Also:

> *Napoli JL, McCormick AM, O'Meara B, Dratz EA. Vitamin A metabolism: alpha-tocopherol modulates tissue retinol levels in vivo, and retinyl palmitate hydrolysis in vitro. Arch Biochem Biophys 230:194-202, 1984*

Vitamin E supplementation may prevent the side effects of high doses of vitamin A (*Graf N et al. Retinoids in the treatment of acute promyelocytic leukemia: review of the literature. Klin Pediatr 207:43-7, 1995; Weiser H, Probst HP, Bachmann H. Vitamin E prevents side effects of high doses of vitamin A in chicks. Ann N Y Acad Sci 669:396-8, 1992*).

> **Review Article:** Vitamin E protects vitamin A from oxidation in both the intestinal lumen and in the tissues, and by joining with it within the membranous parts of cells in performing its functions (*Tappel AL. Nutrition Today July-August 1973*).

- Zinc

Despite an adequate vitamin A intake, a low zinc diet may be associated with signs of vitamin A deficiency (*Rogers S. AAEM Newsletter, Winter, 1988; Smith JC Jr. The vitamin A - zinc connection. Ann N Y Acad Sci 355:62, 1980*):

1. Zinc is crucial for the activity of the enzyme alcohol dehydrogenase - which converts retinol (the ingested form of vitamin A) into retinaldehyde, the first usable breakdown product.

2. A zinc deficiency impairs the synthesis of retinol-binding protein which is necessary to release vitamin A from liver stores into the blood (*Smith JC Jr et al. Zinc: a trace element essential in vitamin A metabolism. Science 181:954-5, 1973; Smith J et al. The effect of zinc deficiency on the metabolism of retinol-binding protein in the rat. J Lab Clin Med 84:692-7, 1974*).

Vitamin B$_6$

MAY BE INFLUENCED BY

- Magnesium

Magnesium and vitamin B$_6$ deficiency produce comparable clinical disorders, and treatment with either magnesium or B$_6$, or both, have been found effective in several clinical conditions in which one or the other has been investigated (*Seelig MS. Magnesium requirements in human nutrition. Magnesium Bull 3(Suppl 1a):26-47, 1981*).

- Riboflavin

Necessary for the proper utilization of vitamin B6 (*Sauberlich HE. Interactions of thiamin, riboflavin and other B-vitamins. Ann N Y Acad Sci 355:80-97, 1980*).

- Vitamin C

Depletion increases vitamin B6 excretion (*Sauberlich HE. Interactions of thiamin, riboflavin and other B-vitamins. Ann N Y Acad Sci 355:80-97, 1980*).

- Vitamin E

Combined supplementation may have a beneficial synergistic effect on cell membrane function.

Experimental Study: Adult male volunteers belonging to a low socioeconomic class were studied. Administration of vitamin B6 alone showed a statistically insignificant increase in erythrocyte membrane Na^+-K^+-ATPase activity, while vitamin E alone produced only a transient increase in total and ouabain insensitive Na^+-K^+-ATPase activity. Combined administration, however, resulted in a significant increase in both total and true Na^+-K^+-ATPase activity (*Nadiger HA, Rao*

AS, Sadasivudu B. *Effects of simultaneous administration of vitamin E and pyridoxine on erythrocyte membrane (sodium, potassium) - ATPase activity. Int J Vitam Nutr Res 54(4):307-11, 1984).*

Vitamin B$_{12}$

MAY BE INFLUENCED BY

- Folic Acid

High dose folate therapy may decrease serum vitamin B$_{12}$ levels; thus B$_{12}$ supplementation or regular monitoring is indicated (*Hunter R et al. Effect of folic-acid supplement on serum-vitamin-B$_{12}$ levels in patients on anticonvulsants. Lancet ii:50, 1969*).

In patients with untreated cobalamin deficiency, dosages of folate >1 mg daily may ameliorate the anemia of pernicious anemia, but in about half the patients the neuropathy develops or progresses (*Chanarin I. Adverse effects of increased dietary folate. Relation to measures to reduce the incidence of neural tube defects. Clin Invest Med 17(3):131-7, 1994*).

- Lithium

Lithium may be involved in the transport and distribution of vitamin B$_{12}$, since hair lithium and cobalt concentrations show a highly significant direct association (*Schrauzer GN, Shrestha KP, Flores-Arce MF. Lithium in scalp hair of adults, students, and violent criminals. Biol Trace Elem Res 34(2):161-76, 1992*).

- Potassium

Prolonged-release potassium supplements can diminish the intestinal absorption of B$_{12}$ preparations (*Drug Evaluations Subscription. Chicago, American Medical Association, Vol III, Section 19, Chapter 5, Spring, 1993*).

- Vitamin B$_6$

Deficiency causes decreased vitamin B$_{12}$ absorption and reduced B$_{12}$ levels in serum and liver (*Sauberlich HE. Interactions of thiamin, riboflavin and other B-vitamins. Ann N Y Acad Sci 355:80-97, 1980*).

- Vitamin C

A report that vitamin C causes the degradation of vitamin B$_{12}$ (*Herbert V, Jacob E. Destruction of vitamin B$_{12}$ by ascorbic acid. JAMA 230(2):241-2, 1974*) was unconfirmed in 2 independent laboratories (*Newmark HL, Scheiner JM, Marcus M, Prabhudesai M. Ascorbic acid and vitamin B$_{12}$. JAMA 242(21):2319-20, 1979; Newmark HL, Scheiner JM, Marcus M, Prabhudesai M. Stability of vitamin B$_{12}$ in the presence of ascorbic acid. Am J Clin Nutr 29(6):645-9, 1976*) who suggested that the degradation of vitamin B$_{12}$ was due to failure of the original investigators to properly protect the extracted B$_{12}$ in the assay procedure.

<u>Vitamin C</u>

MAY BE INFLUENCED BY

- <u>Copper</u>

While the action of all metals increases the rate of destruction of vitamin C, exposure of vitamin C to copper is particularly destructive to it (*deMan JM. <u>Principles of Food Chemistry</u>. Second Edition. Reinhold, New York, Van Nostrand, 1990*).

- <u>Flavonoids</u>

While flavonoids can enhance the bioavailability of vitamin C, the dosages of flavonoids available in commercial preparations are generally too low to be effective.

Negative Experimental Double-blind Study: Ascorbic acid alone was compared under randomized double-blind conditions to a commercial preparation of ascorbic acid plus hesperidin-rutin-buckwheat citrus flavonoids having a ratio (weight per weight) of flavonoids to vitamin C of 0.05 to 1 (which is typical of commercial sources). Following ingestion by 9 healthy subjects, measurements of plasma and urinary vitamin C were comparable, as were 24-hr. vitamin C urinary excretions (*Johnston CS, Luo B. Comparison of the absorption and excretion of three commercially available sources of vitamin C. <u>J Am Diet Assoc</u> 94(7):779-81, 1994*).

Experimental Study: Healthy subjects received solutions of either vitamin C alone or vitamin C plus flavonoids with a 4 to 1 weight per weight ratio of flavonoids to vitamin C. The addition of flavonoids was found to enhance the bioavailability of vitamin C as it was more readily absorbed and remained longer in the body (*Vinson JA, Bose P. Comparative bioavailability of synthetic and natural vitamin C in guinea pigs. <u>Nutr Rep Int</u> 27:875-80, 1983*).

Experimental Study: Compared to the ingestion of vitamin C alone, the addition of 25 mg flavonoids to 500 mg vitamin C (ratio of 1 to 20) increased urinary vitamin C excretion in 5 young male volunteers, suggesting that oral absorption of vitamin C was enhanced (*Jones E, Hughes RE. <u>IRCS Med Sci</u> 12:320, 1984*).

Animal Experimental Study: Guinea pigs received solutions of either vitamin C alone or vitamin C plus flavonoids with a 0.7 to 1 weight per weight ratio of flavonoids to vitamin C. The addition of flavonoids was found to enhance the bioavailability of vitamin C as it was more readily absorbed and remained longer in the body (*Vinson JA, Bose P. Comparative bioavailability of synthetic and natural vitamin C in guinea pigs. <u>Nutr Rep Int</u> 27:875-80, 1983*).

See Also:

Vinson JA, Bose P. Bioavailability of synthetic ascorbic acid and a citrus extract. <u>Ann N Y Acad Sci</u> 498:525-6, 1987

- Glutathione

Acts together with vitamin C to alleviate various oxidant stresses (*Jacob R. The integrated antioxidant system. Nutr Res 15:755-66, 1995*).

- Iron

While the action of all metals increases the rate of destruction of vitamin C, exposure of vitamin C to iron is particularly destructive to it (*deMan JM. Principles of Food Chemistry. Second Edition. Reinhold, New York, Van Nostrand, 1990*).

- Vitamin B6

Depletion is accompanied by reduced whole blood vitamin C levels (*Sauberlich HE. Interactions of thiamin, riboflavin and other B-vitamins. Ann N Y Acad Sci 355:80-97, 1980*).

Vitamin D

MAY BE INFLUENCED BY

- Calcium

Diets deficient in calcium stimulate parathyroid hormone secretion which increases the degradation of 25-hydroxy vitamin D leading to a secondary vitamin D deficiency (*Siu-Caldera ML, Allen LH, O'Brien KO, et al. Diets deficient in calcium increase the degradation of 25(OH) vitamin D. Abstract. J Am Coll Nutr 12:618, 1993*).

- Phosphorus

Phosphorus intake strongly influences vitamin D metabolism.

> **Experimental Study:** The circadian rhythm of serum phosphorus along with the production rate of 1,25-dihydroxyvitamin D was monitored in 6 healthy men receiving 1,500 mg dietary phosphorus/70 kg body wt./d, then restricted to 500 mg, then supplemented to 2,000 mg. Dietary phosphorus was found to be an important determinant of serum phosphorus concentration throughout most of the day, and diet-induced changes in serum phosphorus levels mediated the changes in the production rate of 1,25-$(OH)_2D$ (*Portale AA et al. Dietary intake of phosphorus modulates the circadian rhythm in serum concentration of phosphorus. J Clin Invest 80:1147-54, 1987*).

> **Experimental Study:** Increases and reductions in oral phosphorus intake in healthy men were found to induce rapidly occurring, large, inverse, and persisting changes in serum 1,25-dihydroxyvitamin D levels due to phosphorus-induced changes in the rate of vitamin D production (*Portale A. Oral intake of phosphorus can determine the serum concentration of 1,25-dihydroxyvitamin D by determining its production rate in humans. J Clin Invest 77:7-12, 1986*).

- Vitamin E

Deficiency inhibits vitamin D metabolism in the liver and kidneys *(Sergeev IN, Arkhapchev YP, Spirichev VB. The role of vitamin E in the metabolism and reception of vitamin D. Biochimiya-Engl Tr 55:1483-7, 1990).*

Vitamin E

MAY BE INFLUENCED BY

- Beta-Carotene

Interact synergistically to inhibit lipid peroxidation *(Palozza P, Krinsky NI. B-carotene and alpha-tocopherol are synergistic antioxidants. Arch Biochem Biophys 297(1):184-7, 1992).*

Supplementation with beta-carotene alone may fail to increase plasma vitamin E levels or may even lower them.

Experimental Double-blind Study: 500 pts. received daily supplements of 25 mg beta carotene, 1 gm vitamin C plus 400 mg vitamin E, or all 3 vitamins. After 9 mo., subjects given beta carotene alone had increased beta carotene levels and <u>unchanged</u> vitamin E status, while subjects given vitamin E supplements showed improved vitamin E status and unchanged beta carotene levels. Supplementation with all 3 vitamins improved all measured vitamin levels *(Nierenberg D, Stukel T, Mott L, et al. Steady-state serum concentration of alpha tocopherol not altered by supplementation with oral beta carotene. J Natl Cancer Inst 86:117-20, 1994).*

Experimental Double-blind Study: 45 normal volunteers randomly received either placebo or 15, 30, 45, or 60 mg of oral beta-carotene daily. There was a progressive <u>decrease</u> in plasma alpha-tocopherol. Results were significant between 6 and 9 mo. of dosing in all dosage groups. The greatest decrease was during the last month when it totaled 40% from baseline *(Xu MJ, Plezia PM, Alberts DS, et al. Reduction in plasma or skin alpha-tocopherol concentration with long-term oral administration of beta-carotene in humans and mice. J Natl Cancer Inst 84(20):1559-65, 1992).*

- and Vitamin A

Combined supplementation may increase serum vitamin E levels.

Experimental Study: In a study of 1319 participants enrolled in the Carotene and Retinol Efficacy Trial who had taken 30 mg beta-carotene and 25,000 IU vitamin A for up to 6 yrs., there was a small but statistically significant increase in serum alpha-tocopherol levels, and no evidence of a decrease in serum alpha-tocopherol levels in any of the sub-gps. examined *(Goodman GE, Metch BJ, Omenn GS. The effect of long-term beta-carotene and vitamin A administration on serum concentrations of alpha-tocopherol. Cancer Epidemiol Biomark Prev 3:429-32, 1994).*

Supplementation with the combination of vitamin E and beta-carotene may produce a greater increase in plasma vitamin E levels than that produced by vitamin E supplementation alone.

> **Experimental Study:** 91 volunteers were fed vitamin E 800 mg/day beta-carotene 30 mg/day and ascorbic acid 1000 mg/day in various combinations for 14 days each. Beta-carotene supplementation significantly increased circulating vitamin E above that seen when vitamin E was ingested alone; however, the combination of all three nutrients failed to significantly increase plasma vitamin E. Adding beta-carotene or ascorbic acid to vitamin E supplementation seems a practical means of increasing the antioxidant potential of vitamin E (*Baker H, DeAngelis B, Baker E, et al. Human plasma patterns during 14 days ingestion of vitamin E, beta-carotene, ascorbic acid, and their various combinations. J Am Coll Nutr 15(2):159-63, 1996*).

- Coenzyme Q$_{10}$

Reduces the phenoxyl radical of vitamin E and recycles it back to alpha-tocopherol (*Stoyanovsky D, Osipov A, Quinn P, et al. Ubiquinone-dependent recycling of vitamin-E radicals by superoxide. Arch Biochem 323(2):343-51, 1995*).

- Glutathione

Protects vitamin E from oxidation (*Palamanda J, Kehrer J. Involvement of vitamin-E and protein thiols in the inhibition of microsomal lipid-peroxidation by glutathione. Lipids 28:427-31, 1993*).

- inorganic (ferric) Iron

Oxidizes vitamin E in the intestines, causing its inactivation.

> *Note: Ferrous iron, which is the form of iron commonly used for supplementation, does not oxidize vitamin E.*

- Selenium

Deficiency syndromes of both vitamin E and selenium overlap and most can be treated successfully with either nutrient due to their closely-related mechanisms of action (*Combs GF. Assessment of vitamin E status in animals and man. Proc Nutr Soc 40:187-94, 1981*).

- Vitamin A

High doses may suppress the level of vitamin E by as much as 40% (*Meyskins FL. Coming of age - the chemoprevention of cancer. N Engl J Med 323(12):825-7, 1990*).

- Vitamin B$_6$

Combined supplementation may have a beneficial synergistic effect on cell membrane function.

Experimental Study: Adult male volunteers belonging to a low socioeconomic class were studied. Administration of vitamin B_6 alone showed a statistically insignificant increase in erythrocyte membrane Na^+-K^+-ATPase activity, while vitamin E alone produced only a transient increase in total and ouabain insensitive Na^+-K^+-ATPase activity. Combined administration, however, resulted in a significant increase in both total and true Na^+-K^+-ATPase activity (*Nadiger HA, Rao AS, Sadasivudu B. Effects of simultaneous administration of vitamin E and pyridoxine on erythrocyte membrane (sodium, potassium) - ATPase activity. Int J Vitam Nutr Res 54(4):307-11, 1984*).

- Vitamin C

Sufficient levels are required to regenerate tocopherol from the tocopheroxyl radical so that vitamin E can be maximally effective (*Bendich A et al. The anti-oxidant role of vitamin C. Adv Free Rad Biol Med 2:419-44, 1986; Niki E, Noguchi N, Tsuchihashi H, Gotoh N. Interaction among vitamin C, vitamin E, and β-carotene. Am J Clin Nutr 62(suppl):1322S-6S, 1995*).

Supplementation with the combination of vitamin E and vitamin C may produce a greater increase in plasma vitamin E levels than that produced by vitamin E supplementation alone.

Experimental Study: 91 volunteers were fed vitamin E 800 mg/day beta-carotene 30 mg/day and ascorbic acid 1000 mg/day in various combinations for 14 days each. Ascorbic acid supplementation significantly increased circulating vitamin E above that seen when vitamin E was ingested alone; however, the combination of all three nutrients failed to significantly increase plasma vitamin E. Adding beta-carotene or ascorbic acid to vitamin E supplementation seems a practical means of increasing the antioxidant potential of vitamin E (*Baker H, DeAngelis B, Baker E, et al. Human plasma patterns during 14 days ingestion of vitamin E, beta-carotene, ascorbic acid, and their various combinations. J Am Coll Nutr 15(2):159-63, 1996*).

- Zinc

Deficiency may worsen the effects of vitamin E deficiency.

Animal Experimental Study: Dietary zinc deficiency in rats resulted in a significant decrease in plasma vitamin E concentrations compared to controls. While zinc deficiency also resulted in significant decreases in plasma levels of zinc, retinol, triglyceride and cholesterol, the decrease in plasma vitamin E levels was out of proportion to the decrease in plasma triglyceride and cholesterol concentrations; thus it resulted in a significant reduction in the plasma vitamin E to plasma cholesterol ratio. Vitamin E supplementation increased plasma vitamin E in both zinc-deficient and zinc-supplemented animals, but the increase in plasma vitamin E concentrations was not as great in the zinc-deficient animals (*Bunk MJ et al. Dietary zinc deficiency decreases plasma concentrations of vitamin E. Proc Soc Exp Biol Med 190:379-84, 1989*).

Animal Experimental Study: In a study of rat fetal development, a combined zinc and vitamin E deficiency led to an accumulation of cell membrane damage that was more than additive, suggesting an interaction of these deficiencies (*Harding AJ et al. Teratogenic effect of vitamin E and zinc deficiency in the 11 day rat embryo. Nutr Rep Int 36:473-82, 1987*).

Vitamin K

MAY BE INFLUENCED BY

- Calcium

Excessive doses of calcium or a calcium to phosphorus ratio above 2:1 due to excess calcium interferes with vitamin K synthesis and/or absorption, causing internal bleeding (*Calcium: How much is too much? Nutr Rev 43(11):345, 1985*).

- Vitamin E

A large intake may reduce intestinal absorption of vitamin K and antagonize the effect of vitamin K on coagulation at the level of prothrombin formation (*Bieri JG et al. Medical uses of vitamin E. N Engl J Med 308(18):1063-71, 1983*).

Zinc

MAY BE INFLUENCED BY

- Calcium

Decreases zinc absorption (*Argiratos V, Samman S. The effect of calcium carbonate and calcium citrate on the absorption of zinc in healthy female subjects. Eur J Clin Nutr 48:198-204, 1994*).

Negative Experimental Study: Adult men with a normal dietary zinc intake received calcium 200 mg, 800 and 2000 mg daily. Increasing calcium intake from 200 mg to the 2 higher levels did not significantly change the urinary or fecal zinc excretions or the zinc balance (*Spencer H, Kramer L, Norris C, Osis D. Effect of calcium and phosphorus on zinc metabolism in man. Am J Clin Nutr 40:1213-18, 1984*).

- Copper

Decreases zinc absorption and increases urinary zinc excretion

Experimental Study: 5 healthy men were fed one level of dietary zinc and 3 levels of dietary copper and studied using stable isotope tracers. Based on the findings, a compartmental model predicted that movement of zinc through the GI tract increased, and zinc absorption decreased slightly, when the highest level of copper was fed, and urinary zinc excretion rate tended to increase (*Scott KC, Turnlund JR. A compartmental model of zinc metabolism in adult men used to study effects of three levels of dietary copper. Am J Physiol 267(1 Pt 1):E165-73, 1994*).

Experimental Study: In a study of the effect of copper supplementation during recovery of infants from acute diarrhea, a significant interference by copper supplementation on zinc absorption was noted (*Castillo-Durán C et al. Oral copper supplementation: effect on copper and zinc balance during acute gastroenteritis in infants. Am J Clin Nutr 51:1088-92, 1990*).

Negative Experimental Study: In a study of healthy adult male humans, high doses of oral copper had no effect on zinc absorption (*Valberg LS et al. Effects of iron, tin, and copper on zinc absorption in humans. Am J Clin Nutr 40:536-51, 1984*).

- Folic Acid

Decreases zinc absorption.

Negative Experimental Placebo-controlled Study: 12 men aged 20-34 consumed a diet containing 3.5 mg or 14.5 mg zinc daily for two 25-day intervals. Results suggest that short-term folic acid supplementation does not adversely affect zinc status (*Kauwell GP, Bailey LB, Gregory JF 3rd, et al. Zinc status is not adversely affected by folic acid supplementation and zinc intake does not impair folate utilization in human subjects. J Nutr 125(1):66-72, 1995*).

Review Article: "Although high concentrations of folate may interfere with the intestinal absorption of zinc in experimental animals, the weight of current evidence indicates that daily oral supplements of 5-15 mg folate do not adversely affect zinc balance in normal humans over periods of 6 mo. to 4 yrs." (*Butterworth CE Jr, Tamura T. Folic acid safety and toxicity: A brief review. Am J Clin Nutr 50:353-8, 1989*).

Negative Experimental Blinded Study: Plasma zinc concentration was not significantly different following supplementation with folic acid 10 mg/d for up to 4 mo. (*Butterworth CE, Hatch K, Cole P, et al. Zinc concentration in plasma and erythrocytes of subjects receiving folic acid supplementation. Am J Clin Nutr 47:484-6, 1988*).

Negative Experimental Study: Studies of zinc absorption and utilization in both humans and rats failed to reveal evidence of inhibition by folic acid (*Keating J, Wada L, Stokstad ELR, King JC. Folic acid: Effect on zinc absorption in humans and in the rat. Am J Clin Nutr 46(5):835-9, 1987*).

Experimental Study: Zinc absorption in 10 healthy subjects was reduced by folate supplements (*Simmer K, Iles CA, James C, Thompson RPH. Are iron-folate supplements harmful? Am J Clin Nutr 45(1):122-5, 1987*).

Experimental Study: 8 men were fed diets containing 150 µg folic acid, and 4 of them also received supplementation with an additional 400 µg of folate daily. Fecal zinc was significantly higher in the supplemented gp. both during the control diet and during a low-zinc diet; no differences were noted in fecal zinc during high zinc intake. During all dietary periods urinary zinc excretion was reduced 50% in the folic acid-supplemented group. These data suggest that folate supplementation may influence zinc homeostasis by forming insoluble chelates which impair absorption (*Milne DB, Canfield WK, Mahalko JR, Sandstead HH. Effect of oral folic acid supplements on zinc, copper, and iron absorption and excretion. Am J Clin Nutr 39(4):535-9, 1984*).

- Iron

When deficient, zinc absorption is enhanced (*Pollack S et al. The absorption of nonferrous metals in iron deficiency. J Clin Invest 44:1470, 1965*).

When iron to zinc ratios are greater than 2 to 1, supplementation may exacerbate subclinical zinc depletion by competitively inhibiting intestinal absorption (*Meadows NJ, Grainger SL, Ruse W, et al. Oral iron and the bioavailability of zinc. Br Med J [Clin Res] 287:1013-14, 1983; Solomons NW, Jacob RA. Studies on the bioavailability of zinc in humans. Effects of heme and non-heme iron on the absorption of zinc. Am J Clin Nutr 34:475-82, 1981*).

> *Note: Although iron inhibits zinc absorption from liquids, increased iron does not significantly impair zinc absorption from foods. However, the long-term effects of increased iron intake on zinc nutrition have not been conclusively elucidated* (Davidsson L, Almgren A, Sandström B, Hurrell RF. Zinc absorption in adult humans: the effect of iron fortification. Br J Nutr 74:417-25, 1995).

Experimental Study: When 55 healthy men and women consumed an iron-containing multimineral supplement on an empty stomach, zinc absorption was inhibited from 74-85%. The effect of iron was somewhat mitigated when both minerals were taken with a meal or when a zinc ligand such was histidine was added (*Sandstrom B, Davidsson L, Cederblad A, Lonnerdal B. Oral iron, dietary ligands and zinc absorption. J Nutr 115(3):411-14, 1985*).

See Also:

> *Newhouse I, Clement D, Lai C. Effects of iron supplementation and discontinuation on serum copper, zinc, calcium and magnesium levels in women. Med Sci Sports 25:562-71, 1993*

> *Hambridge K et al. Acute effects of iron therapy on zinc status during pregnancy. Obstet Gyn 70:593-6, 1987*

> *Aggett PJ et al. The mutual inhibitory effects on their bioavailability of inorganic zinc and iron. Prog Clin Biol Res 129:117-24, 1983*

- Magnesium

Deficiency may affect the bioavailability and tissue distribution of zinc.

Animal Experimental Study: When rats were made magnesium-deficient, blood, but not plasma zinc decreased, while intestinal zinc, zinc balance and femur and kidney zinc increased (*Planells E, Aranda P, Lerma A, Llopis J. Changes in bioavailability and tissue distribution of zinc caused by magnesium deficiency in rats. Br J Nutr 72:315-23, 1994*).

- N-acetylcysteine

While it may increase gastrointestinal absorption of zinc, it forms zinc complexes leading to increased urinary zinc excretion (*Brumas V, Hacht B, Filella M, Gerton G. Can N-acetyl-L-cysteine affect zinc metabolism when used as a paracetamol antidote? Agents Actions 36:278-88, 1992*).

- Phytate

Reduces zinc absorption as zinc-phytate complexes precipitate at the pH of the gastrointestinal tract (*Navert B et al. A reduction of the phytate content of bran by leavening in bread and its effect on zinc absorption in man. Br J Nutr 53:47-53, 1985; Vohra P, Gray GA, Kratzer FH. Phytic acid-metal complexes. Proc Soc Exp Biol Med 120:447-9, 1965*).

- Riboflavin

May enhance zinc solubility and intestinal uptake (*Agte VV, Chiplonkar SA, Gokhale MK. Interaction of riboflavin with zinc bioavailability. Ann N Y Acad Sci 669:314-16, 1992*).

- Vitamin A

Facilitates zinc absorption.

> **Animal Experimental Study:** Vitamin A deficiency reduced the presence of zinc-binding proteins in the intestines and zinc absorption in chicks (*Berzin NI, Bauman VK. Vitamin-A-dependent zinc-binding protein and intestinal absorption of Zn in chicks. Br J Nutr 57(2):255-68, 1987*).

- Vitamin B_6

Deficiency may increase zinc absorption while decreasing serum zinc concentrations, suggesting that zinc is less available for metabolic processes (*Turnlund JR et al. A stable-isotope study of zinc, copper, and iron absorption and retention by young women fed vitamin B-6-deficient diets. Am J Clin Nutr 54:1059-64, 1991*).

Supplementation increases zinc absorption.

> **Animal Experimental Study:** Rats given 40 mg/kg vitamin B_6 absorbed 71% of their dietary zinc while controls receiving 2 mg/kg B_6 daily absorbed only 46% (*Evans GW. Normal and abnormal zinc absorption in man and animals: The tryptophan connection. Nutr Rev 38:137, 1980*).

- Vitamin D

Facilitates zinc utilization (*Worker NA, Migicovsky BB. Effect of vitamin D on the utilization of zinc, cadmium and mercury in the chick. J Nutr 75:222-4, 1961*).

- **Vitamin E**

Deficiency may reduce plasma zinc concentration, possibly due to a redistribution of zinc for antioxidant function, membrane stabilization or prostaglandin production (*Goode HF et al. The effect of dietary vitamin E deficiency on plasma zinc and copper concentrations.* <u>Clin Nutr</u> *10:233-5, 1991*).

Deficiency may worsen the effects of zinc deficiency, possibly due to the effect of each upon reducing lipid peroxidation (*Harding AJ et al. Teratogenic effect of vitamin E and zinc deficiency in the 11 day rat embryo.* <u>Nutr Rep Int</u> *36:473-82, 1987*).

Supplementation may increase plasma zinc levels (*Meydani SN, Meydani M, Rall LC, et al. Assessment of the safety of high-dose, short-term supplementation with vitamin E in healthy older adults.* <u>Am J Clin Nutr</u> *60:704-9, 1994*).

Chapter Six

DRUG-NUTRIENT INTERACTIONS

Drugs are listed under general classes as well as individually; therefore both listings should be consulted.

I. DRUGS (general)

- and Iron

Iron-drug interactions causing decreased drug bioavailability of clinical significance are common. There is little known about the effects of concurrent therapy with iron supplements for most drugs (*Campbell NR, Hasinoff BB. Iron supplements: a common cause of drug interactions. Br J Clin Pharmacol 31(3):251-5, 1991*).

II. DRUG CLASSES

ACE Inhibitors

- and Lithium

May cause lithium intoxication (*Drug Evaluations Subscription. Chicago, American Medical Association, Vol I, Section 6, Chapter 3, Summer, 1992*).

- and Potassium

May cause hyperkalemia (*Good CB, McDermott L, McCloskey B. Diet and serum potassium in patients on ACE inhibitors. JAMA 274(7):538, 1995*).

Aminoglycosides

- and Calcium

Aminoglycoside-induced renal tubular injury can lead to hypocalcemia combined with hypomagnesemia, hypokalemia and alkalosis (*Mazze RI, Cousins MJ. Combined nephrotoxicity of gentamicin and methoxyflurane anesthesia. A case report. Br J Anesthesiol 45:394, 1973*).

- and Magnesium

Aminoglycoside-induced renal tubular injury can lead to hypomagnesemia combined with hypokalemia, hypocalcemia and alkalosis (*Mazze RI, Cousins MJ. Combined nephrotoxicity of gentamicin and methoxyflurane anesthesia. A case report. Br J Anesthesiol 45:394, 1973*).

- and <u>Potassium</u>

Aminoglycoside-induced renal tubular injury can lead to hypokalemia combined with hypocalcemia, hypomagnesemia and alkalosis *(Mazze RI, Cousins MJ. Combined nephrotoxicity of gentamicin and methoxyflurane anesthesia. A case report. Br J Anesthesiol 45:394, 1973)*.

<u>Antacids</u>

- and <u>Copper</u>

Can cause copper deficiency by precipitating dietary copper at an alkaline pH in the intestines *(Roe DA. Diet and Drug Interactions. New York, Van Nostrand Reinhold, 1989:85-6)*.

- and <u>Folic Acid</u>

Malabsorption of folacin causing low or deficient plasma and erythrocyte folacin levels may occur with prolonged intake *(Roe DA. Diet and Drug Interactions. New York, Van Nostrand Reinhold, 1989:140)*.

- and <u>Potassium</u>

Antacid abuse may cause hypophosphatemia *(Lotz M, Zisman E, Bartter FC. Evidence for a phosphorus-depletion syndrome in man. N Engl J Med 278:409, 1968)*.

<u>Anticonvulsants</u>

- and <u>Carnitine</u>

Lower serum carnitine levels (especially valproic acid) *(Zelnik N, Fridkis I, Gruener N. Reduced carnitine and antiepileptic drugs: causal relationship or co-existence? Acta Paediatr 84:93-5, 1995)*.

- and <u>Folic Acid</u>

While most studies have not found vitamin B_{12} status to be decreased, large doses of folic acid given to these pts. may precipitate clinical B_{12} deficiency, especially if vitamin B_{12} status was already impaired. Thus, serum B_{12} levels should be obtained as part of their management *(Roe DA. Drug-induced Nutritional Deficiencies. Second Edition. Westport, CT, Avi Publishing, 1985:249-59)*.

- and <u>Vitamin B_{12}</u>

May cause vitamin B_{12} depletion or deficiency; thus serum and erythrocyte folate levels and hematological profiles should be obtained and regular intervals and adequate folic acid should be administered to overcome the increased folate requirement *(Roe DA. Drug-induced Nutritional Deficiencies. Second Edition. Westport, CT, Avi Publishing, 1985:249-59)*.

- and <u>Vitamin D</u>

Produce resistance to vitamin D action by causing a direct inhibitory effect on bone mineral metabolism while increasing the requirement for the vitamin *(Christiansen C, Rodbro P, Munck O. Actions of vitamin D_2 and D_3 and 25-0HD$_3$ in anti-convulsant osteomalacia. Br Med J ii:363-5, 1975).*

- and <u>Vitamin E</u>

Significantly lower plasma vitamin E levels by altering absorption, distribution and metabolism; seizure control may improve with supplementation concurrent with 1 or 2 antiepileptic drugs *(Vitamin E Fact Book. VERIS (Vitamin E Research & Information Service, 5325 S. 9th Ave., LaGrange, IL 60525, 1994).*

- and <u>Vitamin K</u>

WARNING: Water-soluble preparations are contraindicated as they can cause hemolytic anemia and transport of bile pigment into the brain (Kernicterus) of the neonate *(Evans AR, Forester RM, Discombe C. Neonatal hemorrhage following maternal anticonvulsant therapy. Lancet i:517-18, 1970).*

Vitamin K administration will prevent hemorrhage in the newborn infants of mothers who have received these drugs during pregnancy *(Mountain KR, Hirsh J, Gallus AS. Neonatal coagulation defect due to anticonvulsant drug treatment in pregnancy. Lancet i:265-8, 1970).*

Anticoagulants

- and <u>Magnesium</u>

Magnesium salts may prolong or intensify the response to oral anticoagulants *(Drug Evaluations Subscription. Chicago, American Medical Association, Volume I, Section 7, Chapter 2, Spring, 1992).*

- and <u>Vitamin E</u>

Megadoses of vitamin E may prolong or intensify the response to oral anticoagulants *(Drug Evaluations Subscription. Chicago, American Medical Association, Volume I, Section 7, Chapter 2, Spring, 1992).*

- and <u>Vitamin K</u>

Increase the risk of excessive calcium excretion (calcium/creatinine ratio >0.5) *(Jie K-SG et al. Effects of vitamin K and oral anticoagulants on urinary calcium excretion. Br J Haematol 83:100-4, 1993).*

Antipsychotics

- and <u>Lithium</u>

Concomitant use of lithium may increase the risk of neurotoxicity *(Drug Evaluations Subscription, Chicago, American Medical Association, Vol I, Section 3, Chapter 2, Winter, 1994).*

Beta-adrenergic Blocking Agents

- and Coenzyme Q10

Antagonistic to CoQ10-enzymes *(Folkers K. Basic chemical research on coenzyme Q10 and integrated clinical research on therapy of diseases, in G Lenaz, Ed. Coenzyme Q. John Wiley & Sons, 1985).*

Calcium Channel Blocking Agents

- and Calcium

It is possible the therapeutic response to the drugs may be reduced by calcium supplements *(Drug Evaluations Subscription. Chicago, American Medical Association, Volume I, Section 7, Chapter 2, Spring, 1992).*

- and Magnesium

Correct magnesium deficiency in patients with variant angina *(Goto K, Yasue H, Okumura K, et al. Magnesium deficiency detected by intravenous loading test in variant angina pectoris. Am J Cardiol 65(11):709-12, 1990).*

Cephalosporins

- and Vitamin K

Vitamin K antagonists that can produce a coagulopathy *(Pakter RL, Russell TR, Mielke H, West D. Coagulopathy associated with the use of moxalactam. JAMA 248:1100, 1982).*

Glucocorticoids

- and Aluminum-containing Antacids

Reduce glucocorticoid bioavailability *(Roe DA. Diet and Drug Interactions. New York, Van Nostrand Reinhold, 1989:84).*

- and Calcium

May lower serum calcium by reducing its absorption *(Roe DA. Drug-induced Nutritional Deficiencies. Second Edition. Westport, CT, Avi Publishing, 1985:163-4).*

Supplementation with calcium (1 gm HS) helps to prevent steroid-induced osteoporosis *(Reid IR, Ibbertson HK. Calcium supplements in the prevention of steroid-induced osteoporosis. Am J Clin Nutr 44:287-90, 1986).*

- and Potassium

Hypokalemia may occur during prolonged, high-dosage corticosteroid therapy *(Thorn GW. Clinical considerations in the use of corticosteroids. N Engl J Med 274:775, 1966).*

- and <u>Selenium</u>

May lower plasma selenium levels (*Peretz A, Neve J, Famaey J. Selenium in rheumatic diseases. <u>Semin Arth Rheum</u> 20:305-16, 1991*).

- and <u>Vitamin D</u>

Decrease vitamin D availability (*Hodges R. Drug-nutrient interaction, in <u>Nutrition in Medical Practice</u>. Philadelphia, W.B. Saunders, 1980:323-31*) and may lower serum 25-hydroxycalciferol levels (*Hahn TJ, Hendin BA, Scharp CR, Haddad JG. Effect of chronic anticonvulsant therapy on serum 25-hydroxycalciferol levels in adults. <u>N Engl J Med</u> 287:900, 1972*).

HMG-CoA Reductase Inhibitors

- and <u>Niacin</u>

The risk of myopathy and life-threatening rhabdomyolysis increases when these drugs are combined with niacin (*Pierce LR et al. Myopathy and rhabdomyolysis associated with lovastatin-gemfibrozil combination therapy. <u>JAMA</u> 264:71-5, 1990*).

Loop Diuretics

- and <u>Magnesium</u>

May cause hypomagnesemia (*Roe DA. <u>Diet and Drug Interactions</u>. New York, Van Nostrand Reinhold, 1989:150*).

- and <u>Potassium</u>

Prolonged or high doses may cause potassium depletion (*Hamdy RC, Tovey J, Perera N. Hypokalemia and diuretics. <u>Br Med J</u> i:1187, 1980; Steen B. Hypokalemia, clinical spectrum, and etiology. <u>Acta Med Scand Suppl</u> 647:61-6, 1981*).

Monamine Oxidase Inhibitors

- and <u>Tyramine</u>

Foods containing tyramine may cause a hypertensive crisis (*Lim D, McKay M. Food-drug interactions. <u>Drug Information Bulletin</u>, UCLA Dept. of Pharmaceutical Services, 15(2), 1995*).

Non-steroidal Anti-inflammatory Drugs

- and <u>Lithium</u>

Share a common excretory pathway in the proximal tubule, thereby diminishing lithium clearance (*<u>Drug Evaluations Subscription</u>. Chicago, American Medical Association, Vol. III, Section 16, Chapter 1, Summer, 1993*).

Oral Contraceptives

- and Calcium

Estrogen may improve the intestinal absorption of calcium (*Caniggia A et al. Intestinal absorption of calcium 47 after treatment with oral oestrogen, gestagens in senile osteoporosis. Br Med J iv:30-2, 1970*).

- and Copper

May increase blood copper levels and ceruloplasmin levels, perhaps by increasing the absorption of dietary copper (*Roe DA. Drug-induced Nutritional Deficiencies. Second Edition. Westport, CT, Avi Publishing, 1985:276*).

- and Folic Acid

Cause depletion of folate and thus women on oral contraceptives should be screened with plasma and erythrocyte folate levels (*Roe DA. Drug-induced Nutritional Deficiencies. Second Edition. Westport, CT, Avi Publishing, 1985:262-7*).

- and Iron

Decrease menstrual blood loss (*Larsson-Cohn U. An appraisal of the clinical effect of three different oral contraceptive agents and their influence on transaminase activity. Acta Obstet Gynecol Scand 45:499-514, 1966*) which may explain why women taking oral contraceptives require slightly less dietary iron (*Theuer RC. Effect of oral contraceptive agents on vitamin and mineral needs: A review. J Reprod Med 8:13-19, 1972*).

- and Riboflavin

Oral contraceptives do not significantly influence riboflavin status and requirements, although several studies that failed to control riboflavin intake have suggested an interaction (*Roe DA. Drug-induced Nutritional Deficiencies. Second Edition. Westport, CT, Avi Publishing, 1985:269-70*).

- and Vitamin A

Increase plasma vitamin A levels (*Gal I, Parkinson C, Craft I. Effects of oral contraceptives on human plasma vitamin-A levels. Br Med J ii:436-8, 1971*); thus oral vitamin A supplements are not recommended in patients receiving oral contraceptives (*Roe DA. Drug-induced Nutritional Deficiencies. Second Edition. Westport, CT, Avi Publishing, 1985:274-5*).

> *Note: Changes in vitamin status have not been found to occur with the low-estrogen preparations currently in use* (*Roe DA. Diet and Drug Interactions. New York, Van Nostrand Reinhold, 1989:84*).

- and Vitamin B6

It is uncertain whether oral contraceptives cause vitamin B_6 depletion. Claims that oral contraceptives may cause B_6 depletion are largely based on changes in erythrocyte transaminase activity and on tryptophan load tests (*Roe DA. Drug-induced Nutritional Deficiencies. Second Edition. Westport, CT, Avi Publishing, 1985:270-3*). While nonusers of oral contraceptives require 1.5 mg daily of the vitamin, users require between 1.5 and 5 mg daily based on measurements of erythrocyte pyridoxal levels, erythrocyte alanine and aspartic aminotransferase activities, and activities of these enzyme systems following stimulation with pyridoxal phosphate (*Donald EA, Bosse TR. The vitamin B6 requirement of oral contraceptive users. II. Assessment by tryptophan metabolites, vitamin B6, and pyridoxic levels in urine. Am J Clin Nutr 32:1024-32, 1979*).

> *Note: Changes in vitamin status have not been found to occur with the low-estrogen preparations currently in use (Roe DA. Diet and Drug Interactions. New York, Van Nostrand Reinhold, 1989:84).*

- and Vitamin B12

May reduce serum vitamin B12 levels (*Shojania AM, Hornady G, Barnes PH. The effect of oral contraceptives on folate metabolism. Am J Obstet Gynecol 111:782-91, 1971*).

> *Note: Changes in vitamin status have not been found to occur with the low-estrogen preparations currently in use (Roe DA. Diet and Drug Interactions. New York, Van Nostrand Reinhold, 1989:84).*

- and Vitamin C

May reduce ascorbic acid levels in plasma (*Rivers JM, Devine M. Plasma ascorbic acid concentrations and oral contraceptives. Am J Clin Nutr 25:684-9, 1972*), leukocytes and platelets (*Briggs M, Briggs M. Vitamin C requirements and oral contraceptives. Nature (London) 238:277, 1972*).

> *Note: It is unclear whether changes in vitamin C status occur with the low-estrogen preparations currently in use (Roe DA. Diet and Drug Interactions. New York, Van Nostrand Reinhold, 1989:84,139).*

- and Vitamin K

Reduce the need for vitamin K (*Roe DA. Drug-induced Nutritional Deficiencies. Second Edition. Westport, CT, Avi Publishing, 1985:275-6*).

> *Note: Changes in vitamin status have not been found to occur with the low-estrogen preparations currently in use (Roe DA. Diet and Drug Interactions. New York, Van Nostrand Reinhold, 1989:84).*

- and Zinc

May lower plasma zinc levels while raising erythrocyte zinc levels, perhaps due to a redistribution of zinc (*Roe DA. Drug-induced Nutritional Deficiencies. Second Edition. Westport, CT, Avi Publishing, 1985:276*).

Pancreatic Extracts

- and Folic Acid

Form an insoluble complex with folate that reduces folate absorption (*Russell RM, Dutta SK, Oaks EV, et al. Impairment of folic acid absorption by oral pancreatic extracts. Dig Dis Sci 25:369-73, 1980*).

Phenothiazines

- and Coenzyme Q_{10}

Antagonistic to CoQ10-enzymes (*Folkers K. Basic chemical research on coenzyme Q_{10} and integrated clinical research on therapy of diseases, in G Lenaz, Ed. Coenzyme Q. John Wiley & Sons, 1985*). Supplementation may prevent cardiac side effects (*Kishi T, Makino K, Okamoto T, et al, in Y Yamamura, K Folkers, Y Ito, Eds. Biochemical and Clinical Aspects of Coenzyme Q, Volume 2. Amsterdam, Elsevier/North Holland Biomedical Press, 1980:139-57*).

- and Vitamin C

May treat neuroleptic -associated amenorrhea (*Kanofsky JD, Kay SR, Lindenmayer JP, Seifter E. Ascorbic acid action in neuroleptic-associated amenorrhea. Letter. J Clin Psychopharmacol 9(5):388-9, 1989*).

Polymyxins

- and Magnesium

As parenteral magnesium may impair neuromuscular transmission, it could cause respiratory arrest when combined with the polymyxins (*Drug Evaluations Subscription. Chicago, American Medical Association, Vol II, Section 13, Chapter 9, Spring, 1993*).

Sulfonamides

- and Para-amino Benzoic Acid

PABA-containing compounds and local anesthetics derived from PABA (e.g. procaine) may directly inhibit the activity of sulfonamides (*Drug Evaluations Subscription. Chicago, American Medical Association, Vol II, Section 13, Chapter 7, Spring, 1993*).

Sulfonylureas

- and Lithium

Lithium administration may increase the risk of hypoglycemia from the drug (*Drug Evaluations Subscription. Chicago, American Medical Association, Vol II, Section 10, Chapter 3, Winter, 1994*).

- and **Magnesium**

Magnesium hydroxide administration may increase the risk of hypoglycemia from the drug (*Drug Evaluations Subscription*, Chicago, American Medical Association, Vol II, Section 10, Chapter 3, Winter, 1994).

- and **Niacin**

Niacin may increase blood glucose. Concomitant use may thus require an increase in the dose of the sulfonylurea (*Drug Evaluations Subscription*, Chicago, American Medical Association, Vol II, Section 10, Chapter 3, Winter, 1994).

- and **Vitamin E**

Vitamin E supplements suppress hemoglobin glycation; therefore glycemic control may be falsely exaggerated (*Drug Evaluations Subscription*. Chicago, American Medical Association, Vol II, Section 10, Chapter 3, Winter, 1994).

Tetracyclines

- and **Calcium**

With prolonged use, tetracycline can contribute to calcium depletion (*Roe DA. Diet and Drug Interactions*. New York, Van Nostrand Reinhold, 1989:87).

Calcium interferes with tetracycline absorption by chelating the drug (*Drug Evaluations Subscription*. Chicago, American Medical Association, Volume II, Section 13, Chapter 5, Winter, 1993).

- and **Iron**

Concurrent iron ingestion causes a marked decrease in the bioavailability of the drug and its derivatives (*Campbell NR, Hasinoff BB. Iron supplements: a common cause of drug interactions. Br J Clin Pharmacol 31(3):251-5, 1991*).

- and **Magnesium**

Magnesium interferes with tetracycline absorption by chelating the drug (*Drug Evaluations Subscription*. Chicago, American Medical Association, Volume II, Section 13, Chapter 5, Winter, 1993).

- and **Potassium**

May cause hypokalemia due to its nephrotoxic side effects (*Mavromatis F. Tetracycline nephropathy. Case reports with renal biopsy. JAMA 193:191, 1965*).

- and **Vitamin B$_6$**

Impairs vitamin B$_6$ absorption (*Robinson C, Weigly E. Basic Nutrition and Diet Therapy. New York, MacMillan, 1984:46-54*).

- and <u>Vitamin B$_{12}$</u>

Impairs vitamin B$_{12}$ absorption (*Robinson C, Weigly E. Basic Nutrition and Diet Therapy. New York, MacMillan, 1984:46-54*).

- and <u>Zinc</u>

Zinc interferes with tetracycline absorption by chelating the drug (*Drug Evaluations Subscription. Chicago, American Medical Association, Volume II, Section 13, Chapter 5, Winter, 1993*).

<u>Thiazide Diuretics</u>

- and <u>Calcium</u>

Hypercalcemia, which is usually transient, and hypocalciuria occasionally occur with both chlorthiazide and hydrochlorthiazide (*Duarte GC et al. Thiazide-induced hypercalcemia. N Engl J Med 284:828-30, 1971*). In addition to increasing the protein-bound fraction of serum calcium, thiazides increase calcium absorption in the distal convoluted tubule and, by contracting the plasma volume, enhance proximal calcium reabsorption. However true hypercalcemia (increased ionized calcium) is a rare complication usually associated with latent primary hyperparathyroidism (*Drug Evaluations Subscription. Chicago, American Medical Association, Vol II, Section 8, Chapter 1, Winter, 1993*).

- and <u>Lithium</u>

May increase serum lithium levels (*Drug Evaluations Subscription. Chicago, American Medical Association, Vol II, Section 8, Chapter 1, Winter, 1993*).

- and <u>Magnesium</u>

May induce an intracellular magnesium deficiency even despite a normal serum level (*Dorup I, Skajaa K, Thybo NK. Oral magnesium supplementation restores the concentrations of magnesium, potassium and sodium-potassium pumps in skeletal muscle of patients receiving diuretic treatment. J Intern Med 233:177-23, 1993; Saito K, Hattori K, Omatsu T, et al. Effects of oral magnesium on blood pressure and red cell sodium transport in patients receiving long-term thiazide diuretics for hypertension. Am J Hypertens 1(3 Pt 3):71S-74S, 1988*).

> *Note: Magnesium may have a regulatory role in the maintenance of cellular potassium concentration and may be required in addition to potassium supplementation for patients treated with diuretics. Supplementation may be required for at least 6 months before complete normalization can be expected* (*Dorup I, Skajaa K, Thybo HK. Oral magnesium supplementation restores the concentrations of magnesium, potassium and sodium-potassium pumps in skeletal muscle of patients receiving diuretic treatment. J Intern Med 233:177-23, 1993*).

- and Potassium

May induce a potassium deficiency in muscle tissue even despite a normal serum level *(Dorup I, Skajaa K, Thybo NK. Oral magnesium supplementation restores the concentrations of magnesium, potassium and sodium-potassium pumps in skeletal muscle of patients receiving diuretic treatment. J Intern Med 233:177-23, 1993).*

- and Sodium

May cause hyponatremia which develops slowly and will usually resolve rapidly with discontinuance of the drug unless the patient is drinking large volumes of water *(Ashraf N, Locksley R, Arieff AI. Thiazine-induced hyponatremia associated with death or neurological damage in outpatients. Am J Med 70:1163, 1981).*

- and Vitamin D

May cause hypercalcemia *(Drug Evaluations Subscription. Chicago, American Medical Association, Vol II, Section 8, Chapter 1, Winter, 1993).*

Thyroid Hormones

- and Lithium

Patients on lithium will require a higher dosage of thyroid hormone *(Drug Evaluations Subscription. Chicago, American Medical Association, Vol II, Section 10, Chapter 2, Summer, 1993).*

Tricyclic Antidepressants

- and Coenzyme Q_{10}

Antagonistic to CoQ10-enzymes *(Folkers K. Basic chemical research on coenzyme Q_{10} and integrated clinical research on therapy of diseases, in G Lenaz, Ed. Coenzyme Q. John Wiley & Sons, 1985).* Supplementation may prevent cardiac side effects *(Kishi T, Makino K, Okamoto T, et al, in Y Yamamura, K Folkers, Y Ito, Eds. Biochemical and Clinical Aspects of Coenzyme Q. Volume 2. Amsterdam, Elsevier/North Holland Biomedical Press, 1980:139-57).*

- and Riboflavin

Decrease riboflavin absorption *(Goodman L, Gilman A, Eds. The Pharmacological Basis of Therapeutics (6th Ed.). New York, MacMillan Co., 1980:1331-46; 1551-601).*

III. SPECIFIC DRUGS

Adriamycin

- and Coenzyme Q10

Adriamycin inhibits CoQ_{10}-enzymes; thus its cardiotoxicity appears to be at least partly related to its effects on CoQ_{10} and CoQ_{10} supplementation may prevent its cardiotoxicity *(Folkers K. Basic chemical research on coenzyme Q10 and integrated clinical research on therapy of diseases, in G Lenaz, Ed. Coenzyme Q. John Wiley & Sons, 1985).*

- and Niacin

Animal work suggests that supplementation with niacin may reduce cardiotoxicity without interfering with the antitumor activity of the drug *(Schmitt-Gräff A, Scheulen ME. Prevention of adriamycin cardiotoxicity by niacin, isocitrate or N-acetyl-cysteine in mice. A morphological study. Pathol Res Pract 181(2):168-74, 1986).*

> *Note: The relationship of animal studies to human clinical cardiac toxicity is unclear (Ellison NM, Londer H. Vitamins E and C and their relationship to cancer, in GR Newell, NM Ellison, Eds. Nutrition and Cancer: Etiology and Treatment. New York, Raven Press, 1981).*

- and Vitamin C

Animal work suggests that supplementation with vitamin C may reduce toxicity without affecting with the antitumor activity of the drug *(Shimpo K et al. Ascorbic acid and adriamycin toxicity. Am J Clin Nutr 54:1298S-1301S, 1991).*

> *Note: The relationship of animal studies to human clinical cardiac toxicity is unclear (Ellison NM, Londer H. Vitamins E and C and their relationship to cancer, in GR Newell, NM Ellison, Eds. Nutrition and Cancer: Etiology and Treatment. New York, Raven Press, 1981).*

- and Vitamin E

Animal work suggests that supplementation with vitamin E may reduce cardiac and skin toxicity *(Prasad KN et al. Vitamin E increases the growth inhibitory and differentiating effects of tumor therapeutic agents on neuroblastoma and glioma cells in culture. Proc Soc Exp Biol Med 164(2):158-63, 1980).*

> *Note: The relationship of animal studies to human clinical cardiac toxicity is unclear as vitamin E administration has not prevented drug toxicity in cancer patients (Ellison NM, Londer H. Vitamins E and C and their relationship to cancer, in GR Newell, NM Ellison, Eds. Nutrition and Cancer: Etiology and Treatment. New York, Raven Press, 1981).*

Alprenolol

- and Potassium

May cause dose-dependent increases in serum potassium (*Pederson EB, Kornerup HJ. Relationship between plasma aldosterone concentration and plasma potassium in patients with essential hypertension during alprenolol treatment. Acta Med Scand 200:263, 1976*).

Aluminum Hydroxide

- and Phosphorus

Combines with phosphates in the intestines leading to the excretion of aluminum phosphates. Excessive use may result in symptomatic phosphate depletion marked by hypophosphatemia (plasma phosphate <0.35 mmol/L). Uncommonly, osteomalacia may develop (*Harvey SC. Gastric antacids and digestants, in LS Goodman, A Gilman, Eds. The Pharmacological Basis of Therapeutics. 3rd Edition. New York, Macmillan, 1965; Lotz M, Zisman E, Bartter C. Evidence for a phosphorus depletion syndrome in man. N Engl J Med 278:409-15, 1978*).

- and Vitamin A

May impair vitamin A absorption (*Robinson C, Weigly E. Basic Nutrition and Diet Therapy. New York, MacMillan, 1984:46-54*).

Aminopterin

- and Folic Acid

Impairs folate absorption (*Robinson C, Weigly E. Basic Nutrition and Diet Therapy. New York, MacMillan, 1984:46-54*).

Impairs folate availability (*Hackman R, Hurley L. Drug-nutrient interaction in teratogens, in D Roe, T Campbell, Eds. Drugs and Nutrients: The Interactive Effects. New York, Marcel Decker, 1984:299-329*).

- and Vitamin B$_{12}$

Impairs vitamin B$_{12}$ absorption (*Robinson C, Weigly E. Basic Nutrition and Diet Therapy. New York, MacMillan, 1984:46-54*).

Amiodarone

- and Vitamin E

Supplementation reduces pulmonary toxicity (*Kachel DL et al. Amiodarone-induced injury of human pulmonary artery endothelial cells: protection by alpha-tocopherol. J Pharmacol Exp Ther 254:1107-12, 1990*).

Amitriptylene

- and Sodium

May cause dilutional hyponatremia (*Luzecky MH, Burman KD, Schultz ER. The syndrome of inappropriate secretion of antidiuretic hormone associated with amitriptylene administration. South Med J 67:495, 1974*).

Amphotericin B

- and Potassium

May cause hypokalemia due to its nephrotoxic side effects (*Drutz DJ, Fan JH, Tai TY, et al. Hypokalemic rhabdomyolysis and myoglobinuria following amphotericin B therapy. JAMA 211:824-6, 1970*).

Aspirin

- and Folic Acid

May decrease serum folate levels and reduce the binding of folate to serum proteins by competing for binding sites (*Alter HJ, Zvaifler MJ, Rath CE. Interrelationship of rheumatoid arthritis, folic acid and aspirin. Blood 38:405-16, 1971; Lawrence VA, Loewenstein JE, Eichner ER. Aspirin and folate binding: in vivo and in vitro studies of serum binding and urinary excretion of endogenous folate. J Lab Clin Med 103:944-8, 1984*).

- and Iron

Prolonged use can cause iron-deficiency anemia by inducing blood loss from the gastrointestinal tract (*Leonards JH, Levy G. Gastrointestinal blood loss during prolonged aspirin administration. New Engl J Med 289:1020-22, 1973*).

- and Potassium

High-dose therapy can produce hypokalemia (*Smith MJH, Smith PK, Eds. The Salicylates: A Critical Bibliographic Review. New York, Interscience, 1966*).

- and Vitamin C

The drug most likely to produce ascorbic acid tissue depletion in normal individuals (*Coffey G, Wilson CWM. Ascorbic acid deficiency and aspirin-induced haematemesis. Br Med J i:208, 1975*).

Promotes the urinary excretion of ascorbic acid (*Daniels Al, Everson GJ. Influence of acetylsalicylic acid (aspirin) on urinary excretion of ascorbic acid. Proc Soc Exp Biol Med 35:20-4, 1936-7*).

Bisacodyl

- and Potassium

May induce potassium depletion (*Fleming BJ, Genuth SM, Gould AB, Kaminokowski MD. Laxative induced hypokalemia, sodium depletion, and hyperreninemia. Effects of potassium and sodium replacement on the renin angiotensin system. Ann Intern Med 83:60-2, 1975*).

Bleomycin

- and Vitamin E

Animal work suggests that supplementation may reduce drug-induced lung fibrosis (*Prasad KN et al. Vitamin E increases the growth inhibitory and differentiating effects of tumor therapeutic agents on neuroblastoma and glioma cells in culture. Proc Soc Exp Biol Med 164(2):158-63, 1980*).

Calomel

- and Phosphorus

Chronic usage of drugs containing inorganic mercury may result in osteomalacia due to phosphate depletion (*Roe DA. Drug-induced Nutritional Deficiencies. Second Edition. Westport, CT, Avi Publishing, 1985:175-7*).

Captopril

- and Iron

Concurrent iron ingestion decreases the bioavailability of the drug by forming a stable complex with it (*Campbell NR, Hasinoff BB. Iron supplements: a common cause of drug interactions. Br J Clin Pharmacol 31(3):251-5, 1991*).

- and Magnesium

Increases lymphocyte magnesium levels, at least in patients with low levels (*O'Keffe S et al. Effect of captopril therapy on lymphocyte potassium and magnesium concentrations in patients with congestive heart failure. Cardiology 80:100-5, 1992*).

- and Potassium

Increases lymphocyte potassium levels, at least in patients with low levels (*O'Keffe S et al. Effect of captopril therapy on lymphocyte potassium and magnesium concentrations in patients with congestive heart failure. Cardiology 80:100-5, 1992*).

- and Sodium

May cause hyponatremia; may have an anti-aldosterone effect (*Nicholls MG, Espiner EA, Ikram H, Maslowski AH. Hyponatremia in congestive heart failure during treatment with captopril. Br Med J 281:909, 1980*).

Carbamazepine

- and Folic Acid

Impair folates absorption *(Hendal J et al. The effects of carbamazepine and valproate on folate metabolism. Acta Neurol Scand 69(4):226-31, 1984)*.

- and Niacinamide

In children, large doses of niacinamide may increase carbamazepine plasma concentrations *(Drug Evaluations Subscription. Chicago, American Medical Association, Vol I, Section 4, Chapter 1, Fall, 1992)*.

- and Sodium

May cause dilutional hyponatremia *(Rado JP. Water intoxication during carbamazepine treatment. Br Med J 3:479, 1973)*.

Carbenicillin

- and Sodium

May cause hypernatremia as a toxic side effect *(Brumfit W, Percival A. Clinical and laboratory studies with carbenicillin. Lancet i:1289, 1967)*.

Carbenoxolone

- and Potassium

May cause hypokalemia due to its mineralocorticoid-like action *(Lewis JR. Carbenoxolone sodium in the treatment of peptic ulcer. A review. JAMA 229:460, 1974)*.

Carbidopa

- and Iron

Concurrent iron ingestion causes a marked decrease in the bioavailability of the drug *(Campbell NR, Hasinoff BB. Iron supplements: a common cause of drug interactions. Br J Clin Pharmacol 31(3):251-5, 1991)*.

Chloramphenicol

- and Folic Acid

Drug may delay the response of a megaloblastic anemia due to folate deficiency to folate supplementation *(Drug Evaluations Subscription. Chicago, American Medical Association, Vol II, Section 13, Chapter 5, Summer, 1992)*.

- and **Iron**

> Drug may delay the response of anemia due to iron deficiency to folate supplementation
> (*Drug Evaluations Subscription.* Chicago, American Medical Association, Vol II, Section 13, Chapter 5, Summer, 1992).

- and **Vitamin B$_{12}$**

> Drug may delay the response of a megaloblastic anemia due to vitamin B$_{12}$ deficiency to
> folate supplementation (*Drug Evaluations Subscription.* Chicago, American Medical Association, Vol II, Section
> 13, Chapter 5, Summer, 1992).

Chlorpropamide

- and **Sodium**

> May cause hyponatremia due to its antidiuretic effect (*Luethi A, Studer H. Antidiuretic action of
> chlorpropamide and tolbutamide. Minn Med 52:33, 1969*).

Cholestyramine

- and **Carotenoids**

> Reduces serum levels of beta-carotene and lycopene by impairing absorption and as well as
> by lowering serum cholesterol (*Elinder LS, Hadell K, Johansson J, et al. Probucol treatment decreases serum
> concentrations of diet-derived antioxidants. Arterioscler Thromb Vasc Biol 15(8):1057-63, 1995; Mackey SF et al. Effect of
> lipid-lowering drugs on plasma levels of vitamin A-related compounds. Cardiovas Dis Epidemiol ABS:21, 1991*).

- and **Fat**

> Impairs fat absorption (*Roe DA. Drug-induced Nutritional Deficiencies. Second Edition. Westport, CT, Avi
> Publishing, 1985:158-9*).

- and **Folic Acid**

> Malabsorption of folacin causing low or deficient plasma and erythrocyte folacin levels
> may occur with prolonged intake (*West RJ, Lloyd JK. The effect of cholestyramine on intestinal absorption. Gut
> 16:93, 1975*).

- and **Iron**

> Impairs iron absorption (*Roe DA. Drug-induced Nutritional Deficiencies. Second Edition. Westport, CT, Avi
> Publishing, 1985:158-9*).

- and **Vitamin A**

> Impairs vitamin A absorption (*Longnecker JB, Basu SG. Effects of cholestyramine on absorption of amino acids
> and vitamin A in man. Fed Proc 24:375, 1965*).

- and <u>Vitamin B12</u>

Impairs vitamin B12 absorption *(Coronato A, Glass GBJ. Depression of the intestinal uptake of radio-vitamin B12 by cholestyramine. <u>Proc Soc Exp Biol Med</u> 142:1341-4, 1973).*

- and <u>Vitamin D</u>

Impairs vitamin D absorption *(Roe D. Risk factors in drug-induced nutritional deficiencies, in D Roe, T Campbell, Eds. <u>Drugs and Nutrients: The Interactive Effects</u>. New York, Marcel Decker, 1984:505-23).*

- and <u>Vitamin E</u>

Reduces serum vitamin E by impairing absorption and as well as by lowering serum cholesterol *(Elinder LS, Hadell K, Johansson J, et al. Probucol treatment decreases serum concentrations of diet-derived antioxidants. <u>Arterioscler Thromb Vasc Biol</u> 15(8):1057-63, 1995; West RJ, Lloyd JK. The effect of cholestyramine on intestinal absorption. <u>Gut</u> 16:93, 1975).*

- and <u>Vitamin K</u>

Impairs vitamin K absorption *(Roe D. Risk factors in drug-induced nutritional deficiencies, in D Roe, T Campbell, Eds. <u>Drugs and Nutrients: The Interactive Effects</u>. New York, Marcel Decker, 1984:505-23).*

<u>Cimetidine</u>

- and <u>Folic Acid</u>

Reduces folate absorption *(Russell R, Golner B, Krasinski S. Effect of acid lowering agents on folic acid absorption. <u>Fed Proc</u> 46:1159, 1987).*

- and <u>Vitamin B12</u>

Impairs animal protein-bound vitamin B12 absorption by inhibiting gastric acid and pepsin secretion, preventing B12 from being freed from its protein binder during digestion *(Streeter AM, Goulston KJ, Bathur FA, et al. Cimetidine and malabsorption of cobalamin. <u>Dig Dis Sci</u> 27:13-16, 1982).*

- and <u>Vitamin D</u>

Reduces hepatic vitamin D 25-hydroxylase activity *(Bengoa JM, Bolt MJG, Rosenberg IH. Hepatic vitamin D 25-hydroxylase inhibition by cimetidine and isoniazid. <u>J Lab Clin Med</u> 104:546-52, 1984).*

<u>Ciprofloxacin</u>

and <u>Calcium</u>

Concurrent calcium ingestion causes a marked decrease in the bioavailability of the drug *(Lim D, McKay M. Food-drug interactions. <u>Drug Information Bulletin</u>, UCLA Dept. of Pharmaceutical Services, 15(2), 1995).*

- and **Iron**

Concurrent iron ingestion causes a marked decrease in the bioavailability of the drug
(Campbell NR, Hasinoff BB. Iron supplements: a common cause of drug interactions. Br J Clin Pharmacol 31(3):251-5, 1991).

- and **Zinc**

Concurrent zinc ingestion causes a marked decrease in the bioavailability of the drug *(Lim D, McKay M. Food-drug interactions. Drug Information Bulletin, UCLA Dept. of Pharmaceutical Services, 15(2), 1995).*

Cisplatin

- and **Magnesium**

The drug impairs the renal tubular ability to conserve magnesium which may persist for months or even years after it is discontinued *(Toffaletti J. Electrolytes, divalent cations, and blood gases (magnesium). Analyt Chem 63(12):192R-4R, 1991).*

Clofibrate

- and **Vitamin B$_{12}$**

Impairs vitamin B$_{12}$ absorption *(Robinson C, Weigly E. Basic Nutrition and Diet Therapy. New York, MacMillan, 1984:46-54).*

- and **Vitamin E**

Diminishes carrier lipoprotein for vitamin E *(Vitamin E Fact Book. VERIS (Vitamin E Research & Information Service, 5325 S. 9th Ave., LaGrange, IL 60525, 1994).*

Colchicine

- and **Beta-Carotene**

Impairs beta-carotene absorption *(Robinson C, Weigly E. Basic Nutrition and Diet Therapy. New York, MacMillan, 1984:46-54).*

and **Fat**

Impairs fat absorption *(Roe DA. Drug-induced Nutritional Deficiencies. Second Edition. Westport, CT, Avi Publishing, 1985:159-60).*

and **Lactose**

Impairs lactose absorption *(Roe DA. Drug-induced Nutritional Deficiencies. Second Edition. Westport, CT, Avi Publishing, 1985:159-60).*

and **Potassium**

Impairs potassium absorption (*Roe DA. Drug-induced Nutritional Deficiencies. Second Edition. Westport, CT, Avi Publishing, 1985:159-60*).

and **Sodium**

Impairs sodium absorption (*Roe DA. Drug-induced Nutritional Deficiencies. Second Edition. Westport, CT, Avi Publishing, 1985:159-60*).

- and **Vitamin B$_{12}$**

Impairs vitamin B$_{12}$ absorption (*Robinson C, Weigly E. Basic Nutrition and Diet Therapy. New York, MacMillan, 1984:46-54*).

Colestipol

- and **Beta-Carotene**

Long-term therapy may lower beta-carotene levels (*Mackey S et al. Effect of lipid-lowering medications on plasma levels of vitamin A-related compounds. Circulation 83:736, 1991*).

- and **Folic Acid**

Impairs folate absorption (*Roe D. Risk factors in drug-induced nutritional deficiencies, in D Roe, T Campbell, Eds. Drugs and Nutrients: The Interactive Effects. New York, Marcel Decker, 1984:505-23*).

- and **Vitamin A**

Impairs vitamin A absorption (*Schwarz KB, Goldstein PD, Witztum JL, Schonfeld G. Fat soluble vitamin concentrations in hypercholesterolemic children treated with colestipol. Pediatrics 65:243-50, 1980*).

- and **Vitamin D**

Impairs vitamin D absorption (*Roe D. Risk factors in drug-induced nutritional deficiencies, in D Roe, T Campbell, Eds. Drugs and Nutrients: The Interactive Effects. New York, Marcel Decker, 1984:505-23*).

- and **Vitamin E**

Impairs vitamin E absorption (*Roe D. Risk factors in drug-induced nutritional deficiencies, in D Roe, T Campbell, Eds. Drugs and Nutrients: The Interactive Effects. New York, Marcel Decker, 1984:505-23*).

- and **Vitamin K**

Impairs vitamin K absorption (*Roe D. Risk factors in drug-induced nutritional deficiencies, in D Roe, T Campbell, Eds. Drugs and Nutrients: The Interactive Effects. New York, Marcel Decker, 1984:505-23*).

Cyclophosphamide

- and Sodium

May cause dilutional hyponatremia *(Steele TH, Seipiek AA, Block JB. Antidiuretic response to cyclophosphamide in man. J Pharm Exp Therap 185:245, 1973).*

Cycloserine

- and Vitamin B$_6$

Impairs vitamin B$_6$ availability *(Roe D. Risk factors in drug-induced nutritional deficiencies, in D Roe, T Campbell, Eds. Drugs and Nutrients: The Interactive Effects. New York, Marcel Decker, 1984:505-23; 288-9).*

Cyclosporin

- and Magnesium

Increases urinary magnesium loss *(Toffaletti J. Electrolytes, divalent cations, and blood gases (magnesium). Analyt Chem 63(12):192R-4R, 1991).*

Diazoxide

- and Sodium

May cause hypernatremia by increasing the proximal tubular reabsorption of sodium *(Bartorelli CN, Gargano N, Leonetti G, Zanchetti A. Hypotensive and renal effects of diazoxide: A sodium-retaining benzothiadiazine compound. Circulation 27:895-903, 1963).*

Dicoumarol

See also **Warfarin**

- and Aluminum-containing Antacids

Reduce the drug's availability *(Roe DA. Diet and Drug Interactions. New York, Van Nostrand Reinhold, 1989:84).*

- and Vitamin C

Large doses diminish the drug's anticoagulant effect *(Owen CA Jr, Tyce GM, Flock EV, McCall JT. Heparin-ascorbic acid antagonism. Mayo Clin Proc 45:140, 1970; Rosenthal G. Interaction of ascorbic acid and warfarin. JAMA 215:1671, 1971).*

- and Vitamin E

Large doses of vitamin E can potentiate the drug's effects, thus increasing the risk of hemorrhage *(Corrigan JJ Jr, Marcus FI. Coagulopathy associated with vitamin E ingestion. JAMA 230:1300-1, 1974).*

- and <u>Vitamin K</u>

Interferes with the regeneration of vitamin K_1 from its biologically inactive form *(Bell RG. Metabolism of vitamin K and prothrombin synthesis; anti-coagulants and the vitamin K-epoxide cycle. Fed Proc 37:2599-604, 1978).*

Digoxin

- and <u>Aluminum-containing Antacids</u>

Reduce digoxin bioavailability *(Roe DA. Diet and Drug Interactions. New York, Van Nostrand Reinhold, 1989:84).*

- and <u>Calcium</u>

Increases renal calcium clearance *(Kupfer S, Kosovsky JD. Effects of cardiac glycosides on renal tubular transport of calcium, magnesium, inorganic phosphate and glucose in the dog. J Clin Invest 44:1132-43, 1965).*

- and <u>Magnesium</u>

By decreasing intracellular magnesium, the drug causes increased urinary magnesium loss *(Toffaletti J. Electrolytes, divalent cations, and blood gases (magnesium). Analyt Chem 63(12):192R-4R, 1991).*

Magnesium deficiency promotes digoxin-induced dysrhythmias, and inhibits the efficacy of digoxin in controlling atrial fibrillation *(Toffaletti J. Electrolytes, divalent cations, and blood gases (magnesium). Analyt Chem 63(12):192R-4R, 1991).*

<u>Diphenylhydantoin</u>   *See* <u>Phenytoin</u>

<u>Disopyramide phosphate</u>

- and <u>Magnesium</u>

May induce a magnesium deficiency *(Tzivoni D, Keren A. Suppression of ventricular arrhythmias by magnesium. Am J Cardiol 65(20):1397-9, 1990).*

<u>Disulfiram</u>

- and <u>Vitamin B_6</u>

Supplementation with pyridoxine 500 mg daily prevents the drug's hypercholesterolemic effect *(Major LF, Gover PF. Effects of disulfiram and pyridoxine on serum cholesterol. Ann Intern Med 88(1):53-6, 1978).*

L-Dopa

- and Vitamin B$_6$

Impairs vitamin B$_6$ bioavailability (*Hodges R. Drug-nutrient interaction, in Nutrition in Medical Practice. Philadelphia, W.B. Saunders, 1980:323-31*) although plasma and erythrocyte pyridoxal-5-phosphate levels may be increased (*Mars H. Effect of chronic levodopa treatment on pyridoxine metabolism. Neurology 25(3):263-6, 1975*).

> **WARNING:** Supplementation with vitamin B$_6$ may counteract the effects of L-dopa unless the drug is given currently with carbidopa (*AMA Drug Evaluations, Fifth Edition. Chicago, American Medical Association, 1983*).

Doxorubicin

- and Coenzyme Q$_{10}$

Supplementation may double its anti-tumor activity (*Yamanaka N, Kato T, Hishida K, et al, in Y Yamamura, K Folkers, Y Ito, Eds. Biochemical and Clinical Aspects of Coenzyme Q, Volume 2. Amsterdam, Elsevier/North Holland Biomedical Press, 1980:213-24*).

Adverse effects upon heart function may be due to its inhibitory effects on coenzyme Q$_{10}$-dependent enzyme systems (*Iwamoto Y, Hansen IL, Porter TH, Folkers K. Inhibition of coenzyme Q$_{10}$-enzymes, succinoxidase and NADH-oxidase, by adriamycin and other quinones having antitumor activity. Biochem Biophys Res Commun 58:633, 1974*).

Supplementation may reduce cardiac side effects from adriamycin therapy (*Okuma K et al. [Protective effect of coenzyme Q$_{10}$ in cardiotoxicity induced by adriamycin.] Gan To Kagaku Ryoho 11(3):502-8, 1984; Folkers K, Baker L, Richardson PC, et al. New progress on the biomedical and clinical research on Coenzyme Q, in K Folkers, Y Yamamura, Eds. Biomedical and Clinical Aspects of Coenzyme Q, Volume 3. Amsterdam, Elsevier/North Holland Biomedical Press, 1981:399-412*).

Dymelor

- and Coenzyme Q$_{10}$

May promote CoQ$_{10}$ deficiency and inhibit the CoQ$_{10}$ enzyme NADH-oxidase (*Kishi T, Kishi H, Watanabe T, Folkers K. Bioenergetics in clinical medicine. XI. Studies on CoQ and diabetes mellitus. J Med 7:307-21, 1976*).

Edetate Calcium Disodium (EDTA)

- and Calcium

May lower calcium in hypercalcemia (*Milne MD. Drug interactions and the kidney, in LE Cluff, JC Petrie, Eds. Clinical Effects of Interaction between Drugs. New York, American Elsevier, 1974*).

- and <u>Zinc</u>

Given IV, may cause excessive loss of zinc in the urine *(Fell GS et al. Urinary zinc levels as an indication of muscle catabolism. <u>Lancet</u> i:280-2, 1973)*.

<u>Erythromycin</u>

- and <u>Vitamin B Complex</u>

Parenteral dosage forms of erythromycin may be physically and/or chemically incompatible with solutions containing vitamin B complex *(<u>Drug Evaluations Subscription</u>. Chicago, American Medical Association, Vol II, Section 13, Chapter 4, Spring, 1993)*.

- and <u>Vitamin C</u>

Parenteral dosage forms of erythromycin may be physically and/or chemically incompatible with solutions containing ascorbic acid *(<u>Drug Evaluations Subscription</u>. Chicago, American Medical Association, Vol II, Section 13, Chapter 4, Spring, 1993)*.

<u>Estrogen</u>

- and <u>Folic Acid</u>

Impairs folate absorption *(Holtzapple P, Schwartz S. Drug-induced maldigestion and malabsorption, in D Roe, T Campbell, Eds. <u>Drugs and Nutrients: The Interactive Effects</u>. New York, Marcel Decker, 1984:475-83)*.

- and <u>Vitamin B$_6$</u>

Impairs vitamin B$_6$ absorption *(Goodhart R, Shils M, Eds. <u>Modern Nutrition in Health and Disease</u>. Philadelphia, Lea and Febiger, 1980)*.

<u>Ethacrynic Acid</u>

- and <u>Calcium</u>

Increases urinary calcium excretion *(D'Arcy PF, Griffin JP. <u>Iatrogenic Diseases</u>. London, Oxford U. Press, 1972; Demartini FE, Briscoe AM, Ragan C. Effect of ethacrynic acid on calcium and magnesium excretion. <u>Proc Soc Exp Biol Med</u> 124:320-4, 1967)*.

- and <u>Magnesium</u>

Increases urinary magnesium excretion *(Demartini FE, Briscoe AM, Ragan C. Effect of ethacrynic acid on calcium and magnesium excretion. <u>Proc Soc Exp Biol Med</u> 124:320-4, 1967)*.

- and <u>Potassium</u>

> Prolonged or high doses may cause potassium depletion *(Hamdy RC, Tovey J, Perera N. Hypokalemia and diuretics. <u>Br Med J</u> i:1187, 1980; Steen B. Hypokalemia, clinical spectrum, and etiology. <u>Acta Med Scand Suppl</u> 647:61-6, 1981).*

<u>Ethambutol</u>

- and <u>Zinc</u>

> Chelates zinc *(Roe DA. <u>Drug-induced Nutritional Deficiencies</u>. Second Edition. Westport, CT, Avi Publishing, 1985:288).*

<u>Ethionamide</u>

- and <u>Vitamin B6</u>

> May produce a vitamin B6 deficiency *(Roe DA. <u>Drug-induced Nutritional Deficiencies</u>. Second Edition. Westport, CT, Avi Publishing, 1985:154-7).*

<u>Etretinate</u>

- and <u>Calcium</u>

> May cause hypercalcemia *(Roe DA. <u>Diet and Drug Interactions</u>. New York, Van Nostrand Reinhold, 1989:150).*

<u>5-Fluorouracil</u>

- and <u>Thiamine</u>

> Inhibits the conversion of thiamine to thiamine pyrophosphate *(Basu TK, Dickerson JWT. The thiamin status of patients with cancer as determined by the red cell transketolase activity. <u>J Vitam Nutr Res</u> 44:53, 1974).*

<u>Furosemide</u>

- and <u>Calcium</u>

> Produces calciuria *(D'Arcy PF, Griffin JP. <u>Iatrogenic Diseases</u>. London, Oxford U. Press, 1972).*

- and <u>Magnesium</u>

> May cause hypomagnesemia secondary to urinary hyperexcretion of magnesium *(Roe DA. <u>Diet and Drug Interactions</u>. New York, Van Nostrand Reinhold, 1989:150-1).*

- and <u>Potassium</u>

Prolonged or high doses may cause potassium depletion (*Hamdy RC, Tovey J, Perera N. Hypokalemia and diuretics. Br Med J i:1187, 1980; Steen B. Hypokalemia, clinical spectrum, and etiology. Acta Med Scand Suppl 647:61-6, 1981*).

- and <u>Thiamine</u>

May cause thiamine deficiency by increasing urinary losses (*Seligmann H et al. Thiamine deficiency in patients with congestive heart failure receiving long-term furosemide therapy: a pilot study. Am J Med 91(2):151-5, 1991*).

Supplementation may improve cardiac function in patients with congestive heart failure receiving the medication (*Shimon I et al. Improved left ventricular function after thiamine supplementation in patients with congestive heart failure receiving long-term furosemide therapy. Am J Med 98:485-9, 1995*).

<u>Gentamycin</u> *See* '<u>Aminoglycosides</u>'

<u>Glutethimide</u>

- and <u>Vitamin D</u>

Hypothesized to increase the turnover rate of vitamin D, causing depletion of vitamin stores and impairment of vitamin D-dependent calcium absorption (*Greenwood RH, Prunty FTG, Silver J. Osteomalacia after prolonged glutethimide administration. Br Med J i:643-5, 1973*).

<u>Glyburide</u>

- and <u>Coenzyme Q$_{10}$</u>

May promote CoQ$_{10}$ deficiency and inhibit the CoQ$_{10}$ enzyme NADH-oxidase (*Kishi T, Kishi H, Watanabe T, Folkers K. Bioenergetics in clinical medicine. XI. Studies on CoQ and diabetes mellitus. J Med 7:307-21, 1976*).

<u>Gold</u>

- and <u>Selenium</u>

Decreases the bioavailability of selenium (*Peretz A, Neve J, Famaey J. Selenium in rheumatic diseases. Semin Arth Rheum 20:305-16, 1991*).

<u>Hydralazine</u>

- and <u>Vitamin B$_6$</u>

A vitamin B$_6$ antagonist that may cause symptoms of B$_6$ deficiency in about 10% of patients (*Raskin NH, Rishman RA. Pyridoxine-deficiency neuropathy due to hydralazine. New Engl J Med 273:1182-5, 1965*).

Hydrazine

- and Vitamin B$_6$

Impairs vitamin B$_6$ absorption (*Tuckerman M, Turco S. Human Nutrition. Philadelphia, Lea and Febiger, 1983:215-22*).

Ifosfamide

- and N-acetylcysteine

NAC may prevent hemorrhagic cystitis due to drug administration (*Watson RA. Ifosfamide: Chemotherapy with new promise and new problems for the urologist. Urology 24(5):465-8, 1984*).

Indomethacin

- and Folic Acid

Impairs folate absorption (*Hodges R. Drug-nutrient interaction, in Nutrition in Medical Practice. Philadelphia, W.B. Saunders, 1980:323-31*).

- and Vitamin C

Impairs vitamin C absorption (*Hodges R. Drug-nutrient interaction, in Nutrition in Medical Practice. Philadelphia, W.B. Saunders, 1980:323-31*).

Isoniazid (INH)

- and Aluminum-containing Antacids

Reduce isoniazid bioavailability (*Roe DA. Diet and Drug Interactions. New York, Van Nostrand Reinhold, 1989:84*).

- and Calcium

Reduces synthesis of the active forms of vitamin D that are necessary for calcium absorption; thus there is risk of metabolic bone disease with long-term use (*Brodie MJ, Boobis AR, Hillyard CJ, et al. Effect of isoniazid on vitamin D metabolism and hepatic homooxygenase activity. Clin Pharmacol Ther 30:363-7, 1981*).

- and Niacin

Isoniazid inhibits the conversion of tryptophan to niacin. Patients on a marginally niacin-deficient diet may develop pellagra (*DiLorenzo PA. Pellagra-like syndrome associated with isoniazid therapy. Acta Dermatol Venereol 47:318-22, 1967*).

- and <u>Vitamin B$_6$</u>

Causes vitamin B$_6$ depletion which may be manifested by a peripheral neuropathy as it forms a Schiff base with pyridoxal phosphate, resulting in excessive urinary excretion (*Roe DA. <u>Drug-induced Nutritional Deficiencies</u>. Second Edition. Westport, CT, Avi Publishing, 1985:178-9; 281-7*).

- and <u>Vitamin D</u>

Reduces synthesis of the active forms of vitamin D that are necessary for calcium absorption; thus there is risk of metabolic bone disease with long-term use (*Bengoa JM, Bolt MJG, Rosenberg IH. Hepatic vitamin D 25-hydroxylase inhibition by cimetidine and isoniazid. <u>J Lab Clin Med</u> 104:546-52, 1984; Brodie MJ, Boobis AR, Hillyard CJ, et al. Effect of isoniazid on vitamin D metabolism and hepatic homooxygenase activity. <u>Clin Pharmacol Ther</u> 30:363-7, 1981*).

- and <u>Vitamin E</u>

Decreases vitamin E absorption (*<u>Vitamin E Fact Book</u>. VERIS (Vitamin E Research & Information Service, 5325 S. 9th Ave., LaGrange, IL 60525, 1994*).

<u>Isotretinoin</u>

- and <u>Calcium</u>

May cause hypercalcemia (*Roe DA. <u>Diet and Drug Interactions</u>. New York, Van Nostrand Reinhold, 1989:150*).

- and <u>Vitamin A</u>

Avoid concurrent use due to additive side effects (*<u>Drug Evaluations Subscription</u>. Chicago, American Medical Association, Vol II, Section 11, Chapter 1, Summer, 1993*).

<u>Levodopa</u>

- and <u>Protein</u>

Competition with dietary proteins may decrease drug absorption (*Lim D, McKay M. Food-drug interactions. <u>Drug Information Bulletin</u>, UCLA Dept. of Pharmaceutical Services, 15(2), 1995*).

- and <u>Vitamin B$_6$</u>

Large vitamin B6 intake may decrease the effect of the drug (*Lim D, McKay M. Food-drug interactions. <u>Drug Information Bulletin</u>, UCLA Dept. of Pharmaceutical Services, 15(2), 1995*).

<u>Lithium Carbonate</u>

- and <u>Magnesium</u>

May cause hypermagnesemia (*Nielson J. Magnesium-lithium studies. 1. Serum and erythrocyte magnesium in patients with manic states during lithium treatment. <u>Acta Psychiatr Scand</u> 40:190, 1964*).

Lovastatin

- and Coenzyme Q$_{10}$

Reduces CoQ$_{10}$ levels *(Folkers K et al. Lovastatin decreases Coenzyme Q levels in humans. Proc Natl Acad Sci U S A 87:8931-4, 1990).*

> *Note: Vitamin E supplementation has been suggested to offset the loss of Coenzyme Q (Harold Baum, head, School of Life, Basic Medical and Health Sciences, King's College, London - reported in New Scientist, May 24, 1991, p. 24).*

Concurrent CoQ$_{10}$ supplementation may benefit cardiac function *(Folkers K, Langsjoen P, Eds., in K Folkers, GP Littarru, T Yamagami, Eds. Biochemical and Clinical Aspects of Coenzyme Q, Volume 6. Amsterdam, Elsevier Science Publ, 1991:449-52).*

- and Fiber

Fibers such as oat bran and pectin may reduce gastrointestinal absorption of the drug and thus increase LDL cholesterol levels *(Richter WO, Jacob B, Schwandt P. Interaction between fibre and lovastatin. Letter. Lancet 338:706, 1991).*

Magnesium Hydroxide

- and Phosphorus

Combines with phosphates in the intestines leading to the excretion of magnesium phosphates. Excessive use may result in symptomatic phosphate depletion marked by hypophosphatemia (plasma phosphate <0.35 mmol/L). Uncommonly, osteomalacia may develop *(Harvey SC. Gastric antacids and digestants, in LS Goodman, A Gilman, Eds. The Pharmacological Basis of Therapeutics. 3rd Edition. New York, MacMillan, 1965; Lotz M, Zisman E, Bartter C. Evidence for a phosphorus depletion syndrome in man. N Engl J Med 278:409-15, 1978).*

Mannitol

- and Potassium

Hypertonic infusions may increase serum potassium levels *(Moreno M, Murphy C, Goldsmith C. Increase in serum potassium resulting from the administration of hypertonic mannitol or other solutions. J Lab Clin Med 73:291-8, 1969).*

- and Sodium

Infusion by cause hyponatremia because the infused molecules remain within the vascular compartment and raise plasma osmolality, resulting in an expansion of the blood volume and associated lowering of sodium *(Roe DA. Diet and Drug Interactions. New York, Van Nostrand Reinhold, 1989:146).*

Metformin

- and Vitamin B$_{12}$

Impairs vitamin B$_{12}$ absorption (*Hodges R. Drug-nutrient interaction, in Nutrition in Medical Practice. Philadelphia, W.B. Saunders, 1980:323-31*).

Methotrexate

- and Calcium

Long-term use may cause malabsorption with steatorrhea and secondary calcium depletion (*Roe DA. Drugs and nutrient absorption, in M. Winick, Ed. Nutrition and Drugs. New York, Wiley, 1983*).

- and Folic Acid

Methotrexate displaces folate from its binding to the folate reductase enzyme, resulting in its elimination; thus folinic acid, which reverses the cytotoxic effect of the drug, is given afterwards to cancer patients in order to prevent bone marrow depression and intestinal toxicity (*Roe DA. Drug-induced Nutritional Deficiencies. Second Edition. Westport, CT, Avi Publishing, 1985:178-9; 303*). For rheumatoid arthritics, folate can be given coincident with drug therapy without impairing methotrexate's efficacy (*Morgan SL, Baggott JE, Vaughn WH, et al. Supplementation with folic acid during methotrexate therapy for rheumatoid arthritis: a double-blind, placebo-controlled trial. Ann Intern Med 121:833-41, 1994*).

- and Riboflavin

Inhibits the uptake of the drug into malignant cells (*DiPalma JR, Ritchie DM. Vitamin toxicity. Ann Rev Pharm Tox 17:133, 1977*).

Methyldopa

- and Iron

Concurrent iron ingestion causes a marked decrease in the bioavailability of the drug (*Campbell NR, Hasinoff BB. Iron supplements: a common cause of drug interactions. Br J Clin Pharmacol 31(3):251-5, 1991*).

- and Lithium

Confusion, disorientation and tremor may result from an interaction between them (*Drug Evaluations Subscription. Chicago, American Medical Association, Vol I, Section 6, Chapter 4, Winter, 1994*).

Mineral Oil

- and Beta-Carotene

Impairs beta-carotene absorption (*Curtis AC, Balmer RS. The prevention of carotene absorption. JAMA 113:1785-8, 1939*).

- and Vitamin A

Impairs vitamin A absorption (*Morgan JW. The harmful effects of mineral oil (liquid petrolatum) purgatives. JAMA 117:1335-6, 1941*).

- and Vitamin D

Impairs vitamin D absorption (*Morgan JW. The harmful effects of mineral oil (liquid petrolatum) purgatives. JAMA 117:1335-6, 1941*).

- and Vitamin E

Impairs vitamin E absorption (*Vitamin E Fact Book. VERIS (Vitamin E Research & Information Service, 5325 S. 9th Ave., LaGrange, IL 60525, 1994*).

- and Vitamin K

Impairs vitamin K absorption (*Morgan JW. The harmful effects of mineral oil (liquid petrolatum) purgatives. JAMA 117:1335-6, 1941*).

Neomycin

- and Beta-Carotene

Impairs beta-carotene absorption (*Robinson C, Weigly E. Basic Nutrition and Diet Therapy. New York, MacMillan, 1984:46-54*).

and Calcium

Impairs calcium absorption (*Roe DA. Drug-induced Nutritional Deficiencies. Second Edition. Westport, CT, Avi Publishing, 1985:157-8*).

- and Fat

Impairs fat absorption (*Roe DA. Drug-induced Nutritional Deficiencies. Second Edition. Westport, CT, Avi Publishing, 1985:157-8*).

- and Iron

Impairs iron absorption (*Roe DA. Drug-induced Nutritional Deficiencies. Second Edition. Westport, CT, Avi Publishing, 1985:157-8*).

- and Lactose

Impairs lactose absorption (*Roe DA. Drug-induced Nutritional Deficiencies. Second Edition. Westport, CT, Avi Publishing, 1985:157-8*).

- and Magnesium

May cause hypomagnesemia secondary to maldigestion (*Roe DA. Diet and Drug Interactions. New York, Van Nostrand Reinhold, 1989:151*).

- and Nitrogen

Impairs nitrogen absorption (*Roe DA. Drug-induced Nutritional Deficiencies. Second Edition. Westport, CT, Avi Publishing, 1985:157-87*).

- and Potassium

Impairs potassium absorption (*Roe DA. Drug-induced Nutritional Deficiencies. Second Edition. Westport, CT, Avi Publishing, 1985:157-8*).

- and Sodium

Impairs sodium absorption (*Roe DA. Drug-induced Nutritional Deficiencies. Second Edition. Westport, CT, Avi Publishing, 1985:157-8*).

- and Sucrose

Impairs sucrose absorption (*Roe DA. Drug-induced Nutritional Deficiencies. Second Edition. Westport, CT, Avi Publishing, 1985:157-8*).

- and Vitamin A

Impairs vitamin A absorption (*Tuckerman M, Turco S. Human Nutrition. Philadelphia, Lea and Febiger, 1983:215-22*).

- and Vitamin B$_{12}$

Impairs vitamin B$_{12}$ absorption (*Tuckerman M, Turco S. Human Nutrition. Philadelphia, Lea and Febiger, 1983:215-22*).

- and <u>**Vitamin K**</u>

Impairs vitamin K absorption (*Robinson C, Weigly E. <u>Basic Nutrition and Diet Therapy</u>. New York, MacMillan, 1984:46-54*).

<u>Nitroglycerin</u>

- and <u>**N-acetyl Cysteine**</u>

NAC supplementation following nitroglycerin ingestion may potentiate temporal artery dilation and a headache response (*Iverson HK. N-acetylcysteine enhances nitroglycerin-induced headache and cranial artery response. <u>Clin Pharmacol Ther</u> 52:125-33, 1992*).

<u>Nitrous Oxide</u>

- and <u>**Vitamin B$_{12}$**</u>

Interferes with vitamin B$_{12}$ metabolism causing megaloblastosis (*Amess JA, Burman JF, Rees GM, et al. Megaloblastic haemopoiesis in patients receiving nitrous oxide. <u>Lancet</u> ii:339-42, 1978; Deacon R, Perry J, Lumb J, Chanarin I. Selective inactivation of vitamin B$_{12}$ in rats by nitrous oxide. <u>Lancet</u> ii:1023-4, 1978*).

<u>Omeprazole</u>

- and <u>**Vitamin B$_{12}$**</u>

Acutely depresses B$_{12}$ absorption (*Marcuard SP et al. Omeprazole therapy causes malabsorption of cyanocobalamin (vitamin B$_{12}$). <u>Ann Intern Med</u> 120:211-15, 1994; Saltzman JR, Kemp JA, Golner BB, et al. Effect of hypochlorhydria due to omeprazole treatment or atrophic gastritis on protein-bound vitamin B$_{12}$ absorption. <u>J Am Coll Nutr</u> 13(6):584-91, 1994*).

<u>Para-aminosalicylic Acid (PAS)</u>

- and <u>**Fat**</u>

Impairs fat absorption (*Roe DA. <u>Drug-induced Nutritional Deficiencies.</u> Second Edition. Westport, CT, Avi Publishing, 1985:157-8*).

- and <u>**Folic Acid**</u>

Malabsorption of folacin causing low or deficient plasma and erythrocyte folacin levels may occur with prolonged intake (*Roe DA. <u>Diet and Drug Interactions</u>. New York, Van Nostrand Reinhold, 1989:140*).

- and <u>**Vitamin B$_{12}$**</u>

Impairs vitamin B$_{12}$ absorption (*Robinson C, Weigly E. <u>Basic Nutrition and Diet Therapy</u>. New York, MacMillan, 1984:46-54*).

D-Penicillamine

- and Copper

Increases urinary copper excretion *(McCall JT et al. Comparative metabolism of copper and zinc in patients with Wilson's disease (hepatolenticular degeneration). Am J Med Sci 254:13-23, 1967).*

- and Iron

Concurrent iron ingestion causes a marked decrease in the bioavailability of the drug *(Campbell NR, Hasinoff BB. Iron supplements: a common cause of drug interactions. Br J Clin Pharmacol 31(3):251-5, 1991).*

- and Vitamin B_6

Impairs vitamin B_6 availability *(Rumsby PC, Shepherd DM. The effect of penicillamine on vitamin B_6 function in man. Biochem Pharmacol 30:3051-3, 1981).*

- and Zinc

Increases urinary zinc excretion while increasing zinc absorption *(McCall JT et al. Comparative metabolism of copper and zinc in patients with Wilson's disease (hepatolenticular degeneration). Am J Med Sci 254:13-23, 1967).*

May cause zinc deficiency *(Multicentre Trial Group. Controlled trial of D(-)penicillamine in severe rheumatoid arthritis. Lancet i:275-80, 1973).*

Pentamidine

- and Folic Acid

May occasionally depress serum folate levels *(Weston KA, Perera DR, Schultz MG. Pentamidine isethionate in the treatment of pneumocystis carinii pneumonia. Ann Intern Med 73:695-702, 1970).*

Phenformin

- and Coenzyme Q_{10}

May promote CoQ_{10} deficiency and inhibit the CoQ_{10} enzyme NADH-oxidase *(Kishi T, Kishi H, Watanabe T, Folkers K. Bioenergetics in clinical medicine. XI. Studies on CoQ and diabetes mellitus. J Med 7:307-21, 1976).*

- and Vitamin B_{12}

Impairs vitamin B_{12} absorption *(Hodges R. Drug-nutrient interaction, in Nutrition in Medical Practice. Philadelphia, W.B. Saunders, 1980:323-31).*

Phenobarbital

- and Calcium

Long-term use reduces calcium absorption *(Wahl TO, Gobrity AH, Lukert BP. Long-term anticonvulsant therapy and intestinal calcium absorption. Clin Pharmacol Ther 30:506-12, 1981).*

- and Folic Acid

Plasma and erythrocyte folacin levels may be lowered *(Reynolds EH, Milner G, Matthews DM, Chanarin I. Anti-convulsant therapy, megaloblastic haematopoiesis, and folic acid metabolism. Quart J Med 35:521-37, 1966).*

- and Vitamin D

Impairs vitamin D availability *(Holmes R, Kummerow F. The relationship of adequate and excessive intake of vitamin D to health and disease. J Am Coll Nutr 2:173-99, 1983).*

Phenolphthalein

- and Calcium

Impairs calcium absorption *(Roe DA. Drug-induced Nutritional Deficiencies. Second Edition. Westport, CT, Avi Publishing, 1985:154-7).*

- and Potassium

May induce potassium depletion *(Fleming BJ, Genuth SM, Gould AB, Kaminokowski MD. Laxative induced hypokalemia, sodium depletion, and hyperreninemia. Effects of potassium and sodium replacement on the renin angiotensin system. Ann Intern Med 83:60-2, 1975).*

- and Vitamin D

Impairs vitamin D absorption *(Roe DA. Drug-induced Nutritional Deficiencies. Second Edition. Westport, CT, Avi Publishing, 1985:154-7).*

Phenylbutazone

- and Folic Acid

Impairs folate absorption *(Hodges R. Drug-nutrient interaction, in Nutrition in Medical Practice. Philadelphia, W.B. Saunders, 1980:323-31).*

Phenytoin

- and Aluminum-containing Antacids

Reduce phenytoin bioavailability (*Roe DA. Diet and Drug Interactions. New York, Van Nostrand Reinhold, 1989;84*).

- and Calcium

Long-term use reduces calcium absorption (*Wahl TO, Gobrity AH, Lukert BP. Long-term anticonvulsant therapy and intestinal calcium absorption. Clin Pharmacol Ther 30:506-12, 1981*).

- and Folic Acid

Impairs folate absorption (*Roe D. Risk factors in drug-induced nutritional deficiencies, in D Roe, T Campbell, Eds. Drugs and Nutrients: The Interactive Effects. New York, Marcel Decker, 1984:505-23*) which may induce a biochemical or clinical folate deficiency (*Hoffbrand AV, Nicheles RF. Mechanisms of folate deficiency in patients receiving phenytoin. Lancet ii:528-30, 1968*).

Folates may interfere with both the intestinal absorption and the central nervous system effects of phenytoin (*Colman N, Herbert V. Folate metabolism in brain, in S Kumar, Ed. Biochemistry of Brain. New York, Pergamon Press, 1980:103-25*).

- and Vitamin B_{12}

Impairs vitamin B_{12} absorption (*Roe D. Risk factors in drug-induced nutritional deficiencies, in D Roe, T Campbell, Eds. Drugs and Nutrients: The Interactive Effects. New York, Marcel Decker, 1984:505-23*).

- and Vitamin D

Impairs vitamin D availability (*Holmes R, Kummerow F. The relationship of adequate and excessive intake of vitamin D to health and disease. J Am Coll Nutr 2:173-99, 1983*) and may induce a vitamin D deficiency with secondary calcium malabsorption as evidenced by rickets or osteomalacia (*Roe DA. Drug-induced Nutritional Deficiencies. Second Edition. Westport, CT, ARI Publishing, 1985:164-6; 249*).

- and Vitamin K

Impairs vitamin K availability in infants (*Roe D. Risk factors in drug-induced nutritional deficiencies, in D Roe, T Campbell, Eds. Drugs and Nutrients: The Interactive Effects. New York, Marcel Decker, 1984:505-23*).

Potassium Chloride

- and Vitamin B_{12}

Impairs vitamin B_{12} absorption (*Palva IP, Salokannel SJ, Timonen T, Palva HLA. Drug-induced malabsorption of vitamin B_{12}. IV. Malabsorption and deficiency of B_{12} during treatment with slow-release potassium chloride. Acta Med Scand 191:355-7, 1972*).

Primidone

- and Folic Acid

May induce a biochemical or clinical folate deficiency *(Roe DA. Drug-induced Nutritional Deficiencies. Second Edition. Westport, CT, ARI Publishing, 1985:249).*

- and Vitamin D

May induce a vitamin D deficiency as evidenced by rickets or osteomalacia *(Roe DA. Drug-induced Nutritional Deficiencies. Second Edition. Westport, CT, ARI Publishing, 1985:249).*

Probucol

- and Carotenoids

Reduces serum levels of beta-carotene and lycopene, most probably due to reductions in lipoprotein particle size and to competition with these substances for incorporation into VLDL during its assembly in the liver *(Elinder LS, Hadell K, Johansson J, et al. Probucol treatment decreases serum concentrations of diet-derived antioxidants. Arterioscler Thromb Vasc Biol 15(8):1057-63, 1995).*

- and Vitamin E

Reduces serum vitamin E levels secondary to cholesterol and triglyceride lowering *(Elinder LS, Hadell K, Johansson J, et al. Probucol treatment decreases serum concentrations of diet-derived antioxidants. Arterioscler Thromb Vasc Biol 15(8):1057-63, 1995).*

Procarbazine

- and Vitamin B$_6$

In animals, causes lowering of plasma pyridoxal phosphate; however, pyridoxine supplementation does not reverse its neurotoxicity in humans *(Chabner BA, DeVita VT, Considine N, Oliverio VT. Plasma pyridoxal phosphate depletion by the carcinostatic procarbazine. Proc Soc Exp Biol Med 132:1119, 1969; Pratt WB, Ruddon RW. The Anticancer Drugs. Oxford, Oxford U. Press, 1979:249).*

Progesterone

- and Folic Acid

Impairs folate absorption *(Holtzapple P, Schwartz S. Drug-induced maldigestion and malabsorption, in D Roe, T Campbell, Eds. Drugs and Nutrients: The Interactive Effects. New York, Marcel Decker, 1984:475-83).*

- and Vitamin B$_6$

Impairs vitamin B$_6$ availability *(Goodhart R, Shils M, Eds. Modern Nutrition in Health and Disease. Philadelphia, Lea and Febiger, 1980:892-1240).*

Pyrazinamide

- and Vitamin B₆

May produce a vitamin B_6 deficiency *(Roe DA. Drug-induced Nutritional Deficiencies. Second Edition. Westport, CT, Avi Publishing, 1985:200).*

Pyrimethamine

- and Folic Acid

Impairs folate availability *(Tuckerman M, Turco S. Human Nutrition. Philadelphia, Lea and Febiger, 1983:215-22).*

Quinidine sulfate

- and Aluminum-containing Antacids

Reduce quinidine bioavailability *(Roe DA. Diet and Drug Interactions. New York, Van Nostrand Reinhold, 1989:84).*

- and Magnesium

May induce a magnesium deficiency *(Tzivoni D, Keren A. Suppression of ventricular arrhythmias by magnesium. Am J Cardiol 65(20):1397-9, 1990).*

Rantidine

and Vitamin B₁₂

Impairs protein-bound vitamin B_{12} absorption by inhibiting gastric acid secretion, preventing B_{12} from being freed from its protein binder during digestion *(Streeter AM, Goulston KJ, Bathur FA, et al. Cimetidine and malabsorption of cobalamin. Dig Dis Sci 27:13-16, 1982).*

- and Zinc

Reduces zinc absorption (300 mg/d for 3 days) *(Sturniolo GC et al. Inhibition of gastric acid secretion reduces zinc absorption in man. J Am Coll Nutr 4:372-5, 1991).*

Sodium Bicarbonate

- and Folic Acid

Impairs folate absorption by rendering jejunal pH more alkaline *(Benn A, Swan CJH, Cooke WT, et al. Effect of intraluminal pH on the absorption of pteroylmonoglutamic acid. Br Med J 16:148-50, 1971; Mackenzie JF, Russell RJ. The effect of pH on folic acid absorption. Clin Sci Molec Med 51:363-8, 1976; Roe DA. Drug-induced Nutritional Deficiencies. Second Edition. Westport, CT, Avi Publishing, 1985:154-7).*

Sodium Polystyrene Sulfonate

- and Calcium

Believed to bind with calcium, thus preventing it from combining with bicarbonate in the small intestine and resulting in systemic alkalosis (*Hansten PD. Drug Interactions, Edition 4. Philadelphia, Lea & Febiger, 1979*).

- and Magnesium

Believed to bind with magnesium, thus preventing it from combining with bicarbonate in the small intestine and resulting in systemic alkalosis (*Hansten PD. Drug Interactions, Edition 4. Philadelphia, Lea & Febiger, 1979*).

Sodium Sulfate

- and Potassium

Infusion may cause hypokalemia (*Sherwood LM. Hypernatremia during sodium sulfate therapy. Letter. N Engl J Med 277:314, 1967*).

- and Sodium

Infusion may cause hypernatremia (*Sherwood LM. Hypernatremia during sodium sulfate therapy. Letter. N Engl J Med 277:314, 1967*).

Spironolactone

- and Potassium

A potassium-sparing diuretic that may cause hypokalemia by blocking distal tubular sodium-potassium exchange (*Herman E, Rado JP. Fatal hyperkalemic paralysis associated with spironolactone. Arch Neurol 15:74, 1966*).

- and Sodium

May cause hyponatremia with an associated rise in serum potassium levels; may have an anti-aldosterone effect (*Roe DA. Diet and Drug Interactions. New York, Van Nostrand Reinhold, 1989:146*).

Strophanthin

- and Calcium

Increases renal calcium clearance (*Kupfer S, Kosovsky JD. Effects of cardiac glycosides on renal tubular transport of calcium, magnesium, inorganic phosphate and glucose in the dog. J Clin Invest 44:1132-43, 1965*).

- and <u>**Magnesium**</u>

Increases renal calcium clearance *(Kupfer S, Kosovsky JD. Effects of cardiac glycosides on renal tubular transport of calcium, magnesium, inorganic phosphate and glucose in the dog. <u>J Clin Invest</u> 44:1132-43, 1965)*.

<u>Succinyl choline</u>

- and <u>**Potassium**</u>

May increase serum potassium levels *(Gronert GA. Potassium response to succinylcholine. Letter. <u>JAMA</u> 211:300, 1970)*.

<u>Sulfasalazine (salicylazosulfapyridine)</u>

- and <u>**Folic Acid**</u>

Inhibits the intestinal absorption of dietary folacin and inhibits folate-dependent enzymes *(Baum CL, Sulhub J, Rosenberg IH. Antifolate actions of sulfasalazine on intact lymphocytes. <u>J Lab Clin Med</u> 97(6):779-84, 1981; Selhub J, Dhar CJ, Rosenberg IH. Inhibition of folate enzymes by sulfasalazine. <u>J Clin Invest</u> 61:221-4, 1978)*.

<u>Theophylline</u>

- and <u>**Vitamin B$_6$**</u>

A pyridoxal kinase antagonist, theophylline may lower plasma pyridoxal-5^1-phosphate levels while plasma pyridoxal levels are unchanged *(Delport R et al. Vitamin B$_6$ nutritional status in asthma: The effect of theophylline therapy on plasma pyridoxal-5^1-phosphate and pyridoxal levels. <u>Int J Vitam Nutr Res</u> 58(1):67-72, 1988; Ubbink JB et al. The relationship between vitamin B$_6$ metabolism, asthma, and theophylline therapy. <u>Ann N Y Acad Sci</u> 585:285-94, 1990)*.

Vitamin B$_6$ supplementation may reduce tremor and other nervous system side effects of theophylline administration caused by pyridoxal-5-phosphate deficiency *(Bartel PR, Ubbink JB, Delport R, et al. Vitamin B-6 supplementation and theophylline-related effects in humans. <u>Am J Clin Nutr</u> 60:93-9, 1994)*.

<u>Thioridazine</u>

- and <u>**Lithium**</u>

Rarely, the combination has produced severe neurotoxicity *(<u>Drug Evaluations Subscription</u>. Chicago, American Medical Association, Vol I, Section 3, Chapter 2, Winter, 1994)*.

<u>Thiosemicarbizide</u>

- and <u>**Vitamin B$_6$**</u>

May produce a vitamin B$_6$ deficiency *(Roe DA. <u>Drug-induced Nutritional Deficiencies</u>. Second Edition. Westport, CT, Avi Publishing, 1985:154-7)*.

Thyroxine

- and Iron

Concurrent iron ingestion decreases the bioavailability of the drug by forming a stable complex with it (*Campbell NRC et al. Ferrous sulfate reduces thyroxine efficacy in patients with hypothyroidism. Ann Int Med 117(12):1010-13, 1992; Campbell NR, Hasinoff BB. Iron supplements: a common cause of drug interactions. Br J Clin Pharmacol 31(3):251-5, 1991*).

Timolol

- and Potassium

May cause dose-dependent increases in serum potassium (*Pederson OL, Mikkelsen E. Serum potassium and uric acid changes during treatment with timolol alone and in combination with a diuretic. Clin Pharmacol Ther 26:339, 1979*).

Tobacco

- and Beta-carotene

Increases beta-carotene requirement due to increased oxidative stress (*Abbey M, Noakes M, Nestel P. Dietary supplementation with orange and carrot juice in cigarette smokers lowers oxidation products in copper-oxidized low-density lipoproteins. J Am Diet Assoc 95:671-5, 1995*).

- and Folic Acid

Increases folate requirement (*Ortega RM, Lopez-Sobaler AM, Gonzalez-Gross MM, et al. Influence of smoking on folate intake and blood folate concentrations in a group of elderly Spanish men. J Am Coll Nutr 13(1):68-72, 1994*).

- and Vitamin B$_6$

Depresses plasma levels of pyridoxal-5'-phosphate (PLP) and pyridoxal. However, since erythrocyte levels of these forms of vitamin B$_6$ are normal, and because PLP mainly functions as an intracellular coenzyme, the clinical significance of these findings is uncertain (*Vermaak WJH, Ubbink JB, Barnard HC, et al. Vitamin B-6 nutrition status and cigarette smoking. Am J Clin Nutr 51:1058-61, 1990*).

- and Vitamin C

Increases vitamin C requirement due to increased oxidative stress (*Schectman G. Estimating ascorbic acid requirements for cigarette smokers. Ann N Y Acad Sci 686:335-46, 1993*).

- and Vitamin E

Increases vitamin E requirement due to increased oxidative stress (*Van Antwerpen VL, Theron AJ, Richards GA, et al. Vitamin E, pulmonary functions and phagocyte-mediated oxidative stress in smokers and nonsmokers. Free Rad Biol Med 18:935-41, 1995*).

- and <u>Zinc</u>

Reduces tissue zinc levels due to competition with cadmium for binding sites (*Hennig B, McClain C, Diana J. Function of vitamin E and zinc in maintaining endothelial integrity - Implications in atherosclerosis. <u>Ann N Y Acad Sci</u> 686:99-111, 1993*).

Tolazamide

- and <u>Coenzyme Q$_{10}$</u>

May promote CoQ$_{10}$ deficiency and inhibit the CoQ$_{10}$ enzyme NADH-oxidase (*Kishi T, Kishi H, Watanabe T, Folkers K. Bioenergetics in clinical medicine. X I. Studies on CoQ and diabetes mellitus. <u>J Med</u> 7:307-21, 1976*).

Tolbutamide

- and <u>Sodium</u>

May cause hyponatremia due to its antidiuretic effect (*Luethi A, Studer H. Antidiuretic action of chlorpropamide and tolbutamide. <u>Minn Med</u> 52:33, 1969*).

Triamterene

- and <u>Calcium</u>

Produces calciuria (*D'Arcy PF, Griffin JP. <u>Iatrogenic Diseases</u>. London, Oxford U. Press, 1972*).

- and <u>Folic Acid</u>

Impairs folate availability (*Tuckerman M, Turco S. <u>Human Nutrition</u>. Philadelphia, Lea and Febiger, 1983:215-22*).

- and <u>Potassium</u>

A potassium-sparing diuretic that may cause hyperkalemia (*Dorph S, Olgaard A. Effect of triamterene on serum potassium and serum creatinine in long-term treatment with thiazides. <u>Nord Med</u> 79:516, 1968*).

Triazinate

- and <u>Folic Acid</u>

Signs of acute folate deficiency develop at therapeutic doses (*Skeet RT, Cashmore AR, Sawicki WL, Bertino JR. Clinical and pharmacological evaluation of triazinate in humans. <u>Cancer Res</u> 36:48-54, 1976*).

Trientine Hydrochloride

- and Iron

Each inhibits the other's absorption; therefore their administration should be separated by at least 2 hours (*Drug Evaluations Subscription*. *Chicago, American Medical Association, Vol III, Section 19, Chapter 8, Spring, 1992*).

Trimethoprim

- and Folic Acid

Minimal folate deficiency may appear after long-term, high dosage treatment which may be reversed by the administration of folinic acid (*Kahn SB, Fein SA, Brodsky I. Effects of trimethoprim on folate metabolism in man. Clin Pharmacol Therap 9:550-60, 1968*).

Valproate

- and Carnitine

Enhances renal losses of carnitine esters and levels to decrease plasma free carnitine, which may occasionally cause symptoms of carnitine deficiency such as severe cardiac dysfunction (*Bratton SL, Garden AL, Bohan TP, et al. A child with valproic acid-associated carnitine deficiency and carnitine-responsive cardiac dysfunction. J Child Neurol 7(4):413-16, 1992*).

- and Folic Acid

Impairs folate absorption (*Hendal J et al. The effects of carbamazepine and valproate on folate metabolism. Acta Neurol Scand 69(4):226-31, 1984*).

Verapamil

- and Calcium

It is possible the therapeutic response to the drug may be reduced by calcium supplements (*Drug Evaluations Subscription. Chicago, American Medical Association, Volume I, Section 7, Chapter 2, Spring, 1992*).

Vincristine

- and Sodium

May cause dilutional hyponatremia (*Oldam RK, Pomeroy TC. Vincristine-induced syndrome of inappropriate secretion of antidiuretic hormone. South Med J 6:1010, 1972*).

Warfarin

See also **Dicoumarol**

- and **Aluminum-containing Antacids**

Reduce the drug's availability (*Roe DA. Diet and Drug Interactions. New York, Van Nostrand Reinhold, 1989:84*).

- and **Vitamin C**

Large doses diminish the drug's anticoagulant effect (*Owen CA Jr, Tyce GM, Flock EV, McCall JT. Heparin-ascorbic acid antagonism. Mayo Clin Proc 45:140, 1970; Rosenthal G. Interaction of ascorbic acid and warfarin. JAMA 215:1671, 1971*).

- and **Vitamin E**

Very large doses of vitamin E can potentiate the drug's effects, thus increasing the risk of hemorrhage (*Corrigan JJ Jr, Marcus FI. Coagulopathy associated with vitamin E ingestion. JAMA 230:1300-1, 1974*). However, doses of vitamin E up to 1200 IU daily appear to be safe (*Kim JM, White RH. Effect of vitamin E on the anticoagulant response to warfarin. Am J Cardiol 77:545-6, 1996*).

- and **Vitamin K**

Interferes with the regeneration of vitamin K_1 from its biologically inactive form (*Bell RG. Metabolism of vitamin K and prothrombin synthesis; anti-coagulants and the vitamin K-epoxide cycle. Fed Proc 37:2599-604, 1978*) which may cause fluctuation in prothrombin time (*Lim D, McKay M. Food-drug interactions. Drug Information Bulletin, UCLA Dept. of Pharmaceutical Services, 15(2), 1995*).

Zidovudine (AZT)

- and **Copper**

May reduce plasma copper levels (*Baum MK et al. Zidovudine-associated adverse reactions in a longitudinal study of asymptomatic HIV-1 infected homosexual males. J Acquir Immune Defic Syndr 4(12):1218-26, 1991*).

- and **Folic Acid**

May increase red cell folate levels (*Baum MK et al. Zidovudine-associated adverse reactions in a longitudinal study of asymptomatic HIV-1 infected homosexual males. J Acquir Immune Defic Syndr 4(12):1218-26, 1991*).

- and **Vitamin E**

Animal studies suggest that supplementation may increase the drug's therapeutic efficacy (*Gogu SR, Beckman BS, Rangan SRS, Agrawal KC. Increased therapeutic efficacy of zidovudine in combination with vitamin E. Biochem Biophys Res Commun 165(1):401-7, 1989*) while reducing bone marrow toxicity (*Gogu SR et al. Protection of zidovudine-induced toxicity against murine erythroid progenitor cells by vitamin E. Exp Hematol 19(7):649-52, 1991*).

- and **Zinc**

May reduce plasma zinc levels *(Baum MK et al. Zidovudine-associated adverse reactions in a longitudinal study of asymptomatic HIV-1 infected homosexual males. J Acquir Immune Defic Syndr 4(12):1218-26, 1991).*

Chapter Seven

SIGNS AND SYMPTOMS OF HEAVY METAL TOXICITY

Aluminum

Anorexia
Ataxia
Colic
Dementia
Dyspnea (inhalation)
Esophagitis
Gastroenteritis
Hepatic Dysfunction
Nephritis
Pain in Muscles
Psychosis
Weakness

Cadmium

Alopecia
Anemia (iron-deficiency)
Anorexia
Anosmia
Emphysema
Fatigue
Hepatic Dysfunction
Hypertension
Joint Soreness
Nephrocalcinosis
Osteoporosis
Pain in Back and Legs
Skin Dry and Scaly
Teeth Yellow

Lead

Adrenal Dysfunction
Anemia (iron-deficiency)
Anorexia
Anxiety
Concentration Impairment

Confusion
Constipation
Depression
Dizziness
Drowsiness
Fatigue
Headaches
Hypertension
Incoordination
Indigestion
Irritability
Kidney Dysfunction
Memory Impairment
Muscle Weakness and Wasting
Pain in Abdomen
Pain in Bones
Pain in Muscles
Reproductive Dysfunction
Restlessness
Teeth with Blue-Black Lines
   near Base
Tremors

Mercury

Anemia
Anorexia
Ataxia
Colitis
Depression
Dermatitis
Dizziness
Drowsiness
Emotional Instability
Erethism
Fatigue
Headaches
Hearing Impairment
Hypertension

Incoordination
Insomnia
Irritability
Kidney Dysfunction
Memory Impairment
Metallic Taste
Numbness
Paresthesias
Psychosis
Stomatitis
Tremors
Vision Impairment
Weakness

Chapter Eight

TOXIC METAL-NUTRIENT INTERACTIONS

ALUMINUM

MAY INTERFERE WITH NUTRITURE OF -

Calcium

Aluminum from aluminum-containing antacids induces calcium loss by increasing urinary excretion of calcium, thus resulting in a negative calcium balance *(Spencer H, Dramer L. Osteoporosis: calcium, fluoride, and aluminum interactions. J Am Coll Nutr 4:121-8, 1985).*

Copper

Aluminum may reduce copper absorption and affect its distribution in tissues and cells *(Witkowska J, Czerwinska D, Kiepurski A, Roszkowski W. [Harmful elements versus iron, zinc, and copper: their interactions in animals and humans. I. Mercury, tin, nickel, selenium, fluorine and aluminum.] Rocz Panstw Zakl Hig 42(1):15-23, 1991) (in Polish).*

Iron

Aluminum may reduce iron absorption and affect its distribution in tissues and cells *(Witkowska J, Czerwinska D, Kiepurski A, Roszkowski W. [Harmful elements versus iron, zinc, and copper: their interactions in animals and humans. I. Mercury, tin, nickel, selenium, fluorine and aluminum.] Rocz Panstw Zakl Hig 42(1):15-23, 1991) (in Polish).*

Phosphorus

Aluminum blocks the absorption and utilization of phosphate for ATP synthesis (which can cause intramitochondrial phosphate deficiency) *(Allen VG. Influence of aluminum on magnesium metabolism, in BM Altura, J Durlach, MS Seelig, Eds. Magnesium in Cellular Processes and Medicine. Basel, Karger, 1987:50-66).*

Vitamin D

Aluminum, by blocking renal synthesis of 1,25-dihydroxyvitamin D, interferes with vitamin D metabolism *(Moon J. The role of vitamin D in toxic metal absorption: a review. J Am Coll Nutr 13(6):559-69, 1994).*

Zinc

Aluminum may reduce zinc absorption and affect its distribution in tissues and cells (*Witkowska J, Czerwinska D, Kiepurski A, Roszkowski W. [Harmful elements versus iron, zinc, and copper: their interactions in animals and humans. I. Mercury, tin, nickel, selenium, fluorine and aluminum.] Rocz Panstw Zakl Hig 42(1):15-23, 1991) (in Polish).*

TOXICITY MAY BE INFLUENCED BY -

Boron

WARNING: Animal work suggests that aluminum is less toxic when dietary boron is low (*Nielsen FH, Shuler TR, Zimmerman TJ, et al. Dietary magnesium, manganese and boron affect the response of rats to high dietary aluminum. Magnesium 7(3):133-47, 1988).*

Citric Acid

WARNING: Enhances aluminum absorption; therefore should not be taken with aluminum-containing substances, especially when the patient has renal insufficiency (*Domingo JL et al. Effect of ascorbic acid on gastrointestinal aluminum absorption. Letter. Lancet 338:1467, 1991; Fairweather-Tait S, Hickson CK, McGaw B, Reid M. Orange juice enhances aluminum absorption from antacid preparation. Eur J Clin Nutr 48:71-3, 1994).*

Magnesium

Animal work suggests that deficient magnesium nutriture increases aluminum toxicity (*Nielsen FH, Shuler TR, Zimmerman TJ, et al. Dietary magnesium, manganese and boron affect the response of rats to high dietary aluminum. Magnesium 7(3):133-47, 1988).*

Magnesium prevents aluminum from blocking the absorption and utilization of phosphate for ATP synthesis (*Allen VG. Influence of aluminum on magnesium metabolism, in BM Altura, J Durlach, MS Seelig, Eds. Magnesium in Cellular Processes and Medicine. Basel, Karger, 1987:50-66).*

Malic Acid 12-2400 mg daily

One of the most potent aluminum chelators. Of several chelators tested, malic acid resulted in the highest survival ratio in aluminum-intoxicated mice (*Domingo JL, Gomez JM, Llobet JM, Corbella J. Comparative effects of several chelating agents on the toxicity, distribution and excretion of aluminum. Human Toxicol 7:259-62, 1988)* and was the most effective in decreasing brain aluminum levels (*Domingo JL, Gomez M, Llobet JM. Citric, malic and succinic acids as possible alternatives to deferoxamine in aluminum toxicity. J Clin Toxicol 26(1,2):67-79, 1988).*

Silicon

Reduces gastrointestinal absorption by forming a hydroxyaluminosilicate (*Birchall JD. The role of silicon in biology. Chem Brit 26(2):141-4, 1990; Edwardson JA, Moore PB, Ferrier IN, et al. Effect of silicon on gastrointestinal absorption of aluminum. Lancet 342:211-12, 1993*).

Serum silicon levels are directly related to serum aluminum levels; however, the question of whether silicon reduces the bioavailability of absorbed aluminum is unresolved (*Fahal IH, Yaqoob M, Williams PS. Does silicon protect against aluminum toxicity in dialysis patients? Letter. Lancet 343:122-3, 1994*).

Vitamin C

WARNING: Enhances aluminum absorption; therefore should not be taken with aluminum-containing substances, especially when the patient has renal insufficiency (*Domingo JL et al. Effect of ascorbic acid on gastrointestinal aluminum absorption. Letter. Lancet 338:1467, 1991*).

Vitamin D

WARNING: Supplementation increases aluminum absorption (*Moon J. The role of vitamin D in toxic metal absorption: a review. J Am Coll Nutr 13(6):559-69, 1994*).

Zinc

Animal work suggests that inadequate dietary zinc intake increases brain aluminum accumulation (*Wenk GI, Stemmer KI. Suboptimal dietary zinc intake increases aluminum accumulation into the rat brain. Brain Res 288:393-5, 1983*).

CADMIUM

MAY INTERFERE WITH NUTRITURE OF -

Copper

Animal work suggests that cadmium poisoning induces a secondary deficiency of copper (*Mills CF, Dalgarno AC. Nature (London) 239:171, 1972*).

Iron

Animal studies suggest that toxic levels of dietary cadmium interfere with iron absorption and produce an iron deficiency (*Fox MR, Jacobs RM, Jones AO, et al. Effects of vitamin C and iron and cadmium metabolism. Ann N Y Acad Sci 355:249-61, 1980*).

Vitamin D

Cadmium, by blocking renal synthesis of 1,25-dihydroxyvitamin D, interferes with vitamin D metabolism (*Moon J. The role of vitamin D in toxic metal absorption: a review. J Am Coll Nutr 13(6):559-69, 1994*).

Vitamin E

Animal work suggests that cadmium exposure reduces vitamin E levels in blood and tissues (*Shukla GS, Chandra SV. Cadmium toxicity and bioantioxidants: status of vitamin E and ascorbic acid of selected organs in rats. J Appl Toxicol 9:119-22, 1989*).

Zinc

Animal work suggests that dietary cadmium poisoning can induce signs of zinc deficiency (*Supplee WC. Poultry Sci 40:827, 1961*).

TOXICITY MAY BE INFLUENCED BY -

Calcium

Animal work suggests that a low calcium diet increases cadmium toxicity and tissue residues (*Larsson SE, Miscator M. Isr J Med Sci 7:495, 1971*).

Copper

Supplementation reduces cadmium absorption (*MR Spivey Fox, US FDA Division of Nutrition - interviewed by Tom Shealey in Prevention May, 1986:73-7*).

> *Note: Only supplement if copper nutriture is relatively poor.*

Animal work suggests that a dietary copper deficiency increases cadmium toxicity (*Fox MR, Tao SH, Stone CL, Fry BE Jr. Effects of zinc, iron and copper deficiencies on cadmium in the tissues of Japanese quail. Environ Health Perspect 54:57-65, 1984; Hill CH, Matrone G, Payne WL, Barber CW. J Nutr 80:227, 1963*).

Glutathione

Intracellular glutathione may provide a first line of defense against toxicity (*Nutr Rev 46(8):297-9, 1988*).

Iron

Maintenance of modest iron stores appears to be very important in minimizing cadmium absorption (*Fox MR, Jacobs RM, Jones AO, et al. Effects of vitamin C and iron and cadmium metabolism. Ann N Y Acad Sci 355:249-61, 1980*) as iron deficiency in both humans and animals increases cadmium absorption and toxicity (*Flanagan PR, McLellan JS, Haist J, et al.*

Increased dietary cadmium absorption in mice and human subjects with iron deficiency. Gastroenterology 74:841-6, 1974; Hill CH, Matrone G, Payne WL, Barber CW. J Nutr 80:227, 1963).

Iron supplements, particularly in the divalent form, decrease cadmium absorption *(Fox MR, Jacobs RM, Jones AO, et al. Effects of vitamin C and iron and cadmium metabolism. Ann N Y Acad Sci 355:249-61, 1980).*

Note: Only supplement if iron nutriture is relatively poor.

Magnesium

A competitive inhibitor of cadmium *(Guiet-Bara A, Bara M, Durlach J. Magnesium: a competitive inhibitor of lead and cadmium. Ultrastructural studies of the human amniotic epithelial cell. Magnes Res 3(1):31-6, 1990).*

Protein

In rats, a deficiency in dietary protein increases cadmium toxicity and tissue residues *(Gontzea I, Sutzesco P, Cocora D, Lungu D. Arch Sci Physiol 18:211, 1964; Suzuki S, Taguchi T, Yokohashi G. Ind Health 7:155, 1969).*

Selenium

Animal work suggests that concurrent selenium administration may reduce or prevent cadmium toxicity *(Wahba ZZ, Coogan TP, Rhodes SW, Waalkes MP. Protective effects of selenium on cadmium toxicity in rats: role of altered toxicokinetics and metallothionein. J Toxicol Environ Health 38:171-82, 1993).*

Vitamin B Complex

Animal work suggests that concurrent vitamin B complex supplementation may reduce cadmium toxicity by reducing absorption, possibly through forming readily excretable complexes *(Tandon SK, Flora SJ, Behari JR, Ashquin M. Vitamin B complex in treatment of cadmium intoxication. Ann Clin Lab Sci 14(6):487-92, 1984).*

- Vitamin B6

WARNING: Animal work suggests that high supplemental levels of vitamin B6 may aggravate cadmium-induced anemia *(Stowe HR, Goyer RA, Medley P, Cates M. Arch Environ Health 28:209, 1974).*

Vitamin C

Animal work suggests that intake of vitamin C is inversely correlated with cadmium toxicity, probably due to its positive effect on iron metabolism *(Fox MR, Jacobs RM, Jones AO, et al. Effects of vitamin C and iron on cadmium metabolism. Ann N Y Acad Sci 355:249-61, 1980; Hudecová A, Ginter E. the influence of ascorbic acid on lipid peroxidation in guinea pigs intoxicated with cadmium. Food Chem Toxicol 30:1011-3, 1992).* However, supplementation with 1 gm of ascorbic acid daily does not significantly affect hair and blood cadmium levels in normals *(Calabrese EJ, Stoddard A, Leonard DA, Dinardi SR. The effects of vitamin C supplementation on blood and hair levels of cadmium, lead, and mercury. Ann N Y Acad Sci 498:347-53, 1987)*.

Vitamin D

WARNING: Supplementation increases cadmium absorption *(Moon J. The role of vitamin D in toxic metal absorption: a review. J Am Coll Nutr 13(6):559-69, 1994)*.

Vitamin E

Animal work suggests that simultaneous administration of cadmium with vitamin E reduces cadmium-induced biochemical alterations and cadmium accumulation *(Tandon SK, Singh S, Dhawan M. Preventive effect of vitamin E in cadmium intoxication. Biomed Environ Sci 5:39-45, 1992)*.

Zinc

Animal work suggests that dietary zinc deficiency increases cadmium toxicity *(Fox MR, Tao SH, Stone CL, Fry BE Jr. Effects of zinc, iron and copper deficiencies on cadmium in the tissues of Japanese quail. Environ Health Perspect 54:57-65, 1984)*, while concurrent supplementation reduces cadmium absorption *(Jacobs RM, Jones AO, Fox MR, Lener J. Effects of dietary zinc, manganese, and copper on tissue accumulation of cadmium by Japanese quail. Proc Soc Exp Biol Med 172(1):34-8, 1983)*.

LEAD

MAY INTERFERE WITH NUTRITURE OF -

Calcium

Competes with calcium causing critical clinical effects at the cellular and molecular levels, particularly the effects of lead on neurodevelopment and neurofunction *(Goyer RA. Nutrition and metal toxicity. Am J Clin Nutr 61(suppl):646S,50S, 1995)*.

Iron

Competes with iron for absorption *(Goyer RA. Nutrition and metal toxicity. Am J Clin Nutr 61(suppl):646S,50S, 1995)*.

Developing animals exposed to low lead levels slowly accumulate lead in the brain with a concomitant reduction in brain iron *(Miller GD. Interactions between lead and essential elements: behavioral consequences. The Nutrition Report 9(2), 1991)*.

Vitamin D

Lead, by blocking renal synthesis of 1,25 dihydroxyvitamin D, interferes with vitamin D metabolism *(Chesney RW, Rosen JF, DeLuca HF. Disorders of calcium metabolism in children, in G Chiumello, M Sperling, Eds. Recent Progress in Pediatric Endocrinology. New York, Raven Press, 1983:5-24);* thus low serum 1,25 $(OH)_2D_3$ appears to be a sensitive index of lead toxicity *(Moon J. The role of vitamin D in toxic metal absorption: a review. J Am Coll Nutr 13(6):559-69, 1994).*

Zinc

Animal work suggests that lead increases zinc excretion *(Victery W, Thomas D, Shoeps P, Vander AJ Lead increases urinary zinc excretion in rats. Biol Trace Elem Res 4:211-19, 1982).*

Developing animals exposed to low lead levels slowly accumulate lead in the brain with a concomitant reduction in brain zinc *(Miller GD. Interactions between lead and essential elements: behavioral consequences. The Nutrition Report 9(2), 1991).*

TOXICITY MAY BE INFLUENCED BY -

Calcium

Adequate calcium intake reduces the danger of lead poisoning in humans, probably by decreasing lead absorption while increasing renal lead clearance *(Kostial K, Dekanic D, Telisman S, et al. Dietary calcium and blood lead levels in women. Biol Trace Elem Res 28:181-4, 1991; Kuehneman T, Angle C, Manton W, et al. Dietary calcium and environmental correlates of seasonal changes in children's blood lead. Abstract. J Am Coll Nutr 11(5):597-637, 1992; Mahaffey KR, Haseman JD, Goyer RA. Dose-response to lead ingestion in rats on low dietary calcium. J Lab Clin Med 83:92-100, 1973; Mahaffey KR, Treloar S, Banks TA, et al. Differences in dietary intake of calcium, phosphorous and iron of children having normal and elevated blood lead concentrations. J Nutr 106:53, 1976; Sorrell M, Rosen JF. Interactions of lead, calcium, vitamin D, and nutrition in lead-burdened children. Arch Environ Health 32(4):160-4, 1977).*

Animal work suggests that dietary calcium fed at higher than normal levels protects against lead poisoning and tissue deposition *(Bogden JD, Gertner SB, Shristakos S, et al. Dietary calcium modifies concentrations of lead and other metals and renal calbinden in rats. J Nutr 122:1351-60, 1992; Hsu FS, Krook L, Pond WD, Duncan JR. J Nutr 105:112, 1975).*

Copper

Animal work suggests that dietary deficiency increases lead toxicity and the retention of lead in the kidney and liver *(Petering HG, in WG Hockstra, JW Suttie, HE Ganther, W Mertz, Eds. Trace Element Metabolism in Animals. Baltimore, University Park Press, 1974:311).*

Folic acid

Animal work suggests that folic acid is one of the components of the vitamin B complex that reduces lead intoxication and enhances the efficacy of disodium calcium versenate $(Na_2CaEDTA)$ chelation *(Tandon SK, Flora SJ, Singh S. Chelation in metal intoxication. XXIV: Influence on various components of vitamin B complex on the therapeutic efficacy of disodium verseante in lead intoxication. Pharmacol Toxicol 60(1):62-5, 1987).*

Iron

Animal work suggests that a diet low in iron increases lead toxicity (*Levander OA. Lead toxicity and nutritional deficiencies. Environ Health Perspect 29:115-25, 1979; Mahaffey KR. Environ Health Perspect 7:107, 1974*), although results of attempts to demonstrate this relationship in humans have been inconsistent (*Mahaffey KR. Factors modifying susceptibility to lead toxicity, in KR Mahaffey, Ed. Dietary and Environmental Lead: Human Health Effects. New York, Elsevier Science Publications, 1985:373-420*).

Animal work suggests that concurrent iron supplementation reduces lead toxicity (*Hill CH. Interactions of vitamin C with lead and mercury. Ann N Y Acad Sci 355:262-6, 1980*). However, iron supplementation is unable to alter lead excretion following lead poisoning (*Angle CR, Stelmark KL, McIntire MS. Lead and iron deficiency, in DD Hemphill, Ed. Trace Substances in Environmental Health, Volume 9. Columbia, MO, U. of Missouri Press, 1976:377; Mahaffey KR, Rader JI. Metabolic interactions: lead, calcium, and iron. Ann N Y Acad Sci 355:285-97, 1980*).

Note: Only supplement if iron nutriture is relatively poor.

Magnesium

Magnesium is a competitive inhibitor of lead (*Guiet-Bara A, Bara M, Durlach J. Magnesium: a competitive inhibitor of lead and cadmium. Ultrastructural studies of the human amniotic epithelial cell. Magnes Res 3(1):31-6, 1990*).

Phosphorus

Animal work suggests that a diet low in phosphorus increases lead toxicity (*Levander OA. Lead toxicity and nutritional deficiencies. Environ Health Perspect 29:115-25, 1979*).

Protein

Animal work suggests that a deficiency in dietary protein increases lead toxicity and tissue residues (*Gontzea I, Sutzesco P, Cocora D, Lungu D. Arch Sci Physiol 18:211, 1964; Suzuki S, Taguchi T, Yokohashi G. Ind Health 7:155, 1969*). Excessive dietary protein also increases lead toxicity (*Levander OA. Lead toxicity and nutritional deficiencies. Environ Health Perspect 29:115-25, 1979*).

Thiamine

Animal work suggests that concurrent thiamine supplementation may reduce lead poisoning both alone (*Bratton GR, Zmudzki J, Kincaid N, Joyce J. Thiamine as treatment of lead poisoning in ruminants. Mod Vet Pract 62(6):441-6, 1981*) and in combination with the chelating agents calcium ethylenediaminetetraacetic acid (EDTA) (*Rooneratne R, Olkowski A. Lead toxicity chelation therapy: new findings. J Advancement Med 6(4):225-31, 1993*) or calcium disodium EDTA (*Flora SJ, Singh S, Tandon SK. Chelation in metal intoxication XVIII: Combined efficacy of thiamine and calcium disodium versenate on lead toxicity. Life Sci 38(1):67-71, 1986*).

Vitamin B$_6$

Animal work suggests that vitamin B$_6$ is one of the components of the vitamin B complex that reduces lead intoxication and enhances the efficacy of disodium calcium versenate (Na$_2$CaEDTA) chelation *(Tandon SK, Flora SJ, Singh S. Chelation in metal intoxication. XXIV: Influence on various components of vitamin B complex on the therapeutic efficacy of disodium versenate in lead intoxication. Pharmacol Toxicol 60(1):62-5, 1987).*

Vitamin C

Animal work suggests that concurrent vitamin C supplementation may reduce lead toxicity *(Dhawan M, Kachru DN, Tandon SK. Influence of thiamine and ascorbic acid supplementation on the antidotal efficacy of thiol chelators in experimental lead intoxication. Arch Toxicol 62(4):301-4, 1988).* However, supplementation with 1 gm ascorbic acid daily does not significantly affect hair and blood lead levels in normals *(Calabrese EJ, Stoddard A, Leonard DA, Dinardi SR. The effects of vitamin C supplementation on blood and hair levels of cadmium, lead, and mercury. Ann N Y Acad Sci 498:347-53, 1987).*

Animal work suggests that concurrent supplementation with ascorbic acid enhances the efficacy of the thiol metal chelators MFA and DMS in counteracting lead toxicity *(Dhawan M, Kachru DN, Tandon SK. Influence of thiamine and ascorbic acid supplementation on the antidotal efficacy of thiol chelators in experimental lead intoxication. Arch Toxicol 62(4):301-4, 1988).*

- and Thiamine

Animal work suggests that concurrent combined supplementation is more effective than either nutrient alone in reducing lead poisoning *(Flora SJ, Tandon SK. Preventive and therapeutic effects of thiamine, ascorbic acid and their combination in lead intoxication. Acta Pharmacol Toxicol (Copenh) 58(5):374-8, 1986).*

Vitamin D

WARNING: Supplementation increases lead retention in the body, probably due to stimulation of the synthesis of calcium-binding protein *(Levander OA. Nutritional factors in relation to heavy metal toxicants. Fed Proc 36(5):1683-7, 1977).*

Vitamin E

Animal work suggests that vitamin E deficiency increases lead toxicity *(Levander OA, Morris VC, Higgs DJ, Ferretti RJ. J Nutr 105:1481, 1975),* while concurrent vitamin E supplementation reduces the severity of lead intoxication *(Dhawan M, Flora SJ, Tandon SK. Preventive and therapeutic role of vitamin E in chronic plumbism. Biomed Environ Sci 2(4):335-40, 1989).*

Zinc

Deficiency is a risk factor for lead toxicity (*Goyer RA. Lead toxicity: current concerns. Environ Health Perspect 100:177-87, 1993*).

It is uncertain from animal work whether concurrent high dietary zinc levels decrease lead poisoning (*Willoughby RA, MacDonald E, McSherry BJ, Brown G. Can J Comp Med 36:348, 1972*) or increase it (*Hsu FS, Krook L, Pond WG, Duncan JR. J Nutr 105:112, 1975*). Bone lead deposition may be reduced (*Willoughby RA, MacDonald E, McSherry BJ, Brown G. Can J Comp Med 36:348, 1972*), while soft tissue deposition may be increased (*Hsu FS, Krook L, Pond WG, Duncan JR. J Nutr 105:112, 1975; Willoughby RA, MacDonald E, McSherry BJ, Brown G. Can J Comp Med 36:348, 1972*).

- and Thiamine

Animal work suggests that concurrent combined nutritional supplementation is more effective than either nutrient alone in reducing lead poisoning (*Flora SJ, Singh S, Tandon SK. Thiamine and zinc in prevention or therapy of lead intoxication. J Int Med Res 17(1):68-75, 1989*).

MERCURY

MAY INTERFERE WITH NUTRITURE OF -

Copper

Mercury may reduce copper absorption and affect its distribution in tissues and cells (*Witkowska J, Czerwinska D, Kiepurski A, Roszkowski W. [Harmful elements versus iron, zinc, and copper: their interactions in animals and humans. I. Mercury, tin, nickel, selenium, fluorine and aluminum.] Rocz Panstw Zakl Hig 42(1):15-23, 1991*) (*in Polish*).

Iron

Mercury may reduce iron absorption and affect its distribution in tissues and cells (*Witkowska J, Czerwinska D, Kiepurski A, Roszkowski W. [Harmful elements versus iron, zinc, and copper: their interactions in animals and humans. I. Mercury, tin, nickel, selenium, fluorine and aluminum.] Rocz Panstw Zakl Hig 42(1):15-23, 1991*) (*in Polish*).

Riboflavin

Animal work suggests that methylmercury intoxication may cause riboflavin deficiency in the brain (*Sood PP, Vijayalakshimi K. Vitamin status in mice tissues during methylmercury intoxication and detoxification. J Nutr Environ Med 5:133-41, 1995*).

Thiamine

Animal work suggests that <u>methylmercury</u> intoxication may cause tissue thiamine deficiencies (*Sood PP, Vijayalakshimi K. Vitamin status in mice tissues during methylmercury intoxication and detoxification. J Nutr Environ Med 5:133-41, 1995*).

Vitamin B$_6$

Animal work suggests that <u>methylmercury</u> intoxication may cause vitamin B$_6$ deficiency (*Sood PP, Vijayalakshimi K. Vitamin status in mice tissues during methylmercury intoxication and detoxification. J Nutr Environ Med 5:133-41, 1995*).

Vitamin E

Animal work suggests that <u>methylmercury</u> intoxication may cause tissue vitamin E deficiencies (*Sood PP, Vijayalakshimi K. Vitamin status in mice tissues during methylmercury intoxication and detoxification. J Nutr Environ Med 5:133-41, 1995*).

Zinc

Mercury may reduce zinc absorption and affect its distribution in tissues and cells (*Witkowska J, Czerwinska D, Kiepurski A, Roszkowski W. [Harmful elements versus iron, zinc, and copper: their interactions in animals and humans. I. Mercury, tin, nickel, selenium, fluorine and aluminum.] Rocz Panstw Zakl Hig 42(1):15-23, 1991) (in Polish*).

TOXICITY MAY BE INFLUENCED BY -

Alkylglycerols

Animal work suggests that supplementation may reduce tissue deposition of metallic mercury (*Bengt Fredin, Dept. of Physiological Chemistry, U. of Lund, Sweden. Effects of alkoxy-glycerols - Ecomer®- on the accumulation of mercury in rats after a single dose of metallic mercury. Unpublished manuscript, ?1988*).

Supplementation may increase mercury excretion.

Experimental Study: 2 males aged 58 and 35 yrs. with amalgam fillings in their teeth received 0.2 g natural mixed alkylglycerols (Ecomer® 2 caps twice daily) for 14 days. There was a rapid increase in fecal mercury excretion during the first 2-3 days after starting supplementation which then decreased, while urine mercury showed a slight gradual increase (*Bengt Fredin, Dept. of Physiological chemistry, U. of Lund, Sweden. Preliminary observations of rapid effects of Ecomer® on the excretion of Hg in man. (A pilot study) - Unpublished manuscript, 1988*).

Folic acid

WARNING: Animal work suggests that megadoses of folic acid fed concurrently with mercuric chloride (inorganic mercury) increases methylmercury in the liver (*Zorn NE, Smith JT. A relationship between vitamin B $_{12}$, folic acid, ascorbic acid, and mercury uptake and methylation. Life Sci 47(2):167-73, 1990*).

N-Acetylcysteine

In vitro, complexes mercury in the serum (*Lorber A, Baumgartner WA, Bovy RA, et al. Clinical application for heavy metal-complexing potential of N-acetylcysteine. J Clin Pharmacol 13(8):332-6, 1973*).

Animal work suggests that NAC chelates <u>elemental mercury</u>, reducing blood and tissue levels (*Livardjani F, Ledig M, Kopp P, et al. Lung and blood superoxide dismutase activity in mercury vapor exposed rats: effect of N-acetylcysteine treatment. Toxicology 66(3):289-95, 1991*).

A case report suggests that NAC may enhance renal elimination of <u>methylmercury</u> following acute ingestion (*Lund ME, Banner W Jr, Clarkson TW, Berlin M. Treatment of acute methylmercury ingestion by hemodialysis with N-acetylcysteine (Mucomyst) infusion and 2,3 dimercaptopropane sulfonate. J Toxicol Clin Toxicol 22(1):31-49, 1984*).

Pectin

Concurrent administration may reduce mercury poisoning (*Trakhetenberg IM, Talakin IuN, Leskova GE, et al. [Prophylactic use of pectin in occupational mercurialism.] Gig Tr Prof Zabol (7):33-6, 1980) (in Russian*).

Selenium

Nutritional levels protect against the toxicity of both <u>methyl mercury</u> (*Ganther HE, Goudie C, Sunde ML, et al. Science 175:1122, 1972; Ganther HE. Interactions of vitamin E and selenium with mercury and silver. Ann N Y Acad Sci 355:212-26, 1980*) and <u>inorganic mercury</u> (*Burk RF, Foster KA, Greenfield PM, Kiker KW. Proc Soc Exp Biol Med 145:782, 1974; Parizek J, Ostadolova I, Kalouskova J, et al, in W Mertz, WE Cornatzer, Eds. Newer Trace Elements in Nutrition. New York, Dekker, 1971:85*), perhaps due to its antioxidant effect (*Ganther HE. Interactions of vitamin E and selenium with mercury and silver. Ann N Y Acad Sci 355:212-26, 1980*).

See Also:

Whanger PD. Selenium in the treatment of heavy metal poisoning and chemical carcinogenesis. J Trace Elem Electrolytes in Health & Disease 6(4):227-32, 1992

Cuvin-Aralar LA, Furness RW. Mercury and selenium interactions: A review. Ecotoxicol Environ Safety 21:348-64, 1991

Vitamin B12

WARNING: Animal work suggests that megadoses of vitamin B12 fed concurrently with mercuric chloride (inorganic mercury) increases methylmercury in the liver *(Zorn NE, Smith JT. A relationship between vitamin B12, folic acid, ascorbic acid, and mercury uptake and methylation. Life Sci 47(2):167-73, 1990).*

Vitamin C

WARNING: Megadoses may increase tissue retention of mercury *(Blackstone S, Hurley RJ, Hughes RE. Food Cosmet Toxicol 12:511, 1974; Zorn NE, Smith JT. A relationship between vitamin B12, folic acid, ascorbic acid, and mercury uptake and methylation. Life Sci 47(2):167-73, 1990).*

Animal work suggests that concurrent administration of ascorbic acid reduces mercury toxicity *(Hill CH. Interactions of vitamin C with lead and mercury. Ann N Y Acad Sci 355:262-6, 1980).* However, oral supplementation of normal humans with 1 gm daily does not significantly affect hair and blood mercury levels *(Calabrese EJ, Stoddard A, Leonard DA, Dinardi SR. The effects of vitamin C supplementation on blood and hair levels of cadmium, lead, and mercury. Ann N Y Acad Sci 498:347-53, 1987).*

Intravenous administration does not significantly increase urinary excretion of mercury in subjects with low mercury levels from dental amalgam, food, or other sources *(Dirks MJ, Davis DR, Cheraskin E, Jackson JA. Mercury excretion and intravenous ascorbic acid. Arch Environ Health 49(1):49-52, 1994).*

Vitamin E

Animal work suggests that higher than normal dietary levels of vitamin E can decrease the toxicity of methyl mercury *(Welsh SO. The protective effect of vitamin E and N, N'-dephenylenediamine (DPPD) against methylmercury toxicity in the rat. J Nutr 109:1673-81, 1979; Welsh SO, Soares JH Jr. The protective effect of vitamin E and selenium against methyl mercury toxicity in the Japanese quail. Nutr Rep Int 13:43-51, 1976),* perhaps due to its antioxidant effect *(Ganther HE. Interactions of vitamin E and selenium with mercury and silver. Ann N Y Acad Sci 355:212-26, 1980).*

Animal work suggests that inorganic mercury (mercuric chloride) depletes tissues of superoxide dismutase, glutathione peroxidase and catalase, an action that can be prevented by vitamin E supplementation *(Addya S et al. Effects of mercuric chloride on several scavenging enzymes in rat kidney and influence of vitamin E supplementation. Acta Vitaminol Enzymol 6:103-7, 1984).*

Chapter Nine

LABORATORY METHODS FOR NUTRITIONAL EVALUATION

Note: Tests are presented in the rough order of preference, with tests that appear superior listed first.

GENERAL (Protein Energy Malnutrition)

Laboratory indicators *(Wright RA. Commentary: Nutritional assessment. JAMA 244(6), 1980)*:
1. decreased serum albumin concentration in the absence of liver disease (< 3.4 g/dL).
2. decreased serum transferrin (seen in starvation earlier than decreased serum albumin).
3. decreased total lymphocyte count (< 1500/mm^3).
4. decreased 24-hour urine creatinine (roughly proportional to skeletal muscle mass).

Aluminum

Hair analysis, when properly performed, is a reliable measure of tissue levels *(Yokel RA. Clin Chem 28(4):662-5, 1982; Jenkins DW. Toxic Metals in Mammalian Hair and Nails. EPA Report 600/4-79-049 August, 1979 - available through the U.S. Natl Technical Information Service)*. As yet, it cannot be concluded whether aluminum concentrations in hair give a better representation of the body burden than serum aluminum levels do *(De Groot HJ et al. Determination by flameless atomic absorption of aluminum in serum and hair by toxicological monitoring of patients on chronic intermittent haemodialysis. Pharm Weekbl [Sci] 6(1):11-15, 1984)*.

Arsenic

Hair analysis, when properly performed, is a reliable measure of tissue levels *(Jenkins DW. Toxic Metals in Mammalian Hair and Nails. EPA Report 600/4-79-049 August, 1979 - available through the US Natl. Technical Information Service)*.

Urine arsenic levels, like hair levels, increase as intake increases. Blood arsenic levels, however, do not increase until chronic toxicity is reached and give variable results for lower levels of exposure *(Valentine JL et al. Arsenic levels in human blood, urine, and hair in response to exposure via drinking water. Environ Res 20:24-32, 1979)*.

Beta-carotene

Adipose tissue levels appear to be relatively good markers of dietary intake, while plasma concentrations are not reflective of dietary consumption *(Kardinaal A, Van't Veer P, Brants H, et al. Relations between antioxidant vitamins in adipose-tissue, plasma, and diet. Am J Epidemiol 141(5):440-50, 1995)*.

Biotin

There are no sensitive chemical methods for biotin assay, but the flagellate Ochromonas danica, which has a specific and ultrasensitive biotin requirement, has provided a suitable <u>microbiological assay</u> for measuring biotin in blood, serum, urine, brain and liver (*Baker H. Assessment of biotin status: Clinical implications. <u>Ann N Y Acad Sci</u> 447:129-32, 1985*).

The two principal criteria of biotin status are <u>blood and urine levels</u>. Blood levels can show extremely wide variation between individuals, so the significance of low plasma levels is uncertain, especially since biotin deficiency seems rare. In children, however, blood and urine levels are more helpful. For example, levels are lower than normal in infants with seborrheic dermatitis and Leiner's Disease who respond to biotin injections (*Whitehead CC. The assessment of biotin status in man and animals. <u>Proc Nutr Sci</u> 40:165-72, 1981*).

Cadmium

<u>Hair analysis</u>, when properly performed, is a reliable measure of tissue levels (*Jenkins DW. <u>Toxic Metals in Mammalian Hair and Nails</u>. EPA Report 600/4-79-049 August, 1979 - available through the US Natl. Technical Information Service*) and is superior to blood in reflecting long term cadmium exposure (*Thatcher RW et al. Effects of low levels of cadmium and lead on cognitive functioning in children. <u>Arch Environ Health</u> 37:159-65, 1982*).

<u>Blood levels</u> are a poor measure of cadmium toxicity as the metal remains in the blood for only a very brief period of time and thus the levels are always extremely low (*Petering HG et al. Trace element content of hair: Cadmium and lead of human hair. <u>Arch Environ Health</u> 27:327-30, 1973*).

Calcium

<u>Ionized calcium</u>, a measure of unbound serum calcium, is perhaps the most useful measure of calcium balance at present when it is low, but values can be normal in the presence of a negative calcium balance (*Albanese A. <u>Bone Loss: Causes, Detection and Therapy</u>. New York, Alan R. Liss, Inc., 1977*). <u>Total serum calcium</u> is subjected to such close homeostatic regulation that it fails to reflect body calcium status.

See Also:

> *Norris MK. Evaluating serum calcium levels. <u>Nursing</u> 23(2):69, 1993*

<u>Hair analysis</u> is of some value, but its results are limited by the fact that a negative calcium balance may be accompanied by elevated hair levels, and by the lack of established norms for grey hair which is naturally lower in calcium (*Cranton EM. Update on hair element analysis in clinical medicine. <u>J Holistic Med.</u> 7(2):120-34, 1985*).

> *Note: High hair calcium in the presence of a negative calcium balance may be a form of nutritionally-induced secondary hyperparathyroidism related to a low calcium, high phosphorus diet (Bland J. dietary calcium, phosphorus and their relationships to bone formation and parathyroid activity. <u>J John Bastyr College of Naturopathic Medicine</u> 1:3-7, 1979; Margen S, Chu J-Y, Kaufmann NA, Calloway DH. Studies in calcium metabolism: I. The calciuretic effect of dietary protein. <u>Am J Clin Nutr</u> 27:584-9, 1974; Wachman A, Bernstein DS. Diet and osteoporosis. <u>Lancet</u> i:958-9, 1968).*

See Also:

> Gordus A. *Factors affecting the trace metal content of human hair. J Radioanal Chem 15:229-43, 1973*

Carnitine

Plasma and muscle carnitine are closely correlated, while RBC levels may vary independently.

> **Observational Study:** In a study of 25 pts. with normal carnitine metabolism, there was a close correlation between plasma and muscle carnitine, but RBC carnitine seemed to represent a carnitine compartment of its own and is probably less related to mitochondrial fatty acid metabolism than to cell membrane stabilization or buffer function for Na-K-ATPase *(Reichmann H, van Lindeneiner N. Carnitine analysis in normal human red blood cells, plasma, and muscle tissue. Eur Neurol 34(1):40-3, 1994).*

> **Observational Study:** Healthy adult blood was sampled for carnitine content. It appeared that carnitine pools may exist in at least 2 different compartments: plasma and RBC. One may be high and the other low, with different effects seen for each deficiency *(Borum PR et al. Am J Clin Nutr 46:437, 1987).*

Chromium

The most dependable criterion for the diagnosis of chromium deficiency may be the correction of impaired glucose tolerance in response to chromium supplementation, but it requires strict control of dietary intake over an extended period *(Glinsmann WH et al. Plasma chromium after glucose administration. Science 152:1243-5, 1966).*

Although evaluation is hindered by the extremely low levels involved, urinary chromium is a reasonable measure of chromium absorption as the majority of absorbed chromium is excreted in the urine *(Anderson RA, Kozlovsky AS. Chromium intake, absorption and excretion of subjects consuming self-selected diets. Am J Clin Nutr 41:1177-83, 1985).* Repeating urinary chromium after an oral glucose load, according to some authors, may be useful - as the lack of an increase suggests exhaustion of biologically important chromium stores *(Mertz W. Effects and metabolism of glucose tolerance factor, in Present Knowledge in Nutrition. Fourth Edition. Washington, D.C., The Nutrition Foundation, Inc., 1976).* However, urinary chromium excretion may be unaffected by chromium supplementation *(Anderson RA et al. Urinary chromium excretion of human subjects: Effects of chromium supplementation and glucose loading. Am J Clin Nutr 36(6):1184-93, 1982).*

Hair analysis cannot distinguish between contamination by the hexavalent, toxic chromium and the trivalent, nutritional chromium *(Passwater, RA, Cranton EM. Trace Elements, Hair Analysis and Nutrition. New Canaan, CT, Keats Publishing, Inc., 1983:195).* Moreover, because of the low levels involved, hair chromium content has been considered to be too insensitive to identify any but the most severe deficiencies *(Richman S. Chromium, an overview. Anabolism 1-2:5,12, 1984; Hambridge KM. Chromium nutrition in man. Am J Clin Nutr 27:505-14, 1974).* At least one study, however, suggests that hair chromium levels may be a useful index of chromium status:

> **Experimental Placebo-controlled Study:** Initial hair chromium levels were significantly lower in diabetics than in controls and, after chromium supplementation, mean hair

chromium increased by 127 ± 78 ppb in both diabetic and non-diabetic gps., but only by 17 ± 90 ppb in the placebo group (*Hunt AE et al. Effect of chromium supplementation on hair chromium concentration and diabetic status. Nutr Res 5:131-40, 1985*).

In response to a standard glucose load, serum chromium levels may drop one hour later in subjects with presumably inadequate chromium storage. An improvement in the ratio of the serum chromium level one hour after glucose loading to the baseline level (the 'relative chromium response') after chromium supplementation may thus be a measure of improved chromium status (*Lui VJK, Morris S. Relative chromium response as an indicator of chromium status. Am J Clin Nutr 31:972-6, 1978*).

A reliable range for serum chromium is lacking (*Sauberlich HE et al. Laboratory Tests For The Assessment Of Nutritional Status. Florida, CRC Press, 1984*). Chromium supplementation may not affect serum levels (*Polansky MM et al. Serum chromium as an indicator of chromium status of humans. Fed Proc 43, 1984*), and serum chromium is not in equilibrium with tissue stores (*Underwood EJ. Trace Elements in Human and Animal Nutrition. New York, Academic Press, 1977*). Likewise, whole blood chromium has not been shown to reflect tissue stores (*Mertz W. Physiol Rev 49:163-239, 1969*).

Copper

Erythrocyte glutathione peroxidase activity is a sensitive indicator of copper status as are platelet copper, functional activities of platelet cytochrome c oxidase, and clotting factor VIII (*Milne DB, Nielsen FH. Effects of a diet low in copper on copper-status indicators in postmenopausal women. Am J Clin Nutr 63:358-64, 1996*).

Erythrocyte superoxide dismutase activity is an excellent index of copper status (*Hill G, Edes TE. Diabetes and carbohydrates: The copper connection. JAMA 257(19):2593, 1987*). However, its response time to changes in dietary copper intake appears to lag behind changes in serum copper and ceruloplasmin (*Medeiros DM. Copper and its possible role in cardiomyopathies. The Nutrition Report 11(12), December, 1993; Milne DB, Nielsen FH. Effects of a diet low in copper on copper-status indicators in postmenopausal women. Am J Clin Nutr 63:358-64, 1996*).

Confirmation of an elevated body copper burden can be provided by the D-penicillamine challenge test. D-penicillamine 250 mg is given orally every 6 hours away from meals and the urine test is performed on the third day of treatment. Copper urinary excretion usually increases 10-20 fold. In normals, it will be in the range of 500 µg/24h while, in pts. with Wilson's Disease, it will be at least 1,000 µg/24h or even above 2,000 µg/24h (*Walshe JM. The discovery of the therapeutic use of D-penicillamine. J Rheumatol (Suppl 7) 8:3-8, 1981*).

Total erythrocyte copper concentration is widely available. Sixty percent of erythrocyte copper is in superoxide dismutase, while the remainder is in both a readily diffusable pool and a non-dialyzed protein-bound pool (*Halloran SP, in DF Williams, Ed. Copper In Systemic Aspects Of Biocompatability, Vol. 1. Boca Raton FL, CDC Press, 1981:211*).

Hair copper correlates well with liver copper levels, although errors from external contamination of hair (copper-containing fungicides in swimming pools, contaminated water supplies, hair treatments) may occur, and levels are unreliable in the presence of copper-loading liver diseases (*Cranton EM. Update on hair element analysis in clinical medicine. J Holistic Med 7(2):120-34, 1985; Jacob RA. Hair as a biopsy material v. hair metal as an index of hepatic metal in rats: Copper and zinc. Am J Clin Nutr 31:477-80, 1978*). In addition, hair copper may be normal despite gross copper deficiency (*Bradfield RB et al. Preliminary communication: hair copper in copper deficiency. Lancet ii:343-4, 1980*), and hair copper may be elevated in malnutrition (*Weber CW,*

Nelson GW, Vasquez de Vaguera M, Pearson PB. Trace elements in the hair of healthy and malnourished children. J Trop Pediatr 36(5):230-4, 1990).

Serum copper level increases in times of stress, such as when there is inflammation, and thus is unreliable as a measure of copper nutriture (*Medeiros DM. Copper and its possible role in cardiomyopathies. The Nutrition Report 11(12), December, 1993*). Also, 90-95% of serum copper is tightly bound to ceruloplasmin which may make it an insensitive test for marginal deficiencies (*Fisher G. Function and homeostasis of Cu and Zn in mammals. Sci Total Environ 4:373, 1975*). Plasma copper is also relatively insensitive (*Milne DB, Nielsen FH. Effects of a diet low in copper on copper-status indicators in postmenopausal women. Am J Clin Nutr 63:358-64, 1996*).

Whole blood copper level is a combination of approximately equal quantities of copper in the cells and plasma (*Kiem J et al. Sampling and sample preparation of platelets for trace element analysis in nuclear activation techniques in the life sciences, 1978. IAEA, Vienna, 1979:143*); thus, when whole blood copper is depressed, it suggests a deficiency in cells, plasma or both. Normal or elevated whole blood copper may be reflecting an elevation in one blood fraction while another fraction may be normal or even depressed.

Ceruloplasmin, like serum copper, is an acute-phase reactant protein, and thus its levels may vary without regard to copper nutriture (*Hill G, Edes TE. Diabetes and carbohydrates: The copper connection. JAMA 257(19):2593, 1987*).

Folic Acid

"The assessment of . . . folate deficiency should be based on haematological findings of macrocytic anaemia with a right shift of neutrophils, or in the presence of specific neurological symptoms, with or without anaemia" (*Balfour IC, Lane DW. B12/folate assays and macrocytic anaemia. Letter. Lancet 346:446-7, 1995*).

> *Note: "In the evaluation of possible vitamin B9 deficiency, concomitant measurement of plasma B12 is recommended. A low erythrocyte folate level may occur in primary vitamin B12 deficiency, because vitamin B12 is necessary to keep methylfolate in red cells. When serum levels of both vitamins B9 and B12 are low, deficiency of either vitamin may be primary. This is due to the fact that megaloblastic intestinal cells may not absorb properly and, as a result, a secondary deficiency of the other vitamin occurs"* (*Skelton WP III, Skelton NK. Deficiency of vitamins A, B, and C. Something to watch for. Postgrad Med 87(4):293-310, 1990*).

While serum folate tends to reflect *recent* (the past few weeks') dietary intake, red blood cell folate concentration is much less sensitive to short-term variations in folate balance. It is thus is more reliable for indicating risk of development of folate deficiency and can be used as an index of folate depletion (*Anderson SA, Talbot JM. A Review Of Folate Intake, Methodology And Status. Bethesda, MD, Federation of American Societies for Experimental Biology, 1981; Herbert V. Making sense of laboratory test of folate status: folate requirements to sustain normality. Am J Hematol 26:199-207, 1987*).

> **Observational Study:** 50 cases of masked vitamin B12 and folate deficiency detected in an inner-city-area geriatric unit during the course of routine clinical investigation are described. The majority had none of the classical signs of vitamin B12 or folate deficiency, and all had a mean corpuscular volume (MCV) of <100 fl. There was a

significant negative correlation between the MCV and erythrocyte folate *(Craig GM, Elliot C, Hughes KR. Masked vitamin B$_{12}$ and folate deficiency in the elderly. Br J Nutr 54(3):613-19, 1985).*

However, folate depletion in erythrocytes occurs only in the later stages of folic acid deficiency and is usually accompanied by megaloblastic anemia; thus patients with both acquired and inherited folate deficiency may remain moderately deficient for months or years, taking in just enough folate to prevent low red cell folate concentrations and frank anemia *(Botez MI et al. Neurologic disorders responsive to folic acid therapy. Can Med Assoc J 115:217-22, 1976; Herbert V. Experimental nutritional folate deficiency in man. Trans Assoc Am Physicians 75:307, 1962).* Therefore, both RBC and serum folate studies should be done to evaluate for folate deficiency.

> *Note: Microbiological assays remain the standard procedure for measuring total folic acid activity in serum, blood, tissues, and foods. Although a number of commercial radioassay kits are available for measuring folic acid levels in serum and erythrocytes, some uncertainties exist about the validity of the folate values obtained (Sauberlich HE. Newer laboratory methods for assessing nutriture of selected B-complex vitamins. Annu Rev Nutr 4:377-407, 1984).*

Serum folate is highly correlated with cerebrospinal fluid (CSF) folate and better correlated with CSF folate than is erythrocyte folate [as erythrocyte folate is an indicator of folate status in bone marrow erythroblasts about 2 months earlier]. However, it is not known in man whether a low CSF folate is necessarily accompanied by a fall in brain folate level, but experimental studies have suggested that the latter falls last, when stores elsewhere are severely depleted *(Reynolds EH. Interrelationships between the neurology of folate and vitamin B$_{12}$ deficiency, in MI Botez, EH Reynolds, Eds. Folic Acid in Neurology, Psychiatry, and Internal Medicine. New York, Raven Press, 1979).*

In folate deficiency, the urine formiminoglutamic acid (FIGLU) level rises. High FIGLU excretion also occurs, however, in vitamin B$_{12}$ deficiency and in liver disease; thus it is not specific for folate deficiency *(Herbert V. Experimental nutritional folate deficiency in man. Trans Assoc Am Phys 75:307-20, 1962).*

The determination of hypersegmentation of neutrophils is a useful measure of folate deficiency, although it is unreliable during pregnancy and fails to distinguish folate and vitamin B$_{12}$ deficiencies *(Sauberlich HE. Newer laboratory methods for assessing nutriture of selected B-complex vitamins. Annu Rev Nutr 4:377-407, 1984):*

$$\text{Hypersegmentation Index} = \frac{\text{neutrophils with 5 or more 'lobes'}}{\text{neutrophils with 4 'lobes'}} \times 100$$

Normal (serum folate 3.5-16 mg/ml):

mean Hypersegmentation Index: 10.3% (range 2-30%)

Abnormal:

mean Hypersegmentation Index: 62.4% (range 31.5-116%)

(Bills T, Spatz L. Neutrophilic hypersegmentation as an indication of incipient folic acid deficiency. Am J Clin Pathol 68(2):263, 1977).

Note: Supplementation of 5 mg folate daily will usually bring the index to 0%, but higher amounts are sometimes necessary (rule out vitamin B_{12} deficiency and uremia) (Wright J. *The neutrophilic hypersegmentation index ('NHI'): an inexpensive, underutilized test of folate nutrition. Int Clin Nutr Rev 10(4):435-7, 1990*).

Mean corpuscular volume, a measure of erythrocyte size, may be normal in folate deficiency.

Observational Study: 50 cases of masked vitamin B_{12} and folate deficiency detected in an inner-city-area geriatric unit during the course of routine clinical investigation are described. The majority had none of the classical signs of vitamin B_{12} or folate deficiency, and all had a mean corpuscular volume (MCV) of <100 fl (Craig GM, Elliot C, Hughes KR. *Masked vitamin B_{12} and folate deficiency in the elderly. Br J Nutr 54(3):613-19, 1985*).

Hydrochloric Acid Deficiency

In addition to direct measurements of stomach acid, "somewhat increased basal serum gastrin can be found in conditions associated with achlorhydria, such as atrophic gastritis and pernicious anemia (if the antrum is not severely affected)" (Ravel R. *Clinical Laboratory Medicine. Third Edition. Chicago, Year Book Medical Publishers, 1978:399*).

Iodine

Urinary iodine concentration in spontaneous urine samples is the most widely used biochemical indicator for the assessment and monitoring of iodine status. Multi-parameter urine test strips can give falsely raised readings due to interactions with other patches and should thus be avoided (Neubert A, Remer T. *Measurement of urinary iodine concentration. Letter. Lancet 347:1414-15, 1996*).

Iron

Note: In the hospitalized elderly, 75% of anemias are caused by either iron deficiency anemia or anemia of chronic disease (Paine CJ, Polk A, Eichner ER. Analysis of anemia in medical inpatients. Am J Med Sci 268:37-44, 1974). The combination of serum ferritin, plasma transferrin receptors, and erythrocyte sedimentation rate will identify functional iron deficiency in the presence of chronic inflammation in over 80% of cases (Ahluwalia N, Lammi-Keefe CJ, Bendel RB, et al. Iron deficiency and anemia of chronic disease in elderly women: a discriminant-analysis approach for differentiation. Am J Clin Nutr 61:590-6, 1995).

Bone marrow aspiration is the procedure of choice, although it is too invasive for routine use (Finch CA. *Editorial: Evaluation of iron status. JAMA 251(15):2004, 1984*).

Response to iron supplementation (a significant rise in circulating hemoglobin) is considered the ultimate diagnostic test for iron deficiency (Fairbanks VF. *Laboratory testing for iron status. Hosp Pract 26(suppl 3):17-24, 1991; Kim I, Pollitt E, Leibel RL, et al. Application of receiver-operator analysis to diagnostic tests of iron deficiency in man. Pediatr Res 18:916-20, 1984*).

Serum ferritin, an iron storage protein, is an indicator of total body iron storage (Finch CA. *Editorial: Evaluation of iron status. JAMA 251(15):2004, 1984; Frank P, Wang S. Serum iron and total iron binding capacity compared with serum ferritin in assessment of iron deficiency. Clin Chem 27(2):276-9, 1981; Cook JD et al. Serum ferritin as a measure of iron stores in normal subjects. Am J Clin Nutr 27:681-7, 1974).* However, iron in peripheral tissues may be normal even though the ferritin concentration indicates that iron stores are depleted *(Labbe RF. Iron status: from deficiency to toxicity. Clin Chem News, September, 1993, p. 24)* and ferritin may occasionally be normal in confirmed cases of hemochromatosis *(Edwards C, Kushner J. Screening for hemochromatosis. N Engl J Med 328(22):1616-20, 1993).*

> *Note: In children, transferrin saturation, hemoglobin and a peripheral blood smear must be done in conjunction with serum ferritin, as ferritin may be normal despite iron deficiency (Madanat F et al. Serum ferritin in evaluation of iron status in children. Acta Haematol 71:111, 1984).*

The serum transferrin receptor concentration is a recently developed test that may indicate mild tissue iron deficiency. The receptor concentration increases only in response to iron deficiency and reflects the rate of erythropoiesis. This indicator appears to provide a good indicator of tissue iron stones. Combined with serum ferritin levels, which reflect body iron stores *(see above)*, may give a more complete picture of iron status than previously possible. Much interlaboratory standardization is needed before this assay becomes widely available *(Baynes RD, Skikne BS, Cook JD. Circulating transferrin receptors and assessment of iron status. J Nutr Biochem 5:322-30, 1994; Labbe RF. Iron status: from deficiency to toxicity. Clin Chem News, September, 1993, p. 24).*

An iron tolerance test, while not widely used, may be useful in determining mild iron deficiency.

> **Observational Study:** Men with normal iron stores showed little change in plasma iron after ingesting 5, 10 or 20 mg of ferrous sulfate or ferrous fumarate, while plasma iron levels rose significantly when men with a mild iron deficiency took similar doses of iron *(Crosby WH, O'Neill-Cutting MA. A small dose iron tolerance test as an indicator of mild iron deficiency. JAMA 251(15):1986-7, 1984).*

The zinc protoporphyrin/heme ratio is a recently developed test that measures the rate of iron delivery to developing erythrocytes relative to the iron required for hemoglobin formation. If insufficient iron is available, zinc will be utilized to form zinc protoporphyrin which will then bind to a heme site on globin and circulate in mature erythrocytes *(Labbe RF. Iron status: from deficiency to toxicity. Clin Chem News, September, 1993, p. 24).*

The automated blood cell count, when it includes the red cell distribution width (RDW), is an inexpensive yet adequate screening test for iron deficiency, but only in healthy patients *(Bessman JD, McClure S. Detection of iron deficiency anemia. Letter. JAMA 266(12):1649, 1991).*

> *Note: While serum ferritin reflects labile iron stores at a particular instant, an increased RDW reflects iron deficiency long-standing enough to affect erythropoiesis and is an earlier marker of such iron deficiency than a low hemoglobin level or (usually) a low mean corpuscular volume (Bessman JD, McClure S. Red cell distribution width in alcohol abuse and iron deficiency anemia. JAMA 267(8):1070-1, 1992).*

Transferrin saturation is based on the ratio between serum iron and total iron binding capacity. As a measure of the level of mobilized, circulating iron, a low value (<16%) is diagnostic of iron-deficient erythropoiesis. However, it is not always the best indicator of low iron status, especially in children, and may only become abnormal after iron stores have been completely exhausted *(Finch CA. Editorial: Evaluation of iron status. JAMA 251(15):2004, 1984; Labbe RF. Iron status: from deficiency to toxicity. Clin Chem News, September, 1993, p. 24).* It is an excellent indicator of hemochromatosis *(Edwards C, Kushner J. Screening for hemochromatosis. N Engl J Med 328(22):1616-20, 1993),* although it can occasionally be normal in confirmed cases *(Herbert V. Everyone should be tested for iron disorders. J Am Diet Assoc 92(12):1502-9, 1992).*

<u>Serum iron</u> is a poor measure of iron nurture as iron may be deficient despite the lack of anemia and normal serum iron levels. Like transferrin saturation, it may only become abnormal after iron stores have been completely exhausted *(Finch CA. Editorial: Evaluation of iron status. JAMA 251(15):2004, 1984; Frank P, Wang S. Serum iron and total iron binding capacity compared with serum ferritin in assessment of iron deficiency. Clin Chem 27(2):276-9, 1981; Cook JD et al. Serum ferritin as a measure of iron stores in normal subjects. Am J Clin Nutr 27:681-7, 1974).*

<u>Hemoglobin</u> concentration, while simple to perform, is a poor method of identifying iron deficiency and will lead to an underestimation of its prevalence. It reflects only a late stage in the development of iron deficiency, and the degree of iron deficiency anemia does not correlate with the severity of neuropsychological symptoms *(Tershakovec AM, Weller SC. Iron status of inner-city elementary school children: lack of correlation between anemia and iron deficiency. Am J Clin Nutr 54:1071-6, 1991; Tu JB, Shafey H, VenDeweetering C. Iron deficiency in two adolescents with conduct, dysthymic and movement disorders. Can J Psychiatry 39:371-7, 1994).*

> **Observational Study:** 39% of 111 healthy women aged 18-40 were iron-depleted (serum ferritin <20 μg/L), while only 3.6% were anemic as reflected in low hemoglobin values *(Newhouse I, Clement D, Lai C. Effects of iron supplementation and discontinuation on serum copper, zinc, calcium, and magnesium levels in women. Med Sci Sports 25:562-71, 1993).*

<u>Hair iron</u> concentration may be elevated in malnutrition due to disturbed iron metabolism *(Weber CW, Nelson GW, Vasquez de Vaguera M, Pearson PB. Trace elements in the hair of healthy and malnourished children. J Trop Pediatr 36(5):230-4, 1990).*

Lead

<u>Hair analysis,</u> when properly performed, is a reliable measure of tissue levels and the method of choice for diagnosing lead poisoning, although confirmatory studies are necessary *(Foo SC et al. Metals in hair as biological indices for exposure. Int Arch Occup Environ Health 65:S83-86, 1993; Rabinowitz M et al. Delayed appearance of tracer lead in facial hair. Arch Environ Health July/Aug., 1976:220-3).*

<u>Zinc protoporphyrin content</u> is a second choice for diagnosing lead poisoning, while <u>blood lead</u> levels are inadequate as blood rapidly deposits lead into the skeletal tissues and hair *(Passwater, RA, Cranton EM. Trace Elements, Hair Analysis and Nutrition. New Canaan, CT, Keats Publishing, Inc., 1983:195).*

Magnesium

<u>Ionized magnesium</u> can be determined by utilizing nonmagnetic resonance with a new ion-selective electrode specific for magnesium. This electrode, which provides readings in 60-90 seconds, makes it possible to resolve the problem of laboratory diagnosis of magnesium deficiency *(Mimouni FB. The ion-selective magnesium electrode: a new tool for clinicians and investigators. Editorial. J Am Coll Nutr 15(1):4-5, 1996; Seelig MS et al. Low magnesium: a common denominator in pathologic processes in diabetes mellitus, cardiovascular disease and eclampsia. Abstract. J Am Coll Nutr 11(5):597-637, 1992).*

Observational Study: 45 normotensive type II diabetics, 45 hypertensive diabetics and 15 healthy controls were compared. Compared to controls, both diabetic gps. had reduced plasma, erythrocyte and platelet magnesium concentrations, with similar findings in the hypertensive and normotensive diabetics. However, intraplatelet magnesium ion concentrations were significantly lower in the hypertensive diabetics (*Corica F et al. Magnesium levels in plasma, erythrocyte, and platelets in hypertensive and normotensive patients with type II diabetes mellitus. Biol Trace Elem Res 51:130-2, 1996*).

A <u>magnesium challenge test</u> is often the best available method of ascertaining body stores (*Fourth Internat. Sympos. on Magnesium. J Am Coll Nutr 4:303, 1985*) as <u>serum and red cell magnesium levels</u> remain normal unless magnesium depletion is severe (*Rea WJ et al. Magnesium deficiency in patients with chemical sensitivity. Clin Ecology 4(1):17-20, 1986*). However, this method is limited to disease states in which the presumed magnesium deficiency is not due to urinary losses (*Caddell JL et al. The magnesium load test. III. Correlation of clinical and laboratory data in infants from one to six months of age. Clin Pediatr 14:478-88, 1975*).

Protocol: While on a stable intake of magnesium, a baseline urine is obtained and magnesium chloride or magnesium sulfate 0.2 meq/kg IV is given over a 4 hour period. A second urine is begun at challenge and continued over a 24 hour period. Deficiency is defined as <80% excretion of the amt. of challenged magnesium (*Jones JE et al. Magnesium requirements in adults. Med J Clin Nutr 20:632-5, 1967*).

See Also:

> *Gullestad L, Dolva LO, Waage A, et al. Magnesium deficiency diagnosed by an intravenous loading test. Scand J Clin Lab Invest 52(4):245-53, 1992*

> *Ryzen E, Elbaum N, Singer FR, Rude RK. Parenteral magnesium tolerance testing in the evaluation of magnesium deficiency. Magnesium 4:137-47, 1985*

<u>24-hour urinary excretion of magnesium</u> is a sensitive index of magnesium status (*Galland L. Magnesium and inflammatory bowel disease. Magnesium 7(2):78-83, 1988*). A finding of <25 mg/day suggests magnesium depletion (*Lauler DP. Introduction: Magnesium - Coming of age. Am J Cardiol 63(14):1G, 1989*). However, the biological inter- and intra-variables in an apparently normal population are fairly high (36% and 26%, respectively) and urinary magnesium fails to correlate with serum magnesium concentrations (*Djurhuus M et al. Biological variation of serum and urinary magnesium in apparently healthy-males. Scand J Clin Invest 55(6):549-58, 1995*).

Blood magnesium parameters (<u>plasma, serum, red cells, mononuclear blood cells</u>) may fail to correlate with one another (*Ralston MA et al. Magnesium content of serum, circulating mononuclear cells, skeletal muscle, and myocardium in congestive heart failure. Circulation 80(3):573-80, 1989; Yang XY et al. Blood and urine magnesium parameters compared. Abstract. J Am Coll Nutr 8(5):462, 1989*) or with <u>urine excretion and clearance</u> of magnesium (*Yang XY et al. Blood and urine magnesium parameters compared. Abstract. J Am Coll Nutr 8(5):462, 1989*).

<u>Leukocyte and lymphocyte magnesium levels</u> are better correlated with tissue magnesium levels than are serum levels (*Peter WF et al. Leucocyte magnesium concentration as an indicator of myocardial magnesium. Nutr Rep Int 26:105, July 1982; Juan D. Clinical review: The clinical importance of hypomagnesemia. Surgery 5:510-16, 1982*).

Erythrocyte magnesium is less reliable than white blood cell magnesium as magnesium concentrations are 3-4 times as high in reticulocytes as in mature cells and they decline with the age of cells (*Watson WS et al. Magnesium metabolism in blood and the whole body in man using* ^{28}*magnesium.* Metabolism *28:90-5, 1979*). Moreover, erythrocyte magnesium does not correlate with the magnesium content of other cell types (*Alfrey AC et al. Evaluation of body magnesium stores.* J Lab Clin Med *84:153-62, 1974; Elin RJ, Hosseini JM. Magnesium content of mononuclear blood cells.* Clin Chem *31:377-80, 1985*) and is at least partly genetically determined (*Henrotte JB. Genetic regulation of red blood cell magnesium content and major histocompatibility complex.* Magnesium *5:317-27, 1982*). Finally, erythrocyte magnesium may be normal even when plasma magnesium is low (*Elin RJ et al. Erythrocyte and mononuclear blood cell magnesium concentrations are normal in hypomagnesemic patients with chronic renal magnesium wasting.* J Am Coll Nutr *13(5):463-6, 1994*) and no study unequivocally demonstrates that erythrocyte magnesium concentration represents a fair estimate of total body magnesium stores (*Mimouni FB. The ion-selective magnesium electrode: a new tool for clinicians and investigators. Editorial.* J Am Coll Nutr *15(1):4-5, 1996*).

Mononuclear blood cell magnesium has been suggested as a reliable index of magnesium nutritional status as it appears to be more closely related to total body stores than other biochemical indices (*Gallai V et al. Magnesium content of mononuclear blood cells in migraine patients.* Headache *34(3):160-5, 1994*). However, it may be normal even when plasma magnesium is low (*Elin RJ et al. Erythrocyte and mononuclear blood cell magnesium concentrations are normal in hypomagnesemic patients with chronic renal magnesium wasting.* J Am Coll Nutr *13(5):463-6, 1994*) and no study unequivocally demonstrates that its concentration represents a fair estimate of total body magnesium stores (*Mimouni FB. The ion-selective magnesium electrode: a new tool for clinicians and investigators. Editorial.* J Am Coll Nutr *15(1):4-5, 1996*).

Skeletal and myocardial magnesium levels may fail to correlate with one another as well as with blood magnesium parameters (serum and circulating mononuclear cells) (*Ralston MA et al. Magnesium content of serum, circulating mononuclear cells, skeletal muscle, and myocardium in congestive heart failure.* Circulation *80(3):573-80, 1989*).

Serum magnesium may fail to reflect tissue magnesium levels (*L'Estrange JL, Axford R. Study of magnesium and calcium metabolism in lactating ewes fed semi-purified diet low in magnesium.* J Agric Sci *62, 1964; Reinhart RA et al. Myocardial magnesium: relationship to laboratory and clinical variables in patients undergoing cardiac surgery.* J Am Coll Cardiol *17:651-6, 1991; Reinhart RA et al. Intracellular magnesium of mononuclear cells from venous blood of clinically normal subjects.* Clin Chim Acta *167:187-95, 1987; Richardson JA, Welt LG. Hypomagnesemia of vitamin D administration.* Proc Soc Exp Biol Med *118, 1965*).

Observational Study: 47% of 32 pts. admitted to an intensive care unit for chronic obstructive pulmonary disease and acute respiratory failure had low muscle magnesium levels with a normal serum magnesium, and an additional 9.4% had hypomagnesemia with normal muscle magnesium levels. There was no significant correlation between serum and muscle magnesium levels. Compared to pts. with normal muscle magnesium levels, pts. with low muscle magnesium were more likely to have ventricular arrhythmias and prolonged ICU stays (*Fiaccadori E et al. Muscle and serum magnesium in pulmonary intensive care patients.* Crit Care Med *16:751-60, 1988*).

Experimental and Observational Study: Serum magnesium levels for 21 pts. who had undergone intestinal bypass surgery for obesity were not significantly different from those of healthy controls; however there were major differences in muscle magnesium content and urinary magnesium excretion. When a magnesium chloride load test was performed, pts. who retained more than 20% of the load were later shown to have increases in muscle magnesium content (*Holm CN et al. Hum Nutr Clin Nutr 41C:301, 1987*).

Hair magnesium levels are not always reliable as they tend to be elevated when magnesium is being lost from bones and are lower in grey hair (*Cranton EM. Update on hair element analysis in clinical medicine. J Holistic Med 7(2):120-34, 1985*).

Manganese

Whole blood manganese is considered to be a valid indicator of body manganese and soft tissue levels (*Keen CL et al. Whole blood manganese as an indicator of body manganese. N Engl J Med 308:1230, 1983*).

Lymphocyte manganese has been shown to be a reliable indicator of manganese nutriture (*Matsuda A et al. Quantifying manganese in lymphocytes to assess manganese nutritional status. Clin Chem 35(9):1939-41, 1989*).

Both lymphocyte manganese superoxide dismutase and serum manganese concentrations are sensitive to moderate manganese supplementation (*Davis CD, Greger JL. Longitudinal changes of manganese-dependent superoxide dismutase and other indexes of manganese and iron status in women. Am J Clin Nutr 55:747-52, 1992*).

Serum and sweat manganese levels correlate well with the activation of isocitrate dehydrogenase, a simple and inexpensive functional test of manganese nutriture, suggesting that all 3 measures are valid indicators (*Hunnisett A et al. A new functional test of manganese status. J Nutr Med 1:209-15, 1990*).

Hair manganese may be a reliable indicator of body manganese status (*Foo SC, Khoo NY, Heng A, et al. Metals in hair as biological indices for exposure. Int Arch Occup Environ Health 65:S83-86, 1993*), although greying hair has a lower concentration than black hair (*Guillard O et al. Manganese concentration in the hair of greying ("salt and pepper") men reconsidered. Clin Chem 31(7):1251, 1985*).

Mercury

The amount of hair mercury reflects the body burden of mercury (*Airey D. Mercury in human hair due to environment and diet: A review. Environ Health Perspect 52:303-16, 1983; Foo SC, Khoo NY, Heng A, et al. Metals in hair as biological indices for exposure. Int Arch Occup Environ Health 65:S83-86, 1993*).

Blood mercury is useful for assessing recent methyl mercury exposure (*Berglund F et al. [Methyl mercury in fish, a toxologic-epidemiologic evaluation of risks: Report from an expert group.] Nord Hyg T Suppl. 4, 1971 - published in Nord Hyg T Suppl. 3, 1970*), but not for assessing exposure to inorganic mercurials (*Friberg L, Nordberg GF. Inorganic mercury: Relation between exposure and effects, in L Friberg, J Vostal, Eds. Mercury in the Environment. Cleveland, Ohio, Chemical Rubber Co. Press, 1972:113-39*).

Urinary mercury measurements are unreliable as an indication of mercury poisoning (*Ladd AD et al. Absorption and excretion of mercury in man. II. Urinary mercury in relation to duration of exposure. Arch Environ Health 6:480-3, 1963*).

Niacin

Attempts to diagnose deficiency by measuring nicotinic acid in body fluids have proved disappointing; measurements of metabolites have been more meaningful. In general, plasma niacin metabolites are generally less reliable than urinary metabolites (*Jacob RA et al. Biochemical markers for assessment of niacin status in young men: urinary and blood levels of niacin metabolites. J Nutr 119(4):591-8, 1989*).

The urinary excretion of N^1-methylnicotinamide (NMN) and of 2-pyr are reasonably good measures of niacin status (*Jacob RA et al. Biochemical markers for assessment of niacin status in young men: urinary and blood levels of niacin metabolites. J Nutr 119(4):591-8, 1989*). The excretion ratio of 2-pyr to NMN was formerly considered the most reliable indicator (*Sauberlich HE et al. Laboratory Tests for the Assessment of Nutritional Status. Boca Raton, Florida, CRC Press, 1974:70-4*). However, in a recent study, it was less useful than individual measurements of the 2 metabolites (*Jacob RA et al. Biochemical markers for assessment of niacin status in young men: urinary and blood levels of niacin metabolites. J Nutr 119(4):591-8, 1989*).

Erythrocyte nicotinamide adenine nucleotide (NAD) also appears to be a sensitive indicator of niacin nutriture, and a ratio of erythrocyte NAD to erythrocyte nicotinamide nucleotide phosphate (NADP) below 1.0 may identify subjects at risk of developing a niacin deficiency (*Fu CS et al. Biochemical markers for assessment of niacin status in young men: levels of erythrocyte niacin coenzymes and plasma tryptophan. J Nutr 119(12):1949-55, 1989; Jacobson EL. Niacin deficiency and cancer in women. J Am Coll Nutr 12(4):412-16, 1993*).

Nickel

Hair analysis, when properly performed, is a reliable measure of tissue levels when nickel levels are elevated; low hair nickel has no known clinical significance. Due to the possibility of external contamination, blood or urine studies should be performed for confirmation (*Passwater, RA, Cranton EM. Trace Elements, Hair Analysis and Nutrition. New Canaan, Conn., Keats Publishing, Inc., 1983; Jenkins DW. Toxic Metals in Mammalian Hair and Nails. EPA Report 600/4-79-049 August, 1979 - available through the U.S. Natl Technical Information Service*).

Pantothenic Acid

Blood pantothenic acid responds less readily to intake than urinary pantothenic acid although, in general, blood pantothenic acid levels decrease in subjects given a pantothenic acid deficient diet (*Fry PC, Fox HM, Tao HG. Metabolic response to a pantothenic acid deficient diet in humans. J Nutr Sci Vitaminol 22:339-46, 1976*).

Phosphorus

Plasma phosphate is mainly controlled by renal excretion.

Hair phosphorus has little or no relationship to phosphorus metabolism in the body or to dietary phosphorus intake (*Passwater RA, Cranton EM. Trace Elements, Hair Analysis and Nutrition. New Canaan, Connecticut, Keats Publishing, 1983:61*).

Potassium

Red blood cell potassium (or whole blood potassium) is superior to serum potassium level as an index of cellular potassium stores *(Bahemuka M, Hodkinson HM. Red-blood-cell potassium as a practical index of potassium status in elderly patients. Age Ageing 5:24, 1976).*

> **Experimental and Observational Study:** Serum and red blood cell potassium was measured in 17 pts. with EKG abnormalities. Although some of the abnormalities were typical of potassium deficiency, most were non-specific T wave changes which are commonly attributed (without substantiation) to ischemia. Serum potassium levels were normal but RBC potassium levels were below normal in all cases and returned to normal (as did the EKG abnormalities) after treatment with potassium salts *(Sangiori GB et al. Serum potassium levels, red-blood-cell potassium and alterations of the repolarization phase of electrocardiography in old subjects. Age Ageing 13:309, 1984).*

Serum potassium levels are slightly higher than plasma levels.

> **Observational Study:** Serum and plasma potassium levels for 30 pts. were compared using contemporary automated techniques and ion-selective electrodes. The mean difference between serum and plasma potassium levels was 0.18 mmol/l ($p<0.001$) *(Hyman D, Kaplan NM. The difference between serum and plasma potassium. Letter. N Engl J Med September 5, 1985, p. 642).*

Plasma potassium may be falsely increased by up to 1.0 mmol/l by fist-clenching to make the veins more prominent for venipuncture *(Brown JJ et al. Falsely high plasma potassium values in patients with hyperaldosteronism. Br Med J 2:18-20, 1970)*, and anxiety over venipuncture may produce enough hyperventilation-induced respiratory alkalosis to lower the level by that much or more *(Edwards R et al. Acute hypocapneic hypokalemia: An iatrogenic anesthetic complication. Anesth Analg 56:786-92, 1977).*

Hair potassium levels do not reflect dietary intake or body stores *(Passwater RA, Cranton EM. Trace Elements, Hair Analysis and Nutrition. New Canaan, Connecticut, Keats Publishing, 1983:85).*

Riboflavin

The procedure most commonly used to evaluate riboflavin nutriture is the measurement of RBC glutathione reductase (EGR) activity and the stimulation of this activity by flavin adenine dinucleotide (FAD) added *in vitro*. The EGR activity is commonly expressed in terms of "activity coefficient" or in terms of percent stimulation, both of which are derived from the stimulating effect of FAD added *in vitro* to the enzyme reaction. Some animal studies suggest that certain deficiencies, such as thiamine, nicotinic acid and pyridoxine, may reduce the apo-enzyme level *(Sharada D, Bamji MS. Erythrocyte glutathione reductase activity and riboflavin concentration in experimental deficiency of some water soluble vitamins. Int J Vitam Nutr Res 42:43-49, 1972).* Both the age of the subject and the age of the red cell may also influence EGR activity, and the assay may not be valid in subjects with low RBC glucose-6-phosphate dehydrogenase activity *(Sauberlich HE. Newer laboratory methods for assessing nutriture of selected B-complex vitamins. Annu Rev Nutr 4:377-407, 1984).* Also, drugs may affect red cell enzyme activity by altering apoenzyme activities, reducing the life span of the red cell or by interfering with the assay procedure *(Roe DA. Diet and Drug Interactions. New York, Van Nostrand Reinhold, 1989:141).*

Blood riboflavin levels are not necessarily good measures of riboflavin status because of the difficulty in achieving accurate measurements *(Bamjii MS et al. Relationship between biochemical and clinical indices of B-vitamin deficiency. A study in rural school boys. Br J Nutr 41:431-41, 1979)*, although new analytical procedures for measure blood and urinary riboflavin may prove to be useful *(Sauberlich HE. Newer laboratory methods for assessing nutriture of selected B-complex vitamins. Annu Rev Nutr 4:377-407, 1984)*.

Urinary riboflavin excretion depends upon nitrogen balance, kidney function and recent intake *(Heller S et al. Riboflavin status in pregnancy. Am J Clin Nutr 27:1225-30, 1974)*.

Selenium

The only true evidence of selenium deficiency lies in a positive response to selenium therapy *(Neve J et al. Selenium deficiency. Clin Endocrinol Metab 14(3):629-56, 1985)*.

The level of blood glutathione peroxidase has been shown to be a sensitive index of its selenium content in animals and man *(Ganther HE et al. Selenium and glutathione peroxidase in health and disease - a review, in AS Prasad, D Overleas, Eds. Trace Elements in Human Health and Disease, Volume II. New York, Academic Press, 1976:165)*.

Hair selenium is significantly correlated with selenium concentrations in the liver, lung and renal cortex ($p < 0.01$) *(Cheng YD, Zhuang GS, Tan MG, et al. Study of correlation of Se content in human hair and internal organs by INAA. Biol Trace Elem Res 28:737-41 1990)*. It also correlates well with selenium intake, and may be superior to whole blood selenium if organic selenium (L-selenomethionine) is the source of selenium *(Gallagher ML et al. Selenium levels in new growth hair and in whole blood during injection of a selenium supplement for six weeks. Nutr Res 4:577-82, 1984; Valentine, JL et al. Selenium levels in human blood, urine and hair in response to exposure via drinking water. Environ Res 17:347-55, 1978)*. When additional dietary selenium comes from an inorganic source (selenate or selenite), however, hair selenium rises while muscle selenium levels are relatively unchanged *(Salbe AD, Levander OA. Hair and nails as indicators of selenium status in rats fed elevated dietary levels of selenium as L-selenomethionine (SeMet) or sodium selenate (Na_2SeO_4). Fed Proc 46(4), March 5, 1987)*. In addition, selenium-containing shampoos will falsely elevate hair selenium levels.

The value of blood selenium levels as an indicator of selenium nutriture is limited; once adequate selenium intake is achieved, the blood selenium level may not continue to rise with increases in dietary selenium until toxic levels of intake are reached *(Valentine JL et al. Selenium levels in human blood, urine and hair in response to exposure via drinking water. Environ Res 17:347-55, 1978)*.

> **Experimental Study:** 6 healthy volunteers took supplements of 256 mg daily of organic yeast selenium. Blood analysis showed a prompt increase in selenium levels of serum and erythrocytes. Serum levels increased from 88 µg/L to a plateau of 200 µg/L after 7 weeks. Erythrocyte levels commenced to rise at 148 µg/L and rose steadily to 438 µg/L throughout the 26-wk. study. Results suggest that blood selenium is a useful measure of dietary selenium intake *(Tarp U et al. Blood selenium concentrations during long-term supplementation. Nutr Res 6:853-55, 1986)*.

> **Observational Study:** Blood selenium levels failed to correlate with selenium intake except at the extremes *(Lane HW et al. Blood selenium and glutathione peroxidase levels and dietary selenium of free living and institutionalized elderly subjects. Proc Soc Exp Biol Med 173(1):87-95, 1985)*.

Toenail selenium concentration is unaffected by dietary intake in the prior 3 months and appears to provide a time-integrated measure of intake over a period of 26-52 weeks (*Longnecker MP, Stampfer MJ, Morris JS, et al. A 1-y trial of the effect of high-selenium bread on selenium concentrations in blood and toenails. Am J Clin Nutr 57:408-13, 1993*).

Urinary selenium is an inadequate indicator of tissue nutriture (*Neve J et al. Selenium deficiency. Clin Endocrinol Metab 14(3):629-56, 1985*) but may be useful to confirm the findings when blood selenium is being measured (*Valentine JL et al. Selenium levels in human blood, urine and hair in response to exposure via drinking water. Environ Res 17:347-55, 1978*).

Sodium

Serum sodium levels are commonly used as a measure of sodium nutriture. The principal cation of the extracellular fluid, any change in serum sodium is associated with a fluid shift into or out of the cell. Serum levels, however, do not reflect total body sodium content (*Webb WL, Gehi M. Psychosomatics 22(3):199-203, 1981*).

Hair sodium levels do not reflect dietary intake or body stores (*Passwater RA, Cranton EM. Trace Elements, Hair Analysis and Nutrition. New Canaan, Connecticut, Keats Publishing, 1983:85*).

Sulfur

Hair sulfur is a useful diagnostic screen for the evaluation of hair disorders (*Kutner M et al. A critique: Hair sulfur analysis for evaluation of normal and abnormal hair, in AC Brown, Ed. First Human Hair Symposium, Medcom Press*). While low hair sulfur does not appear to correlate with hair loss, and supplementation with sulfur when hair sulfur is low does not appear to stimulate hair growth, alopecia resulting from dietary inadequacies may be reflected by low hair sulfur. In these cases, upon correction of the diet, hair growth is restored and hair sulfur increases (*Brown H, Klauder JV. Sulphur content of hair and of nails in abnormal states. Arch Derm Syphilol 27:584, 1933*).

Taurine

Because plasma and whole-blood taurine are not correlated, assessment of both provides the most accurate estimate of taurine status. Short of that, whole-blood taurine would appear to be the best single measure (*Trautwein EA, Hayes KC. Taurine concentrations in plasma and whole blood in humans: estimation of error from intra- and interindividual variation and sampling technique. Am J Clin Nutr 52:758-64, 1990*).

Thiamine

The most commonly used procedure for assessing thiamine nutriture has been the measurement of Erythrocyte transketolase activity and its stimulation *in vitro* by the addition of thiamine pyrophosphate (TPP effect). Some disease conditions may influence RBC transketolase activity independent of thiamine status. For example, patients in negative nitrogen balance will have diminished RBC transketolase activity due to insufficient apoenzyme to activate transketolase. In addition, low transketolase in diabetes mellitus and polyneuritis does not reflect a thiamine deficit, while patients with pernicious anemia may have elevated transketolase levels unrelated to thiamine status (*Sauberlich HE. Newer laboratory methods for assessing nutriture of selected B-complex vitamins. Annu Rev Nutr 4:377-407, 1984*). Red cell enzyme activities decline as the red cells age, and red cell activity coefficients are elevated with red cell age; thus it has been proposed that interday and interpersonal variability in red cell enzyme activity may be attributed to change in the age structure of the red cell population (*Spooner RJ, Percy RA, Rumley AG. The effect of erythrocyte ageing on some vitamin and mineral dependent enzymes. Clin Biochem 12:289, 1979*). Finally, drugs may affect red cell enzyme activity by altering apoenzyme activities, reducing the life span of the red cell or by interfering with the assay procedure (*Roe DA. Diet and Drug Interactions. New York, Van Nostrand Reinhold, 1989:141*).

> *Note: TPP response should not be used as the sole indicator of marginal thiamine status; thiamine intake as well as other metabolic measures - such as RBC or plasma TPP - should also be used* (*Gans DA, Harper AE. Thiamine status of incarcerated and nonincarcerated adolescent males: dietary intake and thiamin pyrophosphate response. Am J Clin Nutr 53:1471-5, 1991*). *For example, "frequently, no transketolase effect is observable in patients with neuropathies, liver diseases and other ailments even in severe thiamine deficiency"* (*Baker H et al. B-Complex vitamin analyses and their clinical value. J Appl Nutr 41(1):3-12, 1989*).

Erythrocyte thiamine diphosphate levels may be superior to RBC transketolase activity as thiamine diphosphate is more stable in frozen red blood cells, is easier to standardize, and is not subject to the variables present in the transketolase assay (*Baines M, Davies G. The evaluation of erythrocyte thiamine diphosphate as an indicator of thiamine status in man, and its comparison with erythrocyte transketolase activity measurements. Ann Clin Biochem 25:698-705, 1988*).

Several studies have demonstrated a relationship between RBC transketolase activity and urinary thiamine excretion (*Sauberlich HE. Newer laboratory methods for assessing nutriture of selected B-complex vitamins. Annu Rev Nutr 4:377-407, 1984*).

On a thiamine-deficient diet, a decrease in the blood thiamine level is the earliest sign of a thiamine deficiency (*Baker H. Analysis of vitamin status. J Med Soc N J 80:633-6, 1983*). However, blood thiamine determinations have not been satisfactory primarily because of limitations in methodology, as the decreases in blood thiamine during deficiency are not great (*Sauberlich HE. Newer laboratory methods for assessing nutriture of selected B-complex vitamins. Annu Rev Nutr 4:377-407, 1984*).

Vitamin A

A liver biopsy is by far the most accurate method of assessing vitamin A status (*Pitt GAJ. The assessment of vitamin A status. Proc Nutr Sci 40:173, 1981*).

Isotope dilution assay with tetradeuterated vitamin A can validly estimate total body reserves in both the marginal and satisfactory ranges (*Furr HC et al. Vitamin A concentrations in liver determined by isotope dilution assay with tetradeuterated vitamin A and by biopsy in generally healthy adult humans. Am J Clin Nutr 49:713-16, 1989*).

The relative-dose-response test is a reliable means of using measurements of retinol in peripheral circulation to interpret the hepatic reserves of vitamin A. It is based on the principle that, in the retinol-depleted liver, apo-retinol-binding protein (apo-RBP) accumulates in hepatocytes. The availability of excess apo-RBP primes the liver to transport retinol to the nutrient-starved peripheral tissues whenever new vitamin A is acquired from the diet. Thus, an oral challenge with vitamin A provokes a prominent rise in RBP-associated retinol in the circulation in those individuals with minimal hepatic vitamin A reserves (*Bulux J, Carranza, Castañeda C, et al. Studies on the application of the relative-dose-response test for assessing vitamin A status in older adults. Am J Clin Nutr 56:543-7, 1992*).

Plasma retinol is commonly measured to assess vitamin A status. However, due to biological variation within the individual, detecting small differences in plasma retinol concentrations may require up to 12 repeated samplings (*Tangney CC et al. Intra- and interindividual variation in measurements of b-carotene, retinol, and tocopherols in diet and plasma. Am J Clin Nutr 45:764-9, 1987*). Also, acute infections can alter the distribution of retinol in the body (*Arroyave G et al. Decline in serum levels of retinol and retinol binding protein (RBP) during infections. Arch Latinoam Nutr 29:233-60, 1979*).

Finally, when insufficient RBP is available, toxicity due to hypervitaminosis A can occur despite a low concentration of plasma retinol; thus, in addition to plasma retinol concentration, it is important that retinol-binding protein also be measured (*Nutr Rev 40(10), October, 1982*). Although determination of plasma retinol as the retinol-RBP (retinol-binding protein) complex would appear to be a promising method, the major limitation on its value is that plasma retinol concentration is kept reasonably constant to supply vitamin A to the tissues. While there is some relationship between plasma values and liver content, the plasma content only falls substantially if the liver reserves of retinyl esters are effectively exhausted (*Pitt GAJ. The assessment of vitamin A status. Proc Nutr Sci 40:173, 1981*).

In addition, other factors besides vitamin A nutriture can influence plasma retinol levels. If dietary protein is inadequate, or if various diseases are present, insufficient RBP is synthesized by the liver, and the plasma retinol concentration will fall. Estrogens and oral contraceptives can increase plasma retinol-RBP concentrations. Poor growth depresses, and accelerated growth increases, the plasma retinol concentration, and giving retinoids other than retinol can paradoxically depress plasma retinol concentration as a consequence of diminishing tissue demand for retinol (*Pitt GAJ. The assessment of vitamin A status. Proc Nutr Sci 40:173, 1981*).

Vitamin B$_6$

Pyridoxal-5'-phosphate (PLP) and pyridoxal (PL), its hydrolysis product and the ultimate transport form of B$_6$, are the predominant B$_6$ vitamers in the circulation and the measurement of both is recommended. The measurement of erythrocyte PLP and PL may be more informative about vitamin B$_6$ status than plasma measures as a number of physiologic conditions may change the dynamic equilibrium between the various B$_6$ vitamers in the plasma. Also, in acute myocardial infarction, extracellular PLP may be redistributed to the intracellular compartment (*Vermaak WJH et al. Vitamin B-6 nutrition status and cigarette smoking. Am J Clin Nutr 51:1958-61, 1990*).

The urinary pyridoxic acid level may give additional information to that obtained from a combination of pyridoxal phosphate and pyridoxal plasma levels, for example during pregnancy when plasma pyridoxal phosphate is decreased while plasma pyridoxal is increased (*Rogers K, Mohan C. Vitamin B6 metabolism and diabetes. Biochem Med Metab Biol 52:10-17, 1994*).

There are certain difficulties with using vitamin B$_6$-dependent enzyme activities as a measure of B$_6$ status:

1. Some B_6-deficient patients, such as those with liver disease, have high pyridoxal-dependent erythrocyte transaminase levels despite low blood pyridoxine (*Sauberlich HE. Newer laboratory methods for assessing nutriture of selected B-complex vitamins. Annu Rev Nutr 4:377-407, 1984*).

2. The activity of the erythrocyte aminotransferases also increase in thiamine, riboflavin and pantothenate deficiencies and in various disease states (*Baker H. Analysis of vitamin status. J Med Soc N J 80:633-6, 1983*).

3. Erythrocyte glutamate-pyruvate transaminase (alanine aminotransaminase) activity differs significantly among 3 phenotypes despite similar plasma pyridoxal-5'-phosphate levels; thus EGPT activity can only be used to assess vitamin B_6 nutritional status if the GPT phenotype is accounted for (*Ubbink JB et al. Genetic polymorphism of glutamate-pyruvate transaminase (alanine aminotransaminase): Influence on erythrocyte activity as a marker of vitamin B-6 nutritional status. Am J Clin Nutr 50:1420-8, 1989*).

4. Drugs may affect red cell enzyme activity by altering apoenzyme activities, reducing the life span of the red cell or by interfering with the assay procedure (*Roe DA. Diet and Drug Interactions. New York, Van Nostrand Reinhold, 1989:141*).

Xanthurenic acid and kynurenine excretion after a tryptophan load most likely represents an aberrant reaction to the load and has no documented clinical significance. In addition, pregnancy and contraceptive pills may render the test abnormal due to inhibition of kynureninase by estrogens (*Baker H. Analysis of vitamin status. J Med Soc N J 80:633-6, 1983; Sauberlich HE. Newer laboratory methods for assessing nutriture of selected B-complex vitamins. Annu Rev Nutr 4:377-407, 1984*).

Vitamin B_{12}

"The assessment of B_{12} . . . deficiency should be based on haematological findings of macrocytic anaemia with a right shift of neutrophils, or in the presence of specific neurological symptoms, with or without anaemia" (*Balfour IC, Lane DW. B12/folate assays and macrocytic anaemia. Letter. Lancet 346:446-7, 1995*).

> *Note: If vitamin B_{12} deficiency is suspected, folic acid nutriture should also be evaluated since, if levels of both vitamins are low, "deficiency of either vitamin may be primary. This is due to the fact that megaloblastic intestinal cells may not absorb properly and, as a result, a secondary deficiency of the other vitamin occurs"* (*Skelton WP III, Skelton NK. Deficiency of vitamins A, B, and C. Something to watch for. Postgrad Med 87(4):293-310, 1990*).

> *Note: Oral symptoms suggestive of vitamin B_{12} deficiency (e.g. sore tongue, recurrent oral ulcerations, burning mouth) often occur in conjunction with lower serum B_{12} concentrations, gastric parietal cell antibodies and B_{12} malabsorption, but in the absence of anemia* (*Field E, Speechley J, Rugman F, et al. Oral signs and symptoms in patients with undiagnosed vitamin B-12 deficiency. J Oral Pathol 24(10):468-70, 1995*).

The urinary methylmalonic acid assay (by gas chromatography-mass spectrometry) is an excellent indicator of a functional vitamin B_{12} deficiency (*Norman EJ. Letter. Arch Fam Med 4, April, 1995*). However, it may be elevated in other conditions such as benign methylmalonic aciduria (*Ledley FD et al. Benign methylmalonic aciduria. N Engl J Med 311:1015-18, 1984*), and carnitine supplementation may cause MMA levels to decrease (*Roe CR et al. Metabolic response to carnitine in methylmalonic aciduria. Arch Dis Child 58:916-20, 1983*). In order to correct for renal insufficiency and dehydration, the assay must be normalized to creatinine levels *(Norman EJ, Morrison JA. Screening elderly populations for cobalamin (vitamin B_{12}) deficiency using the urinary methylmalonic acid assay by gas chromatography mass spectrometry. Am J Med 94:589-94, 1993).*

> *Note: Since the conversion of methylmalonyl-CoA to succinyl-CoA is catalyzed by vitamin B_{12}, a B_{12} deficiency will inhibit the reaction, leading to an increase in the urinary excretion of methylmalonic acid.*

Observational Study: 18/35 (51%) elderly subjects with elevated urinary MMA had a low serum total cobalamin, 6/33 (18%) had an elevated mean corpuscular volume (MCV), and 3/33 (9%) had a low hematocrit, suggesting that MMA is a more sensitive indicator of vitamin B_{12} deficiency *(Norman EJ, Morrison JA. Screening elderly populations for cobalamin (vitamin B_{12}) deficiency using the urinary methylmalonic acid assay by gas chromatography mass spectrometry. Am J Med 94(6):589-94, 1993).*

Observational Study: 75 pts. with low serum B_{12} levels and 68 normal controls were studied. Of 96 evaluable pts., 7 had clinical deficiency; all had urinary methylmalonic acid levels >5 μg/mg creatinine (sensitivity, 100%). Of the 89 pts. who were not clinically deficient, 88 had urinary methylmalonic acid levels <5 μg/mg creatinine (specificity 99%) *(Matchar DB et al. Isotope-dilution assay for urinary methylmalonic acid in the diagnosis of vitamin B_{12} deficiency. A prospective clinical evaluation. Ann Intern Med 106(5):707-10, 1987).*

Both elevated serum methylmalonic acid and serum homocysteine levels are excellent indicators of cellular vitamin B_{12} deficiency. These tests should be performed on patients who have hematologic, neuropsychiatric or gastrointestinal disorders suggestive of cobalamin deficiency even though their serum cobalamin levels are >221 pmol/L *(Upshaw CB, Carmel R. Approach to a low vitamin B_{12} level. JAMA 272:1233, 1994; Yulin Y et al. Decline of serum cobalamin levels with increasing age among geriatric outpatients. Arch Fam Med 3:918-22, 1994).*

> *Note: The serum methylmalonic acid assay appears especially useful in evaluating vitamin B_{12} status in hepatic disease as serum vitamin B_{12} may be increased (Hagelskjaer L, Rasmussen K. Methylmalonic acid concentration in serum not affected by hepatic disease. Clin Chem 38(4):493-5, 1992).*

Low serum holotranscobalamin II (low vitamin B_{12} on transcobalamin II, the circulating delivery protein) indicates the earliest stage of a negative B_{12} balance that is measurable from the serum *(Herbert V. Staging vitamin B-12 (cobalamin) status in vegetarians. Am J Clin Nutr 59(suppl):1213S-22S, 1994).*

> *Note: Reduced transcobalamin II would raise serum cobalamin levels while lowering intracellular levels (Yulin Y et al. Decline of serum cobalamin levels with increasing age among geriatric outpatients. Arch Fam Med 3:918-22, 1994).*

Despite depressed cerebrospinal fluid vitamin B_{12} levels in the cerebrospinal fluid, serum B_{12} levels are frequently normal *(van Tiggelen CJ, Peperkamp JP, Tertoolen HJ. Assessment of vitamin B_{12} status in CSF. Letter. Am J Psychiatry 141(1):136-7, 1984; van Tiggelen CJM et al. Vitamin B_{12} levels of cerebrospinal fluid in patients with organic mental disorder. J Orthomol Psychiatry 12:305-11, 1983);* thus the cerebrospinal fluid level, although often impractical to obtain, is a better marker of B_{12} deficiency with regard to brain function than serum levels (*Gottfries CG, president of the European College of Neuropsychopharmacology - reported in* Clin Psychiatry News, *September, 1989*).

Most low serum cobalamin levels are due to gastric dysfunction in which protein-bound cobalamin is not digested and can be corrected with oral administration of crystal cobalamin concentrate (*Yulin Y et al. Decline of serum cobalamin levels with increasing age among geriatric outpatients.* Arch Fam Med *3:918-22, 1994*). Serum cobalamin levels may be low despite the absence of hematological and neurological evidence of pernicious anemia and a normal Schilling test.

> *Note: While the* microbiological serum assay *is a reliable indicator of the serum* B_{12} *level* (*Baker H et al. Vitamin analyses in medicine, in RS Goodhart, ME Shils, Eds.* Modern Nutrition in Health and Disease. *Sixth Edition. Philadelphia, Lea & Febiger, 1980:611; Lee DSC, Griffiths BW. B-12 assay methods.* Clin Biochem *18:261-6, 1985),* RIA serum assays *are unreliable because they also measure inactive cobalamin analogues* (*Cohen KL, Donaldson RM Jr. Unreliability of radiodilution assays as screening tests for cobalamin (vitamin B_{12}) deficiency.* JAMA *October 24, 1980, pp. 1942-5; Kolhouse JF et al. Cobalamin analogues are present in human plasma and can mask cobalamin deficiency because current radioisotope dilution assays are not specific for true cobalamin.* N Engl J Med *299:787, 1978*).

Experimental and Observational Study: The mean corpuscular volume (MCV) of erythrocytes from 4 elderly subjects with low serum vitamin B_{12} levels was normal and, for the 3 subjects tested, Schilling tests were normal. However, the deoxyuridine suppression test (DST), a sensitive measure of cellular competence in DNA replication, was abnormal and minimal clinical indications of dysfunction were present. After 6 mo. of cobalamine supplementation, the DST improved (*Carmel R. Reversal by cobalamine therapy of minimal defects in the deoxyuridine suppression test in patients without anemia: further evidence for a subtle metabolic cobalamine deficiency.* J Lab Clin Chem *119:240-4, 1992*).

The Schilling test is a popular test of B_{12} absorption (*Zuckier LS, Chervu LR.* J Nucl Med *25:1032, 1984*) although it may be remain normal when serum B_{12} levels suggest deficiency (see example above) (*Lum MC, Mooradian AD. Vitamin B_{12} deficiency: The Sepulveda GRECC method. No. 14.* Geriatr Med Today *5(10):93-7, 1986*). Because it only tests absorption of free vitamin B_{12}, the Schilling test is often normal despite malabsorption of vitamin B_{12} from food (*Carmel R, Sinow RM, Siegel ME, Samloff IM. Food-cobalamin malabsorption occurs frequently in patients with unexplained low serum cobalamin levels.* Arch Intern Med *148:1715-19, 1988*).

> *Note: The newer dual-isotope variation has the advantage of being independent of urine volume and renal function* (*Lum MC, Mooradian AD. Vitamin B_{12} deficiency: The Sepulveda GRECC method. No. 14.* Geriatr Med Today *5(10):93-7, 1986); however, it is less reliable and exposes the patient to an often unnecessary double dose of radiation* (*Carmel R. Approach to a low vitamin B_{12} level. Questions and Answers.* JAMA *272(16):1233, 1994*).

Experimental and Observational Study: 4 elderly subjects with low serum vitamin B_{12} levels were studied. For the 3 subjects tested, Schilling tests were normal. However, the deoxyuridine suppression test (DST), a sensitive measure of cellular competence in DNA replication, was abnormal and minimal clinical indications of dysfunction were present. After 6 mo. of cobalamine supplementation, the DST improved (*Carmel R. Reversal by cobalamine therapy of minimal defects in the deoxyuridine suppression test in patients without anemia: further evidence for a subtle metabolic cobalamine deficiency.* J Lab Clin Chem *119:240-4, 1992*).

The determination of <u>hypersegmentation of neutrophils</u> is a useful measure of vitamin B_{12} deficiency, although it is unreliable during pregnancy and fails to distinguish between vitamin B_{12} and folate deficiencies (*Sauberlich HE. Newer laboratory methods for assessing nutriture of selected B-complex vitamins. Annu Rev Nutr 4:377-407, 1984*).

An <u>erythrocyte count</u> is of limited value, even for screening, as vitamin B_{12} deficiency may present without anemia. Moreover, even when anemia is present in B_{12} deficiency, it may not be the classic macrocytic type; thus <u>measures of red cell size</u> are also unreliable (*Ralph Green, chairman, department of laboratory hematology, the Cleveland Clinic Foundation - presented at a session of the Am. College of Clinical Pathologists and College of Am. Pathologists and summarized in Helwick C. Red cell is inadequate as red flag for low B-12. Med World News November 1991:33*).

> **Observational Study:** 50 cases of masked vitamin B_{12} and folate deficiency detected in an inner-city-area geriatric unit during the course of routine clinical investigation are described. The majority had none of the classical signs of vitamin B_{12} or folate deficiency, and all had a mean corpuscular volume of <100 fl. Moreover, the MCV failed to correlate with serum vitamin B_{12} levels (*Craig GM, Elliot C, Hughes KR. Masked vitamin B_{12} and folate deficiency in the elderly. Br J Nutr 54(3):613-19, 1985*).

Vitamin C

There is to date no satisfactory assay technique for ascorbic acid status. Once collected, AA readily oxidizes to dehydroascorbic acid and then to diketogulonic acid. The latter step is irreversible but the former may be prevented by acidification of the specimen immediately upon collection. Many factors influence the levels present at any particular time (physiologic status, drug ingestion, etc.) (*Lee W et al. Ascorbic acid status: Biochemical and clinical considerations. Am J Clin Nutr 48:286-90, 1988*).

The <u>ascorbic acid saturation test</u> must be carefully conducted and interpreted with caution, but the results can conclusively exclude scurvy as a diagnosis (*Sauberlich HE. Vitamin C status: Methods and findings. Ann N Y Acad Sci 258:438-49, 1975; Dutra De Oliveira JE et al. Clinical usefulness of the oral ascorbic acid tolerance test in scurvy. Am J Clin Nutr 7:630, 1959*). A 24-hour urine for ascorbic acid is collected daily prior to and following oral supplementation with 1 gm of ascorbic acid daily. Urinary ascorbic acid output will rise until saturation is achieved (*Milner G. Br J Psychiatry 109:294-9, 1963*).

> Normal range: 1-2 days
> Borderline to frank scurvy: 7-10 days

The <u>leukocyte ascorbic acid concentration</u> tends to respond less readily than does the serum level to recent dietary intake and may be more closely related to tissue stores than are serum levels (*Burr ML et al. Plasma and leukocyte ascorbic acid levels in the elderly. Am J Clin Nutr 27:144, 1974*), although it may be normal despite other evidence of vitamin C deficiency (*Thomas AJ et al. Is leucocyte ascorbic acid an unreliable estimate of vitamin C deficiency? Age Ageing 13(4):243-7, 1984*). Factors such as infection, suppressed immunity, myocardial infarction and hyperglycemia may lower these levels, as may such drugs as aspirin, oral contraceptives and hydrocortisone (*Lee W et al. Ascorbic acid status: Biochemical and clinical considerations. Am J Clin Nutr 48:286-90, 1988*).

While <u>serum and plasma ascorbate levels</u> may not always fully reflect vitamin C intakes or the state of tissue ascorbate reserves, within a limited range, serum ascorbate levels show a linear relationship with vitamin C intake, and low serum levels indicate low or inadequate intake with probably only partial reserves present *(Sauberlich HE. Vitamin C status: Methods and findings. Ann N Y Acad Sci 258:438-49, 1975).*

> *Note: Except for high-performance liquid chromatography (HPLC), commonly used analytic procedures for plasma or serum vitamin C cannot distinguish between ascorbic acid and its isomer, erythorbic acid, which is widely used as a food additive, especially in processed meats. Therefore, unless the HPLC-amperometric method is used, plasma or serum vitamin C analyses should be conducted on overnight fasting blood specimens (Sauberlich HE et al. Influence of dietary intakes of erythorbic acid on plasma vitamin C analyses. Am J Clin Nutr 54:1319S-22S, 1991).*

<u>Erythrocyte and whole-blood ascorbic acid levels</u> appear to be less sensitive indicators of vitamin C deficiency than are serum levels *(Sauberlich HE. Vitamin C status: Methods and findings. Ann N Y Acad Sci 258:438-49, 1975).*

<u>Urinary excretion of ascorbic acid</u> declines to undetectable levels in vitamin C depletion and thus could be used to corroborate other findings *(Hodges RE et al. Clinical manifestations of ascorbic acid deficiency in man. Am J Clin Nutr 24:432, 1971).*

The <u>lingual ascorbic acid test</u> is performed as follows. One minim of 1/430 N 2,6 dichlorphenolinodolphenol (dark blue) is dropped upon the dorsum of the tongue and the number of seconds it takes for the color to vanish is recorded. The greater the vitamin C concentration in the tissue, the faster the reduction of the dye to a colorless state *(Cheraskin E, Ringsdorf WM Jr, El-Ashiry G. A lingual vitamin C test. Int J Vitam Res 34(1):31-8, 1964).* The value of the test is controversial.

> **Positive Review Article:** The lingual vitamin C test is a relatively simple, inexpensive, and reasonably accurate screening procedure for the detection of hypovitaminosis C in tissues. Results are consistent and are significantly correlated with intradermal ascorbate levels. Since plasma levels reflect diet more than tissue concentrations, the lingual test correlates better with plasma levels when performed during fasting, although the results of the two tests remain significantly correlated even under non-fasting conditions *(Cheraskin E. Vitamin C and stomatology: a mouthful of evidence. J Orthomol Med 6(3-4):147-54, 1991).*

> **Negative Review Articles:** Results of the lingual ascorbic acid test are not related to changes in ascorbic acid intake and are not consistent with plasma or leukocyte ascorbate concentrations *(Leggott PJ et al. Response of lingual ascorbic acid test and salivary ascorbate levels to changes in ascorbic acid intake. J Dent Res 65(2):131-4, 1986; Ascorbic acid intake and salivary ascorbate levels. Nutr Rev 44(10):328-30, 1986).*

Vitamin D

Cholecalciferol (vitamin D_3) is the natural vitamin, while ergocalciferol (vitamin D_2) is obtained exclusively from the diet. Each is biologically inert until it undergoes successive enzymatic hydroxylations, at C-25 in the liver and at C-1 in the kidney, to produce 1,25-dihydroxyvitamin D.

While intracellular 25-hydroxyvitamin D may serve a specific function, it is unproved and can be regarded as part of the body stores of vitamin D. Measurement of <u>plasma 25-hydroxyvitamin D</u> provides an index of the bodily reserve of the pro-hormone, and measurement of <u>plasma 1,25-dihydroxyvitamin D</u> an index of prevailing biological action, although the level of 1,25-dihydroxyvitamin D can only be interpreted with reference to the subject's mineral nutrition and the prevailing physiological state *(Stanbury SW. Vitamin D: metamorphosis from nutrient to hormonal system. <u>Proc Nutr Soc</u> 40:179-86, 1981).*

Vitamin E

Because absorption, transport and tissue distribution of the vitamin depend upon many factors, the individual requirement varies. Also, as it has no special storage sites, vitamin E cannot be released on demand and thus must be taken up continuously. No reliable and easily accessible bioequivalent of an inadequate or excessive supply is available, as presumed deficiency syndromes develop over long periods, and overt toxicity remains unknown *(Schultz M, Leist M, Petrzika M, et al. Novel urinary metabolite of α-tocopherol, 2,5,7,8-tetramethyl-2(2'-carboxyethyl)-6-hydroxychroman, as an indicator of an adequate vitamin E supply? <u>Am J Clin Nutr</u> 62(suppl):1527S-34S, 1995).*

<u>Adipose tissue levels</u> appear to be relatively good markers of dietary intake *(Kardinaal A, Van't Veer P, Brants H, et al. Relations between antioxidant vitamins in adipose-tissue, plasma, and diet. <u>Am J Epidemiol</u> 141(5):440-50, 1995).*

<u>Platelet tocopherol levels</u> appear to be the best blood measure of the dietary intake of vitamin E *(Lehmann J et al. Vitamin E and relationships among tocopherols in human plasma, platelets, lymphocytes, and red blood cells. <u>Am J Clin Nutr</u> 47:470-4, 1988).*

See Also:

> *Vatasser G et al. Vitamin E concentrations in the human blood plasma and platelets. <u>Am J Clin Nutr</u> 37:1020-4, 1983*

Since <u>plasma and serum vitamin E levels</u> are closely correlated with total serum triglycerides *(Farrell PM, Biere JG. <u>Am J Clin Nutr</u> 28:1381, 1975)*, <u>tocopherol to triglyceride serum ratios</u> should be calculated in assessing tocopherol status when plasma or serum vitamin E is being measured. The normal range of this ratio is 35-120 *(Bland J, Prestbo E. Vitamin E: Comparative absorption studies. <u>Int Clin Nutr Rev</u> 4(2):82-6, 1984).*

> **Note:** *Plasma vitamin E levels are also significantly correlated (p<0.001) with total cholesterol and total lipid (Vandewoude MF, Vandewoude MG. Vitamin E status in an normal population: The influence of age. <u>J Am Coll Nutr</u> 6(4):307-11, 1987).*

Vitamin K

Vitamin K acts as a cofactor in a reaction that converts specific glutamic acid residues present in vitamin D-dependent proteins to γ-carboxyglutamic acid. When the vitamin is even mildly deficient, abnormal, des-γ-carboxy forms of these proteins referred to as PIVKA (protein induced by vitamin K deficiency or antagonism) are secreted in the plasma. <u>A highly sensitive immunological method of direct measurement of PIVKA</u> is an excellent measure of vitamin K nutriture *(Blanchard RA, Furie BC, Jorgensen M, et al. Acquired vitamin K-dependent carboxylation deficiency in liver disease. <u>N Engl J Med</u> 30(5)5:242-8, 1981; Widdershoven J, Kollee L, van Munster P, et al. Biochemical vitamin K deficiency in early infancy:*

diagnostic limitation of conventional coagulation tests. Helv Paediatr Acta 41(3):195-201, 1986). Other sensitive measures for evaluating vitamin K status are undercarboxylated osteocalcin and plasma phylloquinone *(Sokoll LJ, Sadowski JA. Comparison of biochemical indexes for assessing vitamin K nutritional status in a healthy adult population. Am J Clin Nutr 63:566-73, 1996).*

Subclinical deficiency, which may be manifested by changes in bone metabolism, does not usually affect blood clotting parameters. An example is prothrombin time which can still be normal when the prothrombin concentration is only 50% of normal *(Ferland G. Subclinical vitamin K deficiency: recent developments. Nutr Rep 12(1), January, 1994; Suttie JW. Vitamin K and human nutrition. J Am Diet Assoc 92:585-90, 1992; Widdershoven J, Kollee L, van Munster P, et al. Biochemical vitamin K deficiency in early infancy: diagnostic limitation of conventional coagulation tests. Helv Paediatr Acta 41(3):195-201, 1986).*

Zinc

The amount of zinc required to maintain normal zinc status has not been determined, and the evaluation of zinc nutriture has been difficult due to the lack of a marker of zinc status that is both sensitive and specific to changes in dietary intake *(Thomas EA, Bailey LB, Kauwell GA, et al. Erythrocyte metallothionein response to dietary zinc in humans. J Nutr 122:2408-14, 1992).*

The most reliable method of diagnosing zinc deficiency is a therapeutic trial *(Editorial: Another look at zinc. Br Med J 282:1098-9, 1981).* There is an urgent need to find a simple and rapid indicator of zinc deficiency *(Thompson RPH. Assessment of zinc status. Proc Nutr Soc 50:19-28, 1991).*

The zinc tolerance test is perhaps the best available method of determining body zinc nutriture, since serum, salivary, urinary and hair zinc levels may fail to correspond *(Capel ID et al. The assessment of zinc status by the zinc tolerance test in various groups of patients. Clin Biochem 15(5):257-60, 1982).* After a fast, a baseline plasma level is drawn, and an oral loading dose of zinc sulfate 220 mg (50 mg elemental zinc) is given. Two hours later, plasma zinc is redrawn. A two or threefold increase in plasma zinc is indicative of zinc inadequacy *(Capel ID et al. The assessment of zinc status by the zinc tolerance test in various groups of patients. Clin Biochem 15(5):257-60, 1982; Sullivan JF et al. A zinc tolerance test. J Lab Clin Med 93(3):485-92, 1979).*

Neutrophil zinc and alkaline phosphatase activity in neutrophils may be the preferred assays for the diagnosis of zinc deficiency *(Prasad AS. Laboratory diagnosis of zinc deficiency. J Am Coll Nutr 4(6):591-8, 1985).*

Leukocyte zinc is a useful index of body stores which has been shown to correlate with muscle zinc levels *(Jones RB et al. The relationship between leukocyte and muscle zinc in health and disease. Clin Sci 60:237-9, 1981).*

Observational Study: In 23 randomly selected elderly subjects aged 65-85, zinc levels in the plasma and erythrocytes were normal, while zinc levels in the granulocytes and platelets were significantly decreased in 1/3 of the cases compared to younger age controls. Lower zinc levels were associated with a higher incidence of anergy and hypogeusia, decreased interleukin-2 activity of T helper cells, and decreased serum testosterone and dihydrotestosterone levels in the males *(Prasad AS. Zinc in growth and development and spectrum of human zinc deficiency. J Am Coll Nutr 7(5):377-84, 1988).*

Sweat zinc is a useful and sensitive index of zinc status which is more reliable than either hair or serum zinc *(Davies S. Assessment of zinc status. Int Clin Nutr Rev 4(3):122-9, 1984; Howard JMH. Serum, leukocyte, sweat and hair zinc levels - a correlational study. J Nutr Med 1:119-26, 1990).*

Experimental and Observational Study: When the sweat zinc of 7 adult subjects was very low, hair zinc concentration could be low, normal or high while serum zinc was in the low normal range. When zinc supplementation was given, serum zinc became normal within 1-2 days, while sweat zinc took longer to increase to the normal range (*Davies S. Effects of oral zinc supplementation on serum, hair and sweat zinc levels in 7 subjects. Sci Total Environ 42:45-8, 1985*).

The plasma levels of the enzyme 5'-nucleotidase may identify marginal zinc deficiency.

Experimental Study: 15 older adults, mean age 66.6 yrs., consumed a marginally zinc-deficient diet for 15 days followed by 6 days of zinc repletion. Plasma zinc levels were unchanged. Both alkaline phosphatase and erythrocyte metallothionein were unchanged during depletion but showed a small, statistically significant drop after repletion. In contrast, plasma levels of the enzyme 5'-nucleotidase significantly decreased during depletion (p<0.01) and increased after repletion (p<0.05) (*Bales CW, DiSilvestro RA, Currie KL, et al. Marginal zinc deficiency in older adults: responsiveness of zinc status indicators. J Am Coll Nutr 13(5):455-62, 1994*).

Erythrocyte metallothionein levels may identify zinc depletion.

Experimental Study: Metallothionein is a low-molecular-weight protein that selectively binds heavy metals and is involved in the regulation of zinc metabolism. Previous studies have indicated that erythrocyte metallothionein is responsive to acute dietary zinc deficiency and supplementation in humans. 15 males aged 27 ± 3.6 yrs. participated in the 90 day, 4 phase study consisting of acclimation (7 days; low zinc diet: 15 mg Zn/d), treatment (6 wks.; either 3.2, 7.2 or 15.2 mg Zn/d), depletion (12 days; 0.55 mg Zn/d) and supplementation (30 days; self-selected diet plus 50 mg Zn/d). During the treatment phase, erythrocyte metallothionein decreased in the gp. fed 3.2 mg zinc daily relative to the acclimation phase, indicating that the metallothionein response is sensitive to changes in dietary zinc intake at the lower end of normal intakes. During the depletion phase, erythrocyte metallothionein decreased below normal in all gps. (46±10%) and increased during the supplementation phase. Erythrocyte zinc decreased in all gps. during the depletion phase relative to the treatment phase, and then increased during the supplementation phase (*Thomas EA, Bailey LB, Kauwell GA, et al. Erythrocyte metallothionein response to dietary zinc in humans. J Nutr 122:2408-14, 1992*).

Depressed hair zinc levels reliably indicate depletion, but normal or even high values do not rule out low body stores (*Davies S. Assessment of zinc status. Int Clin Nutr Rev 4(3):122-9, 1984; Pekarek RS et al. Abnormal cellular immune responses during acquired zinc deficiency. Am J Clin Nutr 32:1466-71, 1979; Hambridge KM et al. Low levels of zinc in hair, anorexia, poor growth and hypogeusia in children. Pediatr Res 6:808-74, 1971*). In addition, because standard washing procedures are unable to remove exogenous zinc without reducing endogenous zinc levels, hair levels are unreliable when external zinc contamination is likely to have occurred (*Buckley RA, Dreosti I. Am J Clin Nutr 40:840-6, 1984*), and hair zinc may fail to reflect increases in dietary zinc in subjects whose initial zinc status is adequate (*Medeiros DM et al. Failure of oral zinc supplementation to alter hair zinc levels among healthy human volunteers. Nutr Res 7:1109-15, 1987*).

Plasma zinc, which is decreased in moderate to severe zinc deficiency (*Prasad AS. Zinc in growth and development and spectrum of human zinc deficiency. J Am Coll Nutr 7(5):377-84, 1988*), is a poor measure of total body zinc stores (*Barrie SA, Wright JV, Pizzorno JE, et al. Comparative absorption of zinc picolinate, zinc citrate and zinc gluconate in* humans. *Agents Actions 21(1-2:223-8, 1987; Solomons NW. On the assessment of zinc and copper nutriture in man. Am J Clin Nutr 32:856-71, 1979).* A moderately low plasma level may simply reflect mobilization of zinc from plasma to the liver and other tissues as part of the normal response to infection or stress *(Wagner PA. Zinc nutriture in the elderly. Geriatrics 40:111-13,117-8,124-5, 1985).* In addition, plasma zinc concentrations depend upon albumin concentration *(Ainley CC et al. Zinc state in anorexia nervosa. Br Med J [Clin Res] 293:992-3, 1986).* Therefore, plasma zinc determinations should be complemented with zinc determinations in a nucleated tissue, such as liver, muscle or bone *(Abdulla M. How adequate is plasma zinc as an indicator of zinc status? Prog Clin Biol Res 129:171-83, 1983).*

Serum zinc is a poor measure of total body zinc stores *(Solomons NW. On the assessment of zinc and copper nutriture in man. Am J Clin Nutr 32:856-71, 1979).*

Urinary zinc is a poor marker of zinc nutriture. It is probably of greatest value in zinc depletion where it is reduced due to a zinc-sparing effect *(Henkin RI. Zinc in wound healing. Editorial. N Engl J Med 291(13):675-6, 1974).* When zinc nutriture is presumed normal, zinc supplementation of perhaps 100 mg daily is needed before urinary zinc output is increased *(Verus AP, Samman S. Urinary zinc as a marker of zinc intake: results of a supplementation trial in free-living men. Eur J Clin Nutr 48:219-21, 1994).* Moreover, any bodily process that involves the breakdown or rapid turnover of cells (including decreased food intake and starvation) is associated with increased urinary zinc excretion, which may or may not be reflected in serum zinc, and stress from any source, including surgery, may cause a redistribution of bodily zinc causing transient urinary zinc loss for a few days *(Henkin RI. Zinc in wound healing. Editorial. N Engl J Med 291(13):675-6, 1974).*

Combining measurement of the serum zinc concentration with urinary zinc excretion will provide a more accurate assessment than the use of either measure by itself *(Henkin RI. Zinc in wound healing. Editorial. N Engl J Med 291(13):675-6, 1974).*

Erythrocyte zinc, while sometimes low in zinc deficiency, is unreliable as erythrocyte zinc levels are substantially influenced by factors controlling the partitioning of zinc across red cell membranes *(Davies S. Assessment of zinc status. Int Clin Nutr Rev 4(3):122-9, 1984).* In addition, as erythrocytes turn over slowly, their zinc levels do not reflect recent changes in zinc status *(Prasad AS. Laboratory diagnosis of zinc deficiency. J Am Coll Nutr 4(6):591-8, 1985).*

A simple zinc taste test which suggests that there will be a favorable response to zinc supplementation uses a test solution made by dissolving zinc sulfate 1 gm in 1 liter of distilled water (0.1% solution). If the subject tasting 5 -10 ml notes either no taste or a dry and furry taste developing after a few minutes, zinc supplementation is suggested. Adequate zinc nutriture is suggested by an immediate taste which may be strong and unpleasant *(Bryce-Smith D, Simpson RID. Anorexia, depression, and zinc deficiency. Lancet ii:1162, 1984).* This test, however, has not been well-validated and, in its present form, appears to be of limited value *(Nichols J, Morgan J, Taylor A. Postnatal depression and zinc status - a preliminary study. J Nutr Med 3:35-42, 1992).*

INDEX

ORDERING INFORMATION

The following books by Melvyn R. Werbach, M.D. are available by mail directly from *Third Line Press*:

(USE THE HANDY ORDER FORM ON THE NEXT PAGE.)

1. Foundations of Nutritional Medicine   ISBN 0-9618550-6-1

330 pages   8 1/2" x 11"   1997   hard cover   *Price:* $49.95

2. Nutritional Influences on Illness. *Second* Edition   ISBN 0-9618550-3-7

700 pages   8 1/2" x 11"   1993   hard cover   *Price:* $64.95

"I cannot imagine a health care provider who would not gain from appropriating the information in this book . . . ."

James Heffley, Ph.D.
Editor, **Journal of Applied Nutrition**

3. Nutritional Influences on Mental Illness   ISBN 0-9618550-1-0

360 pages   7" x 10"   1991   hard cover   *Price:* $39.95

"A worthy companion to . . . Nutritional Influences on Illness, considered by many a classic for its clarity, breadth and editorial care. . . . This is a book that deserves to be on every professional's shelf within easy reach."

Russell M. Jaffe, M.D., Ph.D.
International Clinical Nutritional Review

4. Botanical Influences on Illness (Michael T. Murray, N.D., co-author)   ISBN 0-9618550-4-5

344 pages   7" x 10"   1994   hard cover   *Price:* $39.95

"This will become a standard reference for practitioners utilizing botanicals, and should be a required reference for those who don't."

Steven Foster
Quarterly Review of Natural Medicine

5. Third Line Medicine: Modern Treatment for Persistent Symptoms

ISBN 0-14-19063-5

215 pages   5" x 7 1/2"   1986   soft cover   *Price:* $10.95

An answer for patients who fail to benefit from mainstream treatments.

"For this clear exposition of what has happened and where we are going, all doctors . . . ought to be grateful."

Abram Hoffer, M.D., Ph.D.
Editor-in-Chief, **Journal of Orthomolecular Medicine**

(over)

THIRD LINE PRESS, INC.
4751 Viviana Drive, Suite 102
Tarzana, California 91356
USA

Phones: (800) 916-0076
(818) 996-0076
FAX: (818) 774-1575
e-mail: tlp@third-line.com

✓ *Please send:*

____ copies of **Foundations of Nutritional Medicine** @ $49.95 $ _____

____ copies of **Nutritional Influences on Illness,** *Second* Edition @ $64.95 $ _____

____ copies of **Nutritional Influences on Mental Illness** @ $39.95 $ _____

____ copies of **Botanical Influences on Illness** @ $39.95 $ _____

____ copies of **Third Line Medicine: Modern Treatment** **for Persistent Symptoms** @ $10.95 $ _____

---

* SHIPPING CHARGES
(add $3.00 for orders outside the US)
1 book $6.00
2 books: $7.00
3 books: $8.50
4-6 books: $10.00

Subtotal $ _____

8.25% tax (California only) $ _____

* Shipping $ _____

QUANTITY PRICES ON REQUEST
Prices subject to change without notice

TOTAL $ _____

✓ *If a check is not enclosed, please charge my:*   Visa ____   MasterCard ____

Card #: _____ - _____ - _____ - _____   Expiring: _____

Signature: _____

OUTSIDE OF THE UNITED STATES

* Beyond North America, shipping charges are for surface shipping (up to 3 months).
* Air mail rates are available on request.
* If payment is *not* made by Visa or MasterCard, your check must be
  in US dollars and drawn on a US bank.

NAME: _____

ADDRESS: _____

_____

_____

PHONE: _____   **FAX:** _____

E-MAIL: _____

330